Pharmacotherapeutic Management of Cardiovascular Disease Complications: A Textbook for Medical Students

Authored by

A. Bharath Kumar

Department of Pharmacy Practice
SRM College of Pharmacy
SRM IST, Kattankulathur 603203
Tamil Nadu,
India

&

M.S. Umashankar

Department of Pharmaceutics
SRM College of Pharmacy
SRM IST, Kattankulathur 603203

Tamil Nadu,
India

Pharmacotherapeutic Management of Cardiovascular Disease Complications: A Textbook for Medical Students

Authors: M.S. Umashankar & A. Bharath Kumar

ISBN (Online): 978-981-14-6821-6

ISBN (Print): 978-981-14-6819-3

ISBN (Paperback): 978-981-14-6820-9

need for a court order if at any point you breach any terms of this License Agreement. In no event will any delay or failure by Bentham Science Publishers in enforcing your compliance with this License Agreement constitute a waiver of any of its rights.

3. You acknowledge that you have read this License Agreement, and agree to be bound by its terms and conditions. To the extent that any other terms and conditions presented on any website of Bentham Science Publishers conflict with, or are inconsistent with, the terms and conditions set out in this License Agreement, you acknowledge that the terms and conditions set out in this License Agreement shall prevail.

Bentham Science Publishers Pte. Ltd.
80 Robinson Road #02-00
Singapore 068898
Singapore
Email: subscriptions@benthamscience.net

BENTHAM
SCIENCE

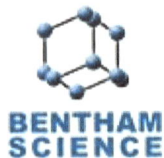

CONTENTS

PREFACE

The book *Pharmacotherapeutic Management of Cardiovascular Disease Complications: A Textbook for Medical Students,* presents promising treatment practices for the management of cardiovascular disease complications in health care settings.

Cardiovascular disease incidence is spontaneously rising all over the world, significantly impacting health care cost with poor health care outcomes. More recently, cardiovascular disease prevention and management, became a foremost health care issue in both developed and developing countries. The current health care statistics reveal 17.3 million deaths due to cardiovascular diseases every year and this will extend to 23.6 million by the year 2030.

The book coauthored by *A. Bharath Kumar and Dr. M.S. Umashankar,* discusses the pharmacotherapeutic management of cardiovascular disease complications, clinical symptoms, pathophysiology, early time diagnosis, control of risk factors and treatment methodology which help medical students to deliver a more promising treatment to patients and minimize the progression of cardiovascular disease, effectively. Chapter 1 provides a brief introduction to anatomy and physiology of the heart. Chapter 2 describes biomarkers' role in the detection of cardiovascular diseases and the pharmacological responses of the drugs. Chapter 3 discusses the diagnostic investigations of cardiovascular diseases via electrocardiogram, echocardiography, MRI scan, CT scan, treadmill test, doppler studies and coronary angiography to determine the severity of cardiovascular diseases. Chapter 4 presents valvular heart disease risk factors, clinical symptoms, diagnosis and management. Chapter 5 describes hyperlipidemia complications, their prevention, new potential targets and treatments. Chapter 6 represents hypertension treatment patterns and uncontrolled blood pressure manifestations. Chapter 7 shows an overview of atherosclerosis, risk factors, clinical symptoms, diagnostic tests and pharmacotherapeutic options for the management. Chapter 8 depicts deep vein thrombosis management, its risk factors, clinical symptoms, diagnostic tests and management. Chapter 9 gives a note on aortic aneurysm prevention and management in health care settings. Chapter 10 describes stroke etiology, diagnosis, prevention and its control. Chapter 11 displays the management of heart failure, etiology, clinical symptoms, and diagnostic investigations and medications.

Chapter 12 discusses cardiac arrhythmia management, classifications, diagnosis, pathophysiology and its management. Chapter 13 confers myocardial infarction risk factors, pathogenesis and current therapeutic options for the management of myocardial infarction. Chapter 14 presents angina pectoris epidemiology, risk factors, pathogenesis, diagnosis, and pharmacotherapeutic management. Chapter 15 discloses congenital heart defects, clinical manifestations, pathogenesis, diagnosis, and management of congenital heart defects. Chapter 16 gives an overview of inflammatory heart disease prevention and management. Chapter 17 discusses the prevalence, pathophysiology, causes, clinical symptoms and commonly prescribed drugs in cardiomyopathy. Chapter 18 discusses risk factors, pathophysiology, clinical symptoms, diagnosis and management of rheumatic heart disease. Chapter 19 explains cardiovascular disease comorbid diabetic complications. Chapter 20 provides detail about cardiovascular disease amid diabetic nephropathy patients. Chapter 21 sheds light on newer technology treatment of cardiovascular disease. Lastly, chapter 22 imposes clinical pharmacists' intervention services in the prevention and management of cardiovascular diseases in a hospital set up.

The authors are very grateful to our respected *Dean (Prof), Dr. K.S. Lakshmi,* for her constant encouragement in writing this book. The efforts of *Ms. Fariya Zulfiqar* (Manager Publications) in the completion of this book are highly appreciated.

CONSENT FOR PUBLICATION

Not applicable.

CONFLICT OF INTEREST

None.

ACKNOWLEDGEMENTS

We thank Dr. K.S. Lakshmi, Dean, SRM College of Pharmacy, SRM Institute of Science and Technology, for her encouragement and support.

A. Bharath Kumar

Department of Pharmacy Practice
SRM College of Pharmacy
SRM IST, Kattankulathur 603203
Tamil Nadu,
India

&

M.S. Umashankar

Department of Pharmaceutics
SRM College of Pharmacy
SRM IST, Kattankulathur 603203
Tamil Nadu,
India

CHAPTER 1

Introduction to Heart Anatomy and Physiology

Abstract: The cardiac system represents the heart and blood vessels. The blood is distributed to multiple organs present in the body. Capillaries are minute blood vessels, allow the gas exchange processes. Veins send blood to the heart from the capillaries. The heart is situated in the thorax, posterior to the sternum and superior surface of the diaphragm. The heart has four chambers, and two atria above and two ventricles below. The oxygenated blood moves to left portion of the heart and enters into the left atria and ventricle. The deoxygenated blood pumped into the right side of the heart and moves into the right ventricle and flows towards the lungs. The heart is covered with three protective layers which include an epicardium, myocardium, and endocardium. The cardiac physiological functions are controlled by a group of electrical impulses. The electrical impulse origin from the sinoatrial node and located on the top side of the right atrium. It causes atria muscle contractions and thereby sends blood into the ventricles. A cardiac cell demonstrated the electrical activity and transmits the cardiac impulses to the heart to maintain the normal heart beating and initiation of the cardiac cycle. The cardiac event causes the opening and closing of valves results in contraction and relaxation of cardiac chambers. The cardiac cycle consists of systole and diastole events, during the systole, ventricles contract and send blood to arteries and during diastole, the ventricle relaxes and collects blood from atria. The electrical activity of the heart originates from SA node and causes atria to initiate contraction of cardiac muscles and supply of blood into the ventricles.

Keywords: Cardiac Cells, Cardiac Cycle, Cardiac Events, Cardiovascular System.

INTRODUCTION

The heart is a muscular organ which is situated in the chest. The contraction of the heart muscles causes the pumping of blood to all vital organs of the body. It distributes the deoxygenated blood to the lungs and collects oxygen thereby sends carbon dioxide to move out of the lungs. The heart and blood vessels are known as the circulatory system. The heat contract about 100,000 times per day and around 5 liters of blood are pumped each minute. A blood vessel sends the blood to reach all parts of the body. Arteries are stained with red due to oxygen rich carry ability and veins are blue colored due to poor oxygen carrying ability and sends the blood to the heart.

M.S. Umashankar & A. Bharath Kumar

Capillaries are tiny blood vessels and inside of tissues exchange of gases can occur. The heart emits about 70 ml of blood during the contraction in an inactive stage which is equivalent to 5.25 liters of fluid per minute and 14,000 liters per day [1, 2].

Location of Heart

The heart is situated in the medial portion of the lungs is called as mediastinum. The heart is separated from the mediastinum through a layer is called pericardium. The dorsal surface of the heart located in vertebrae and sternum. The superior and inferior vena cava, aorta and pulmonary trunk are connected to the heart. The inferior tip of the heart is connected to the left side of the sternum between fourth and fifth ribs. The right portion of the heart is positioned anterior and the left side of the heart was projected towards posterior. The separated part of the apex is attached to the inferior lobe of the left lung is known as notch.

Size and Shape of the Heart

The shape of the heart is similar to a pinecone and heart size is about 12 cm in length, 8 cm in wide, and 6 cm thickness. The human heart weight mostly differs in both sexes. The male heart weight is ranges 300–350 grams and female heart weight is ranges from approximately 250–300 grams.

Chambers and Blood Circulation in the Heart

The heart is divided into four chambers and right and left atrium, acts as a collecting chamber and contraction of cardiac muscles send blood to lower cavity and ventricles distribute blood to all the organs present in the body. Pulmonary value transports blood from the lungs receives oxygen and delivers carbon dioxide. The right ventricle sends deoxygenated blood to the lungs and finally reaches the pulmonary arteries and oxygenated blood moves to pulmonary veins [3, 4].

It pumps the blood to the left atrium and left ventricle consecutively sends oxygenated blood to the aorta. Oxygen, nutrients present in blood can be utilized by the cells during the metabolic pathways. Carbon dioxide and metabolic fragments can move into the blood. Capillaries are combined to form venules and larger veins connected to the superior and inferior vena cava and right atrium. The blood present in the superior and inferior vena cava reaches into right atrium and right ventricle, respectively.

Heart Chambers

The heart comprises four chambers which includes two atria and two ventricles

Receiving chambers: Two atria act as receiving chambers and having an essential role in the pumping of blood.

Discharging chambers: Ventricles are acts as a discharging chamber during its contraction, blood is ejected out of the heart and reaches the blood.

Septum: It divides heart longitudinally into inter ventricular septum and inter atria septum.

Blood Vessels

Aorta: Blood move to the left portion of the heart through the arch of the aorta and sends to body tissues.

Pulmonary veins: The oxygenated blood is consumed by the lungs and returns to the left side of the heart.

Pulmonary arteries: Pulmonary trunk divides right and left pulmonary arteries, and distributes blood to the lungs.

Superior and inferior vena cava: The heart receives oxygen-poor blood from the veins through superior and inferior vena cava and sends to pulmonary circulation.

Heart valves

It consists of four valves and sends the blood into the heart chambers.

Mitral valve: It is present between the left atrium and left ventricle.

Pulmonary valve: It is situated between the right ventricle and the pulmonary artery.

Tricuspid valve: It is positioned between the right atrium and right ventricle.

Aortic valve: It is present between the left ventricle and the aorta.

ANATOMY OF HEART

The heart consists of four chambers It includes atria and ventricle.

Atria: It is present in the two upper cavities of the heart.

Ventricle: It is situated in two lower chambers of the heart.

Left Side of the Heart

Oxygenated blood shifted to the left atrium from pulmonary veins and which results in contraction of the left atrium and leads to the pumping of blood into the left ventricle. The anatomy of heart is shown in Fig. (**1**).

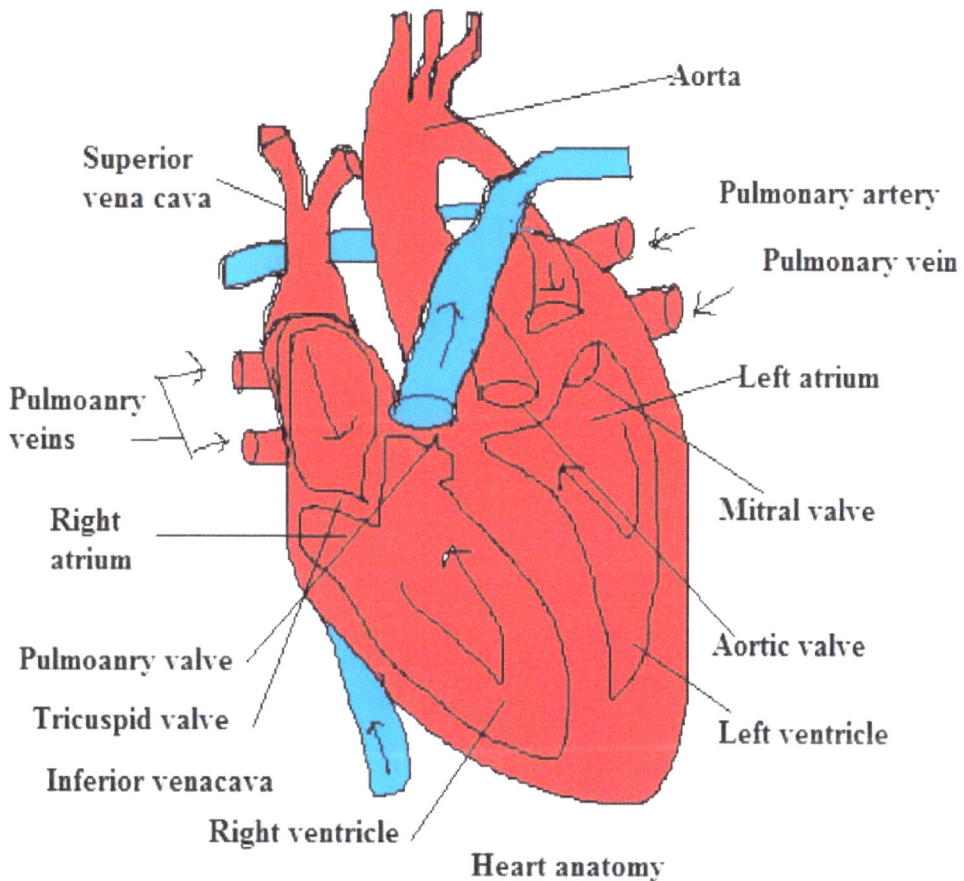

Fig. (1). Heart Anatomy.

Right Side of the Heart

Right atrium collects deoxygenated blood from superior and inferior vena cava. The complete filling of the right ventricle sends blood to the lungs through the pulmonary artery [5 - 8].

The heart wall is covered with three layers It includes

Epicardium: It is a protective layer of the heart and covered with connective tissue.

Myocardium: It is covered with muscles of the heart.

Endocardium: It is located on the inside of the heart and protects heart valves and chambers.

Pericardium: It is enclosed with a thin protective membrane known as the pericardium.

Covering Layers of Heart

The heart is accompanied by three covering layers. It includes pericardium, myocardium, epicardium. The pericardium is connected with strong connective tissue that protects the heart. The pericardium consists of two layers that include parietal pericardium linked to fibrous pericardium and visceral pericardium is attached to the heart. The pericardial cavity is located between epicardium and pericardium. A macroscopic layer consisting of the heart is covered with simple squamous epithelial cells known as mesothelium which is linked to the pericardium. Mesothelium cells produce lubricating serous fluid that can lower the rubbing during heart contractions. The heart wall is covered with three layers, which include epicardium, myocardium, and endocardium. The middle layer is the myocardium which is made of collagenous fibers and contraction of myocardium membrane causes pumping of blood into the heart. The inner layer of the heart is endocardium connected to the myocardium with a small layer of connective tissue. The endocardium is lined with simple squamous epithelium cells and continues with blood vessels. The endothelium cells may the control growth of the cardiac muscle cells which secretes endothelins monitors the concentration and relaxation of the heart [9 - 11].

The Internal Structural Pattern of the Heart

Septa part of the heart: Septa divide the heart into chambers. Septa are the other portion of myocardium cells which are covered with endocardium and situated between the two atria. The inter atria septum is represented with oval-shape called fossaovalis connected to fetal heart called as foramen ovale. It can permit the blood to the fetal heart through the right and left atrium. The foramen ovale can establish the blood circulation pattern to the heart. The inter ventricular septum is placed between two ventricles. The septum is situated between atria; ventricles are named as atrioventricular septum. It allows blood to pass into atria and ventricles towards the lungs and finally reaches into the pulmonary trunk and aorta.

Right Atrium

It collects blood from systemic circulation and sends to the heart. The inferior vena cava receives blood from lower limbs, abdomen and pelvic region of the body. Eventually, superior vena cava drains the blood from coronary artery and move to the systemic circulation. The right atrium is smooth and having prominent ridges. The left atrium has no ridges. The atria collect the venous blood continuously and to prevent the venous flow during the contraction of ventricle. The ventricular filling occurs during the atria relaxation and contraction and blood are pumped into ventricles. The atrium and ventricle valve are controlled by the tricuspid valve.

Left Atrium

The blood can move constantly from pulmonary veins and to the atrium and act as a receiving chamber. The relaxation of the atria and ventricle makes the blood can move into the heart. The completion of the ventricular relaxation phase the contraction of the left atria results in the blood reach into the right ventricle. The left atrium and ventricle valve is guarded by the mitral valve.

Right Ventricle

It receives blood from the right atria and both sides of the tricuspid valve are connected to connective tissue is known as chordae tendineae. There are many chordae tendineae is attached to each side of the tricuspid valve. The chordae tendineae is composed of collagenous fibers, elastic fibers, and endothelium cells. The papillary muscles are enlarging from the ventricular surface and three papillary muscles are located in the right ventricle which is known as anterior, posterior, and septal muscles and connected to the respective valves. Ventricle walls are covered with trabeculae carne and the edges of the cardiac muscles are enclosed with an endocardium layer known as a moderator band which can help during the cardiac conduction process. During the time of right ventricle contraction, the ventricle delivers blood into the pulmonary trunk. The lower surface of the pulmonary trunk and semi lunar valve can prevent the blood backflow from the pulmonary trunk [12 - 15].

Left ventricle

The left side of the ventricle delivers blood to the vascular stream and sends blood to the aorta through semi lunar valve. The valves provide unidirectional blood flow to the heart. The tricuspid valve situated between the right atrium and right ventricle. The pulmonary valve is situated at the base of the pulmonary trunk. The pulmonary valve lined with endothelial cells and connective tissue. The relaxation of ventricles causes returning blood flow into the ventricle. This blood circulation into the pulmonary valve results in producing heart sounds.

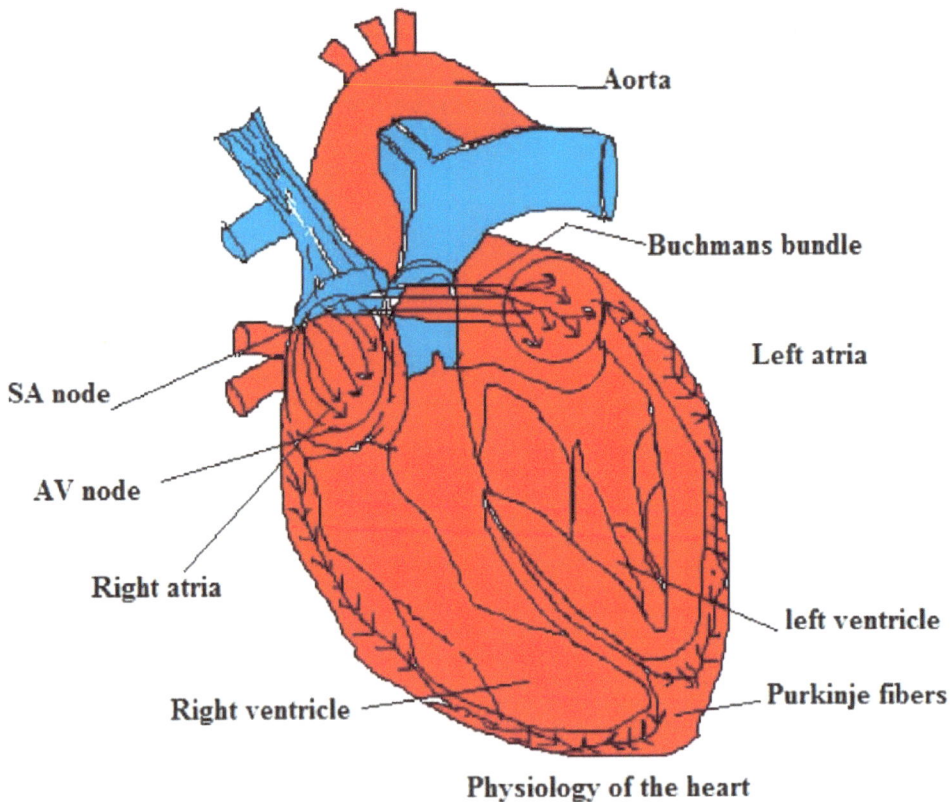

Physiology of the heart

Fig. (2). Physiology of heart.

PHYSIOLOGY OF THE HEART

The heart can continuously pump the blood throughout the body. It is covered by muscular layers which help to contract and relax rhythmical manner during the life time of individuals. The cardiovascular system has four chambers. The upper part of the heart on both sides atrium is located, which can collect the blood from the heart. Atrium sends blood to the ventricle and it delivers blood to the heart during the cardiac contractions. The right side of the heart allows oxygen-poor blood from several portions of the body and transfer to the lungs. The oxygen absorption takes place in the lungs and moves into the systemic circulation. The left side of the heart accepts oxygenated blood from the lungs and distribute to the body [16 - 19]. The physiology of heart is shown in Fig. (**2**).

Systole The contraction of the cardiac muscles in the ventricles is known as systole. The elevated pressure during contraction of the ventricles is known as systolic pressure.

Diastole

The repose of cardiac muscles located in the ventricles is called diastole. The decrease of pressure during ventricular relaxation is known as diastolic pressure.

Conduction System of the Heart

The heart is covered with various muscle tissues. A group of cardiac muscle fibers monitors the contraction and relaxation of the heart to attain the better pumping action of the heart. The sinoatrial node is the natural pacemaker for the heart. Electrical impulse spreads through the atria and ventricles and reaches to cardiac muscle tissue to produce contractions effectively. The electrical impulse extends throughout the atria and produces wave like contractions in the heart. These impulses originate from the sinoatrial node reaches the atrio ventricular node reaches the ventricles and results in contraction of the ventricles. The impulse reaches to the right and left bundle branches to cause contractions of the cardiac muscles to normalize the heart function [20, 21].

Cardiac Cycle

There are three phases are involved in initiation of cardiac cycle which include atrial systole, ventricular systole and relaxation.

Atrial systole Contraction of the atria pushes blood into the ventricles and opening of AV valves and close of semi lunar valves helps for returning blood to the heart.

Ventricular systole In this phase ventricles contracts and sends blood into the aorta. The high pressure in the ventricles causes open of the semi lunar valves and close of AV valves can occur during the ventricular systole and eventually blood moves from the ventricles into the arteries.

Relaxation Phase

The chamber of the heart in diastole position receives blood from veins causes ventricles repolarization. It leads to the initiation of depolarization and contraction of cardiac cells in the heart. The opening of AV valves can allow the blood to freely move to ventricles and closing of semi lunar valves to decrease the back flow of blood from arteries to ventricles.

Blood Supply to Heart

The deoxygenated blood from superior and inferior vena cava moves to the heart. Blood moves into the right atrium, right ventricle and reaches the pulmonary trunk and thereby it reaches the systemic circulation. It carries oxygen and eliminates carbon dioxide from the blood. The blood present in the lungs proceed to the heart through the pulmonary veins reaches to left atrium and leads to contraction of left atrium sends the blood into the aorta and finally, it reaches the heart [22, 23].

Electrocardiogram It is used to measure the conduction nature of the heart through fixing on the skin surface. It will produce a unique pattern of impulses in response to the electrochemical variations occur in the heart. The initial portion of the wave is known as P wave, which occurs a minute raise in voltage of 0.1mv is responsible for the depolarization process.

The other portion of ECG is QRS complex could show changes in Q, R, S waves. QRS complex causes the depolarization of the ventricles at a certain period of ventricular systole. T wave is a small peak that is associated with QRS complex. T wave demonstrates ventricular repolarization at the relaxation stage of the cardiac cycle. Abnormal waves of ECG are utilized to detect cardiovascular diseases such as myocardial infarction, angina pectoris, electrolyte imbalances and heart attack *etc.*,

Heart Sounds

The "lubb" sound comes from the heart during the first heartbeat and which shows a longer duration of the heart sound. It is produced by the closing of AV valves. Dupp sound is shorter which leads to the closing of the semilunar valves. These heartbeats are repeated in a regular pattern to maintain the normal function in the human body [24, 25].

Cardiac Output

It is defined as the volume of blood being pumped by the heart in one minute. Stroke volume is defined as the amount of blood distributed to aorta during the ventricular systole. Heart rate is defined as the number of heart beats per minute.

Cardiac output = Stroke volume x Heart rate.

CONCLUSION

The heart is one of the essential organs of the human body and having four layers and chambers. It shows the complex nature of veins, arteries to deliver deoxygenated and oxygenated blood to various organs present in the human body. The human heart represents a pair of atria and ventricle which can receive and sends blood into ventricles. The exchange of oxygen, carbon dioxide occurs in the lungs and highly oxygenated blood moves to the left atrium, left ventricle and finally reaches the systemic circulation. The heart is situated in mediastinal space within the thoracic cavity and covered with pericardial tissue. The heart wall is covered with three layers which include an outer layer of the epicardium, a thick layer of the myocardium and an inner layer of endocardium. The cardiovascular system plays an essential role in regulating homeostasis conditions in the body. The blood moves from the heart towards arteries, arterioles, and capillaries and the exchange of nutrients and gasses can take place in the arteries and finally returns to venules and veins. The ventricle contractions are caused by the electrophysiological changes during the cardiac function which can be determined by measuring stroke volume and cardiac output. The sphygmomanometer is used to measure the total peripheral resistance, mean arterial pressure in the arterioles. The electrocardiogram is used to detect the cardiovascular disease burden among the high cardiovascular risk profile patients. The heart output is calculated by the rate of venous return from the peripheral tissues. The physiological conditions increase in cardiac output which can lead to raising the venous return. The sympathetic nervous system affects mean systemic pressure and resistance to venous return can affect the cardiac physiological functions. The chronic sympathetic system can decrease renal sodium excretion, increasing blood volume leads to affect the cardiac functions.

REFERENCES

[1]   Gerald D. Buckberg, Navin C. Nanda, Christopher Nguyen, and Mladen J. Kocica. What Is the Heart? Anatomy, Function, Pathophysiology, and Misconceptions. J Cardiovasc Dev Dis 2018; 5(2): 33.
[http://dx.doi.org/10.3390/jcdd5020033]

[2]   Mall FP. On the muscular architecture of the ventricles of the human heart. Am J Anat 1911; 11: 211-78.
[http://dx.doi.org/10.1002/aja.1000110302]

[3]   James TN, Sherf L. Ultrastructure of the human atrioventricular node. Circulation 1968; 37(6): 1049-70.
       [http://dx.doi.org/10.1161/01.CIR.37.6.1049] [PMID: 5653047]

[4]   Stevens C, Remme E, LeGrice I, Hunter P. Ventricular mechanics in diastole: material parameter sensitivity. J Biomech 2003; 36(5): 737-48.
       [http://dx.doi.org/10.1016/S0021-9290(02)00452-9] [PMID: 12695004]

[5]   Anderson RH, Brown NA. The anatomy of the heart revisited. Anat Rec 1996; 246(1): 1-7.
       [http://dx.doi.org/10.1002/(SICI)1097-0185(199609)246:1<1::AID-AR1>3.0.CO;2-Y]   [PMID: 8876818]

[6]   Anderson RH. Clinical anatomy of the aortic root. Heart 2000; 84(6): 670-3.
       [http://dx.doi.org/10.1136/heart.84.6.670] [PMID: 11083753]

[7]   Anderson RH, Ho SY, Brecker SJ. Anatomic basis of cross-sectional echocardiography. Heart 2001; 85(6): 716-20.
       [http://dx.doi.org/10.1136/heart.85.6.716] [PMID: 11359762]

[8]   Hill AJ, Coles JA Jr, Sigg DC, Laske TG, Iaizzo PA. Images of the human coronary sinus ostium obtained from isolated working hearts. Ann Thorac Surg 2003; 76(6): 2108.
       [http://dx.doi.org/10.1016/S0003-4975(03)00268-6] [PMID: 14667663]

[9]   Mall FP. On the muscular architecture of the ventricles of the human heart. Am J Anat 1911; 11: 211-78.
       [http://dx.doi.org/10.1002/aja.1000110302]

[10]   Robb JS, Robb RC. The normal heart: Anatomy and physiology of the structural units. Am Heart J 1942; 23: 455-67.
       [http://dx.doi.org/10.1016/S0002-8703(42)90291-6]

[11]   Buckberg GD. Basic science review: the helix and the heart. J Thorac Cardiovasc Surg 2002; 124(5): 863-83.
       [http://dx.doi.org/10.1067/mtc.2002.122439] [PMID: 12407367]

[12]   Chauvin M, Shah DC, Haïssaguerre M, Marcellin L, Brechenmacher C. The anatomic basis of connections between the coronary sinus musculature and the left atrium in humans. Circulation 2000; 101(6): 647-52.
       [http://dx.doi.org/10.1161/01.CIR.101.6.647] [PMID: 10673257]

[13]   Cook AC, Anderson RH. Attitudinally correct nomenclature. Heart 2002; 87(6): 503-6.
       [http://dx.doi.org/10.1136/heart.87.6.503] [PMID: 12010926]

[14]   Silver MD, Lam JHC, Ranganathan N, Wigle ED. Morphology of the human tricuspid valve. Circulation 1971; 43(3): 333-48.
       [http://dx.doi.org/10.1161/01.CIR.43.3.333] [PMID: 5544987]

[15]   Folkow B, Svanborg A. Physiology of cardiovascular aging. Physiol Rev 1993; 73(4): 725-64.
       [http://dx.doi.org/10.1152/physrev.1993.73.4.725] [PMID: 8105498]

[16]   Liakopoulos OJ, Tomioka H, Buckberg GD, Tan Z, Hristov N, Trummer G. Sequential deformation and physiological considerations in unipolar right or left ventricular pacing. Eur J Cardiothorac Surg 2006; 29 (Suppl. 1): S188-97.
       [http://dx.doi.org/10.1016/j.ejcts.2006.02.053] [PMID: 16563791]

[17]   Anderson RH, Loukas M. The importance of attitudinally appropriate description of cardiac anatomy. Clin Anat 2009; 22(1): 47-51.
       [http://dx.doi.org/10.1002/ca.20741] [PMID: 19097120]

[18]   Loukas M, Groat C, Khangura R, Owens DG, Anderson RH. The normal and abnormal anatomy of the coronary arteries. Clin Anat 2009; 22(1): 114-28.
       [http://dx.doi.org/10.1002/ca.20761] [PMID: 19097062]

[19]   Loukas M, Bilinsky S, Bilinsky E, Matusz P, Anderson RH. The clinical anatomy of the coronary collateral circulation. Clin Anat 2009; 22(1): 146-60.
[http://dx.doi.org/10.1002/ca.20743] [PMID: 19097064]

[20]   Skwarek M, Hreczecha J, Dudziak M, Jerzemowski J, Szpinda M, Grzybiak M. Morphometric features of the right atrioventricular orifice in adult human hearts. Folia Morphol (Warsz) 2008; 67(1): 53-7.
[PMID: 18335414]

[21]   Hildreth V, Anderson RH, Henderson DJ. Autonomic innervation of the developing heart: origins and function. Clin Anat 2009; 22(1): 36-46.
[http://dx.doi.org/10.1002/ca.20695] [PMID: 18846544]

[22]   Becker AE, Anderson RH. Atrioventricular septal defects: What's in a name? J Thorac Cardiovasc Surg 1982; 83(3): 461-9.
[http://dx.doi.org/10.1016/S0022-5223(19)37286-1] [PMID: 7062758]

[23]   Chow LT, Chow SS, Anderson RH, Gosling JA. Innervation of the human cardiac conduction system at birth. Br Heart J 1993; 69(5): 430-5.
[http://dx.doi.org/10.1136/hrt.69.5.430] [PMID: 7686024]

[24]   Skwarek M, Hreczecha J, Grzybiak M, Kosiński A. Remarks on the morphology of the papillary muscles of the right ventricle. Folia Morphol (Warsz) 2005; 64(3): 176-82.
[PMID: 16228952]

[25]   Wafae N, Hayashi H, Gerola LR, Vieira MC. Anatomical study of the human tricuspid valve. Surg Radiol Anat 1990; 12(1): 37-41.
[http://dx.doi.org/10.1007/BF02094123] [PMID: 2345895]

CHAPTER 2

Role of Biomarkers in Detection of Cardiovascular Diseases

Abstract: Cardiovascular diseases cause more deaths in the world. Atherosclerotic plaques cause thrombus formation in the blood vessels leads to impediment in the vascular lumen can create a complete blockage of the blood vessels which increases the risk of developing coronary artery disease. The biomarker is used to assess the biological process and pharmacological responses of the drugs to a targeted intervention. It is used to identify the disease progression burden among the affected population. The cardiovascular biomarkers include B-type natriuretic peptide, urinary NGAL, troponin, C-reactive protein, N-terminal prohormone BNP, myeloperoxidase, lipoprotein-associated phospholipase A2, cytokine IL-37, troponin, fibrinogen, metalloproteinase-1, and cystatin C is used to predict the risk of progression of cardiovascular diseases.

Keywords: Biomarker, Cardiovascular Disease, Coronary Artery Disease, Risk Prediction, Therapeutic Interventions.

INTRODUCTION

Cardiovascular disease is the leading cause of death in the world. Among cardiovascular diseases, atherosclerosis is causing enormous rates of morbidity and mortality in the world. The pathophysiological approaches which explain that the arterial wall thickening due to the formation of atherosclerotic plaques in the blood stream lead to the development of coronary artery disease complications. Atherosclerotic plaques may become complicated due to thrombus formation in the blood vessels and lead to a sudden obstruction of the vascular lumen can create a complete blockage of the blood vessels which can cause the coronary artery disease risk to the individual patients. Depending on the severity of obstruction which may lead to acute coronary syndrome, myocardial infarction, and stroke causes sudden death. The risk factors for cardiovascular disease include hypertension, diabetes mellitus, smoking, and obesity which have led to the development of coronary artery disease risk. The implementation of effective clinical pharmacist care strategies with the health care team in an effective manner can minimize coronary artery disease risk complications [1 - 3].

M.S. Umashankar & A. Bharath Kumar

The cardiovascular risk prediction can depend on the presence of risk factors and novel diagnostic investigations and novel risk markers can use for prediction of cardiovascular risk burden among high-risk population. Recent research findings demonstrate that there is a high incidence of the unexpected rate of acute ischemic events occurring in the community which leads to affect the health related quality of life of individual patients. Biomarkers play a potential role in the identification of disease severity among cardiovascular patients. The National Institute of Health Consortium in 2001 defined biomarker as a characteristic that is objectively measured and evaluated as an indicator of normal biological processes, pathogenic processes and pharmacologic responses to a therapeutic intervention process.

IDEAL CHARACTERISTICS OF BIOMARKERS

Biomarkers should have specific characteristics which include

The biomarker should be very specific to the particular diseases and which is easily detectable in as specified concentrations.

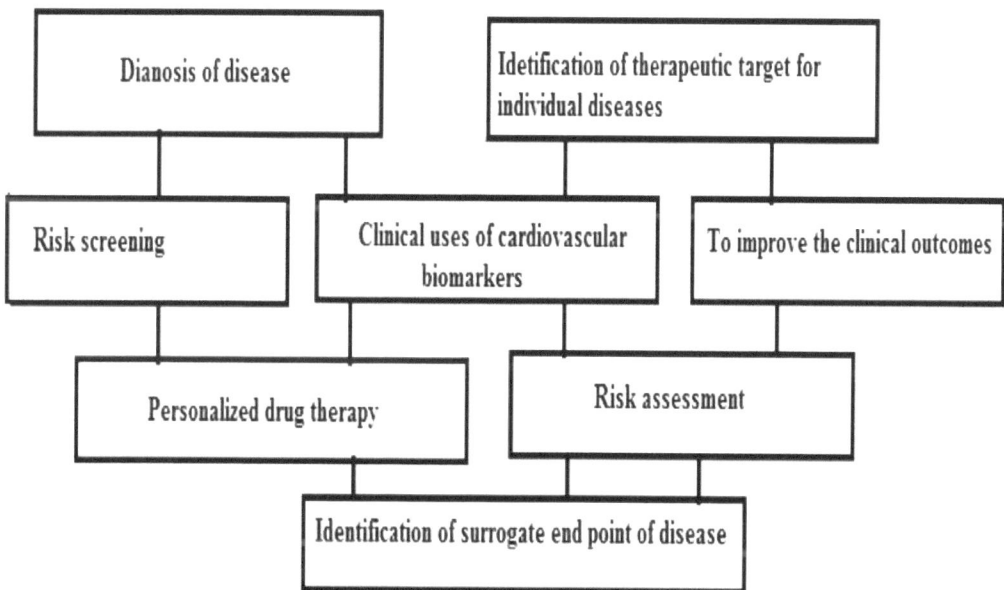

Fig. (1). Clinical uses of biomarkers.

It is used to identify the disease progression burden among the affected population.

The biomarker detection should be fast, simple, easy process and low cost.

The chosen biomarker should possess greater effectiveness preclinical and as well as clinical level.

It can be used for early detection of disease, evaluation of acute and chronic clinical conditions of the diseases.

It is used to stratify the risk and to confirm the diagnosis, selection of appropriate treatment. The clinical uses of biomarkers were shown in Fig. (**1**).

It must have good accuracy and reliability.

It must show the effective impact on early therapeutic intervention.

Biomarkers having an essential role in the evaluation of disease burden and also used to develop the novel drug for treatment for the prevention of various diseases in clinical practice.

Biomarkers are generally representing a biochemical change at a tissue. Therefore they are strongly associated with a pathologic process. The cardiovascular disease biomarkers were shown in Fig. (**2**).

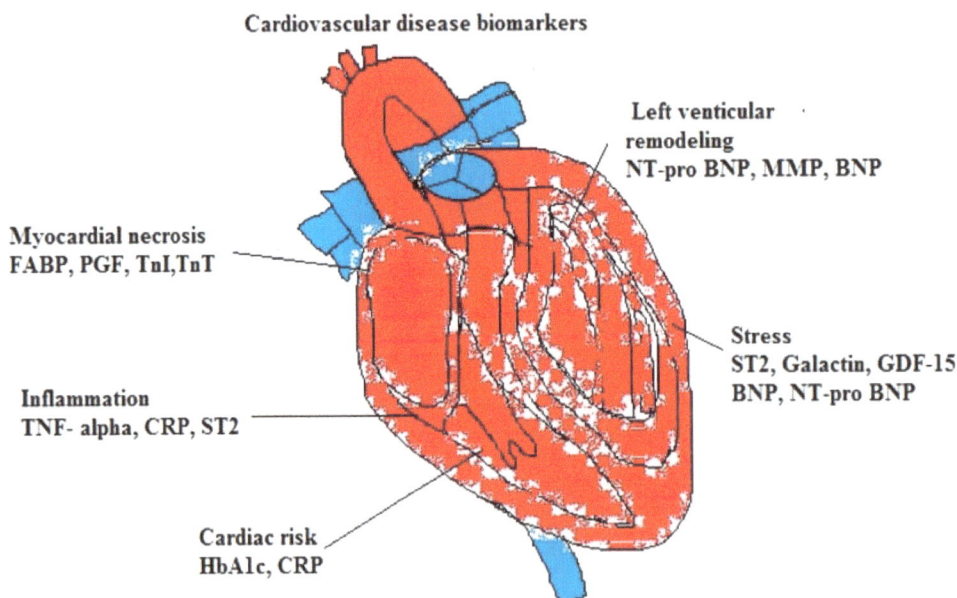

Cardiovascular disease biomarkers

Left venticular remodeling
NT-pro BNP, MMP, BNP

Myocardial necrosis
FABP, PGF, TnI,TnT

Stress
ST2, Galactin, GDF-15
BNP, NT-pro BNP

Inflammation
TNF- alpha, CRP, ST2

Cardiac risk
HbAlc, CRP

Fig. (2). Cardiovascular disease biomarkers.

MYOCARDIUM INJURY RISK PREDICTION BIOMARKERS

Cardiac Troponin

The cardiomyocyte necrosis releases troponin I or T into the systemic circulation of individual patients which is used for the detection of myocardial ischemia conditions. The immune assays are predicted that the assay of troponin T and I are elevated during severe heart failure patients. Therefore, this marker has been used for the detection of established heart failure. Troponin is a complex of three globular contractile regulatory proteins (troponin T, and I) which relies on the thin filament of striated muscle which inhibits the contraction of actin and myosin. Cardiac troponin I (cTnI) and T (cTnT) are the specific proteins for the identification of myocardial damage. During the severe condition of acute myocardial infarction Troponin I and Troponin T are released from necrotic myocardium which predicts the risk complications of the disease. The cardiac tropinin can be detected in peripheral blood and used for the detection of cardiomyocyte damage. These are found to be one of the more sensitive biomarkers for the detection of myocyte injury which is more specific for predicting the risk of myocardial infarction [4].

Troponin T, troponin I, and creatinine kinase-MB are the common markers for the diagnosis of myocardial injury. The increased troponin concentrations are associated with greater risk of developing cardiovascular diseases in the health care.

High-Sensitivity Cardiac Troponin (hs-cTn)

This type of maker is used for assessment of myocardial injury among high-risk group of patients. The abnormal elevation of cardiac troponin levels can predict the high risk profile of cardiovascular disease patients.

Heart-Type Fatty Acid Binding Protein (H-FABP)

It represents a group of transport proteins which allow for the transport of fatty acids through the cell membrane. FABP is tissue specific type. There is another type of FABP includes liver-type FABP (L-FABP), intestinal-type (I-FABP), brain-type FABP (B-FABP), and heart-type FABP (H-FABP). H-FABP is a low molecular weight protein having 132 amino acids and is involved in myocardial fatty-acid metabolism. It is found in abundance in cardiomyocytes and also in small quantities in the brain, kidney, and skeletal tissue, and it levels can increase in ischemic events [5 - 7].

INFLAMMATION PREDICTION BIOMARKERS

High-Sensitivity C-reactive Protein (hs-CRP)

It belongs to the pentraxin family which is a type of immune response protein. The Hs-CRP risk status was categorized into various levels which include low, intermediate and high risk. The interpretation of Hs-CRP results includes CRP level < 1 mg/L are desirable and shows a low systemic inflammatory status. The lower level of atherosclerotic cardiovascular risk level between 1 and 3 mg/L indicates moderate vascular risk and patients presented with CRP levels > 3 mg/L showed higher vascular risk. Patients with CRP levels more than > 10 mg/L may results in the transient infectious process so thereby the test should be repeated within two to three weeks of duration [8 - 12].

Growth-Differentiation Factor-15 (GDF-15)

It is a divergent member of the transforming growth factor-β cytokine family and its activity is expressed by activated macrophages. It is associated with cellular oxidative stress, ischemia. GDF-15 is normally associated with several pathological processes leading to the development of cardiovascular diseases [13 - 16].

Fibrinogen

Fibrinogen is a blood clotting factor which is an acute phase protein synthesized by the liver. It has been involved in platelet aggregation, endothelial injury and mainly involved in thrombus formation. The elevated fibrinogen levels are associated with increased risk of cardiovascular risk events. Fibrinogen is composed of three polypeptide chains which are Aα, Bβ, and γ. Previous research studies have explained that γA/γ′ fibrinogen is associated with increased risk of coronary artery disease, ischemic stroke, peripheral artery disease and, heart failure. Gama globulin is a common risk factor for developing cardiovascular diseases [17].

Uric Acid

Uric acid is the end product of purine metabolism in humans. The increased levels of serum uric levels are associated with the development of cardiovascular diseases. Hyperuricemia is associated with increased oxidative stress, promoting endothelial dysfunction and enhances inflammatory conditions in the body.

PLAQUES RUPTURE ASSESSMENT BIOMARKERS

Myeloperoxidase (MPO)

It is a member of the heme peroxidase family which is produced by polymorphonuclear cells. The leukocytes, neutrophils, and monocytes are released during the inflammatory conditions. Myeloperoxidase is considered to be a majorly contributes to the formation of plaque. It has an inverse correlation with paraoxonase-1 which is bound to high density lipoprotein which suggests that pro-oxidants and anti-oxidants may contribute to the progression of coronary plaque instability [18].

Matrix Metalloproteinases

These are a family of endopeptidases that are secreted by various inflammatory and tumor cells such as zymogens. MMPs have various roles in coronary artery intimal thickening, which destroys the extracellular matrix results in plaque rupture. The matrix metalloproteinases are classified into interstitial collagenases that degrade fibrillar collagen; stromelysins have broader specificity, gelatinases that degrades the collage and macrophage elastase that primarily cleaves the elastin. The MMP-2, MMP-8, and MMP-9 have been recognized as proteases that contribute to atherosclerotic plaque rupture. The high elevation of MMP-2 activity in plaques is associated with a higher rate of subsequent ischemic cardiac and cerebrovascular events [19, 20].

Pregnancy-Associated Plasma Protein-A (PAPP-A)

It is a zinc-binding matrix metalloproteinase which belongs to the metzincin super family of metalloproteinases. These are identified in pregnant women placenta cells. PAPP-A induces the activation of insulin-derived growth factor-1 can cause inflammation and lipid uptake could contribute to atherogenesis and plaque instability. PAPP-A is a promising biomarker tool for risk stratification for acute coronary artery disease.

Platelet Activation Biomarkers

Secretory Phospholipase A2 (sPLA2)

The Secretory phospholipase A2 consist of 10 disulfide-rich isoenzymes includes sPLA2-IB, -IIA, -IIC, -IID, -IIE, -IIF, -III, -V, -X, and –XIIA and these are involved in the various biological process. The sPLA2s, sPLA2-IIA, sPLA2-V, and sPLA2-X having a potential role in atherogenesis and inflammation process of origin.

Lipoprotein-Associated Phospholipase A2

It is a member of the phospholipase A2 super family and is also known as platelet-activating factor acetyl hydrolase and produced by monocytes and macrophages. Lp-PLA2 can modify the LDL particles present in the phospholipids hydrolysis process and results in oxidation. The accumulation of lyso-phosphatidylcholine and oxidized fatty acids in the sub intimal space contributes to the development of the plaque. Lp-PLA2 function is essential for vulnerable plaques formation and the occurrence of acute coronary artery syndrome [21].

Soluble CD40 Ligand (sCD40L)

It belongs to the tumor necrosis factor super family and expressed in various cell types such as lymphocytes, dendritic cells, neutrophils, and macrophages, epithelial cells, vascular smooth muscle cells, and endothelial cells are responsible for the inflammation process. The CD40L with its receptor CD40 having immune modulatory properties. The CD40L is subsequently cleaved for a period of minutes to hours leads to generating soluble fragment (sCD40L) that is responsible for atherosclerotic plaque instability.

BIOMARKERS OF NEUROHORMONAL ACTIVATION

Copeptin It is a glycosylated 39-amino-acid peptide. It is a C-terminal part of the precursor pre-provasopressin. The copeptin is a well established biomarker for the detection of cardiovascular disease. It is a novel hallmark of the activation of the hypothalamus-pituitary-adrenals axis [22].

Mid-Regional-Pro-Adrenomedullin

It is a 52-amino acid ringed peptide with C-terminal amidation, was first found in pheochromocytoma cells in the adrenal medulla. Adreno medulla is a vasodilator synthesized in the adrenal medulla and from the heart, vascular endothelial cells, Adrenomedull levels in the heart may elevate as a result of Fluid. It is a vasodilatory peptide, which is elevated in the circulating levels are having strongly associated with the presence of chronic heart failure.

MYOCARDIAL DYSFUNCTION DETECTION BIOMARKERS ST

It is a member of the interleukin-1 receptor family and present in two different forms which include trans membrane receptor and a soluble decoy receptor. ST-2 is a receptor from interleukin family that exists with two gene forms which include soluble and trans membrane form [23].

Endothelin-1 (ET-1)

It is a 21-amino acid peptide and a potent vasoconstrictor and pro-fibrotic hormone which is secreted by vascular endothelial cells. The elevated ET-1 level is associated with acute heart failure.

Galectin-3

It is a glycoprotein-binding protein is secreted by activated cardiac macrophages. It will participate in the atherogenesis process and enhance the phagocytosis process [24].

Neuregulin-1

It is released from endothelial cells and binds to ErbB receptors on nearby cardiac myocytes to promote cell growth. NRG-1 is the most abundant protein in the cardiac system. The presence of oxidative stress, ischemic conditions the NRG -1 expression can occur in the ErbB cell receptors [25].

BIOMARKERS OF MICRO RNAS (MIRNAS)

These are consisting of short nucleotides and non coding nature of RNA molecules. A sequence of six to eight nucleotides which bind to messenger ribonucleic acid called miRNA targets. It will down regulate the translation at the post expression level and prevents the gene expression through translational repression and mRNA degradation process. The real time polymerase chain reaction has been used for the assessment of miRNA expression levels.

OTHER BIOMARKERS INVOLVED IN THE PREDICTION OF CARDIOVASCULAR DISEASE RISK PREDICTION

Neutrophil Gelatinase-Associated Lipocalin

It is a glycoprotein covalently bound to matrix metaloproteinase-9 and released by renal tubular cells in response to renal inflammatory conditions.

Natriuretic Peptides

It include brain natriuretic peptide, atrial natriuretic peptide and their N-terminal pro-hormones N-terminal pro-atrial natriuretic peptide and N-terminal pro-brain natriuretic peptide levels were elevated in patients presented with left ventricular dysfunction which leads to the development of cardiovascular diseases.

Apelin

It is a 36-amino acid peptide and is an endogenous ligand of G-protein-coupled receptors of apelin receptor. Recently, apelin was recognized as adipokine which is secreted from white adipose tissue. Apelin receptor is located in vascular smooth muscle cells, ventricular cardiomyocytes and intra-myocardial endothelial cells. The apelin can stimulate endothelium-dependent nitric oxide which leads to relaxation of the blood vessels and finally reduces arterial blood pressure. It shows antioxidant effects, lipogenesis, lipolysis and release of free fatty acids have a greater role in reducing the inflammatory process.

Growth Differentiation Factor-15

The abnormal increased levels of GDF-15 levels are associated with the development of various cardiovascular diseases such as hypertrophy, atherosclerosis, heart failure, obesity *etc.* It also inhibits epidermal growth factor receptor activation and NF-kB/JNK/caspase-3 pathway. The abnormal GDF-15 levels can be useful to identify the cardiovascular complications. The GDF-15 is elevated during tissue injury and inflammatory states and increases cardio metabolic risk.

Cyclophilin A

CyPA is secreted from vascular cell components of cells such as endothelial cells and vascular smooth muscle cells. CyPA initiates the expression of adhesion molecules in endothelial cells and induces the apoptosis process. Intracellular and extracellular CyPA can cause intimal thickening and involved in the atherosclerosis process.

Prolactin

Prolactin is a polypeptide which is converted to pituitary hormone and produce lactation in females. It can regulate reproduction, growth and development, immune regulation and metabolism functions. The higher prolactin levels lead to impair glucose secretion. The increased levels of proactin were seen in acute coronary syndromes, pre-eclampsia and heart failure patients.

Heart-type Fatty Acid Binding Protein (H-FABP)

It is a type of transport protein that allows for the transport of fatty acids through the membranes. The various types of FABP include liver-type FABP (L-FABP), heart-type FABP (H-FABP) and intestinal-type (I-FABP). It is a low molecular weight protein comprised of 132 amino acids involved in fatty-acid metabolism. The early stage of progression of myocardial infarction it will be released into cytosol. It is found very small quantities in kidney, and skeletal tissue and brain. The abnormal levels of FABP lead to increase in the risk of ischemic events.

CONCLUSION

The cardiovascular disease mortality rate still increasing from developed and developing countries. The progression of cardiovascular diseases is linked with multiple risk factors that include diabetes mellitus, alcohol, hypertension, smoking, stress and obesity which have led to the development of cardiovascular disease risk. Prompt detection of risk factors, risk screening and novel risk markers can use for prediction of future progression of cardiovascular risk burden among disease population. Currently, several cardiovascular disease biomarkers available which are used as diagnostic and predictive biomarkers used to detect and lower the risk of cardiovascular complications. These biomarkers measurement is easy and within a short period we can assess the disease severity with accurate results. These biomarkers reflect pathophysiological mechanisms associated with cardiovascular disease. It will give significant information about the prognosis of the disease and assists in effective clinical information for better treatment. It is used to assess the surrogate endpoints values in clinical studies which are helpful for the design of advance cardiovascular disease treatment in the clinical practice.

REFERENCES

[1]   Biomarkers and surrogate endpoints: preferred definitions and conceptual framework. Clin Pharmacol Ther 2001; 69(3): 89-95.
       [http://dx.doi.org/10.1067/mcp.2001.113989] [PMID: 11240971]

[2]   Redberg RF, Vogel RA, Criqui MH, Herrington DM, Lima JA, Roman MJ. 34th Bethesda Conference: Task force #3--What is the spectrum of current and emerging techniques for the noninvasive measurement of atherosclerosis? J Am Coll Cardiol 2003; 41(11): 1886-98.
       [http://dx.doi.org/10.1016/S0735-1097(03)00360-7] [PMID: 12798555]

[3]   Hoff J, Wehner W, Nambi V. Troponin in cardiovascular disease prevention: updates and future direction. Curr Atheroscler Rep 2016; 18(3): 12.
       [http://dx.doi.org/10.1007/s11883-016-0566-5] [PMID: 26879078]

[4]   Everett BM, Brooks MM, Vlachos HE, Chaitman BR, Frye RL, Bhatt DL. Troponin and cardiac events in stable ischemic heart disease and diabetes. N Engl J Med 2015; 373(7): 610-20.
       [http://dx.doi.org/10.1056/NEJMoa1415921] [PMID: 26267622]

[5]   McMahon CG, Lamont JV, Curtin E, *et al.* Diagnostic accuracy of heart-type fatty acid-binding protein for the early diagnosis of acute myocardial infarction. Am J Emerg Med 2012; 30(2): 267-74.
       [http://dx.doi.org/10.1016/j.ajem.2010.11.022] [PMID: 21208763]

[6]   Gami BN, Patel DS, Haridas N, Chauhan KP, Shah H, Trivedi A. Utility of heart-type fatty acid binding protein as a new biochemical marker for the early diagnosis of acute coronary syndrome. J Clin Diagn Res 2015; 9(1): BC22-4.
       [http://dx.doi.org/10.7860/JCDR/2015/11006.5451] [PMID: 25737977]

[7]   Otaki Y, Watanabe T, Takahashi H, *et al.* Association of heart-type fatty acid-binding protein with cardiovascular risk factors and all-cause mortality in the general population: the Takahata study. PLoS

One 2014; 9(5): e94834.
[http://dx.doi.org/10.1371/journal.pone.0094834] [PMID: 24847804]

[8]   Bassuk SS, Rifai N, Ridker PM. High-sensitivity C-reactive protein: clinical importance. Curr Probl Cardiol 2004; 29(8): 439-93.
[PMID: 15258556]

[9]   Devaraj S, Xu DY, Jialal I. C-reactive protein increases plasminogen activator inhibitor-1 expression and activity in human aortic endothelial cells: implications for the metabolic syndrome and atherothrombosis. Circulation 2003; 107(3): 398-404.
[http://dx.doi.org/10.1161/01.CIR.0000052617.91920.FD] [PMID: 12551862]

[10]   Kaptoge S, Di Angelantonio E, Lowe G, *et al.* C-reactive protein concentration and risk of coronary heart disease, stroke, and mortality: an individual participant meta-analysis. Lancet 2010; 375(9709): 132-40.
[http://dx.doi.org/10.1016/S0140-6736(09)61717-7] [PMID: 20031199]

[11]   Oemrawsingh RM, Cheng JM, Akkerhuis KM, *et al.* High-sensitivity C-reactive protein predicts 10-year cardiovascular outcome after percutaneous coronary intervention. EuroIntervention 2016; 12(3): 345-51.
[http://dx.doi.org/10.4244/EIJY15M07_04] [PMID: 26158553]

[12]   Lane T, Wassef N, Poole S, *et al.* Infusion of pharmaceutical-grade natural human C-reactive protein is not proinflammatory in healthy adult human volunteers. Circ Res 2014; 114(4): 672-6.
[http://dx.doi.org/10.1161/CIRCRESAHA.114.302770] [PMID: 24337102]

[13]   Daniels LB, Clopton P, Laughlin GA, Maisel AS, Barrett-Connor E. Growth-differentiation factor-15 is a robust, independent predictor of 11-year mortality risk in community-dwelling older adults: the Rancho Bernardo Study. Circulation 2011; 123(19): 2101-10.
[http://dx.doi.org/10.1161/CIRCULATIONAHA.110.979740] [PMID: 21536998]

[14]   Cotter G, Voors AA, Prescott MF, *et al.* Growth differentiation factor 15 (GDF-15) in patients admitted for acute heart failure: results from the RELAX-AHF study. Eur J Heart Fail 2015; 17(11): 1133-43.
[http://dx.doi.org/10.1002/ejhf.331] [PMID: 26333529]

[15]   Wollert KC, Kempf T, Lagerqvist B, *et al.* Growth differentiation factor 15 for risk stratification and selection of an invasive treatment strategy in non ST-elevation acute coronary syndrome. Circulation 2007; 116(14): 1540-8.
[http://dx.doi.org/10.1161/CIRCULATIONAHA.107.697714] [PMID: 17848615]

[16]   Hagström E, James SK, Bertilsson M, *et al.* Growth differentiation factor-15 level predicts major bleeding and cardiovascular events in patients with acute coronary syndromes: results from the PLATO study. Eur Heart J 2016; 37(16): 1325-33.
[http://dx.doi.org/10.1093/eurheartj/ehv491] [PMID: 26417057]

[17]   Becatti M, Marcucci R, Bruschi G, *et al.* Oxidative modification of fibrinogen is associated with altered function and structure in the subacute phase of myocardial infarction. Arterioscler Thromb Vasc Biol 2014; 34(7): 1355-61.
[http://dx.doi.org/10.1161/ATVBAHA.114.303785] [PMID: 24790138]

[18]   Sawicki M, Sypniewska G, Kozinski M, *et al.* Diagnostic efficacy of myeloperoxidase for the detection of acute coronary syndromes. Eur J Clin Invest 2011; 41(6): 667-71.
[http://dx.doi.org/10.1111/j.1365-2362.2010.02457.x] [PMID: 21226709]

[19]   Wang LX, Lü SZ, Zhang WJ, Song XT, Chen H, Zhang LJ. Comparision of high sensitivity C-reactive protein and matrix metalloproteinase 9 in patients with unstable angina between with and without significant coronary artery plaques. Chin Med J (Engl) 2011; 124(11): 1657-61.
[PMID: 21740772]

[20]   Kelly D, Cockerill G, Ng LL, *et al.* Plasma matrix metalloproteinase-9 and left ventricular remodelling after acute myocardial infarction in man: a prospective cohort study. Eur Heart J 2007; 28(6): 711-8.

[http://dx.doi.org/10.1093/eurheartj/ehm003] [PMID: 17339265]

[21]   Packard CJ, O'Reilly DS, Caslake MJ, *et al.* Lipoprotein-associated phospholipase A2 as an independent predictor of coronary heart disease. N Engl J Med 2000; 343(16): 1148-55.
[http://dx.doi.org/10.1056/NEJM200010193431603] [PMID: 11036120]

[22]   Greisenegger S, Segal HC, Burgess AI, Poole DL, Mehta Z, Rothwell PM. Copeptin and long-term risk of recurrent vascular events after transient ischemic attack and ischemic stroke: population-based study. Stroke 2015; 46(11): 3117-23.
[http://dx.doi.org/10.1161/STROKEAHA.115.011021] [PMID: 26451023]

[23]   Schmitz J, Owyang A, Oldham E, *et al.* IL-33, an interleukin-1-like cytokine that signals *via* the IL-1 receptor-related protein ST2 and induces T helper type 2-associated cytokines. Immunity 2005; 23(5): 479-90.
[http://dx.doi.org/10.1016/j.immuni.2005.09.015] [PMID: 16286016]

[24]   Maiolino G, Rossitto G, Pedon L, *et al.* Galectin-3 predicts long-term cardiovascular death in high-risk patients with coronary artery disease. Arterioscler Thromb Vasc Biol 2015; 35(3): 725-32.
[http://dx.doi.org/10.1161/ATVBAHA.114.304964] [PMID: 25614283]

[25]   Geisberg CA, Wang G, Safa RN, *et al.* Circulating neuregulin-1β levels vary according to the angiographic severity of coronary artery disease and ischemia. Coron Artery Dis 2011; 22(8): 577-82.
[http://dx.doi.org/10.1097/MCA.0b013e32834d3346] [PMID: 22027878]

CHAPTER 3

Diagnostic Investigations for Detection of Cardiovascular Diseases

Abstract: Cardiovascular diseases are a group of disorders of the cardiovascular system which include coronary heart disease, hypertension, myocardial infarction, angina pectoris, rheumatic heart disease, and stroke *etc.* Currently, cardiovascular diseases are causing 21.9 percent of total deaths globally and that will rise to 26.3 percent by 2030. The risk factors for cardiovascular disease include hypertension, stress, alcohol, diabetes mellitus, smoking, and obesity which highly impact the development of cardiovascular disease. The cardiovascular disease diagnostic test includes electrocardiogram, echocardiography, MRI scan, CT scan, treadmill test, Doppler studies and coronary angiography tests which are vital for determining the severity of cardiovascular disease among diagnosed patients. Early detection of cardiovascular disease risk factors and regular cardiovascular disease risk screening modalities can lower the alarming incidences of cardiovascular diseases in health care settings.

Keywords: Coronary Angiography, Coronary Heart Disease, Diabetes Mellitus, Echocardiography, Electrocardiogram, Hypertension, Treadmill Test.

INTRODUCTION

Cardiovascular diseases are the disorders of the cardiovascular system which include coronary heart disease, hypertension, myocardial infarction, angina pectoris, rheumatic heart disease, cerebrovascular disease, and other conditions. The presence of various cardiovascular risk factors and lack of screening and treatment approaches can cause higher incidences of cardiovascular mortality and morbidity in clinical settings. Currently, the cardiovascular diseases are causing 21.9 percent of total deaths globally and which will be 26.3 percent by 2030.

The reduction of cardiovascular disease incidences can be lowered by adhering to the medications, approaching healthier lifestyle practices and novel diagnostic approaches can helpful for the reduction of cardiovascular incidences in health care. The American Heart Association guidelines strongly recommend that newer therapeutic approaches and personalization of treatment modalities can use for successful management of coronary artery disease complications in the clinical

M.S. Umashankar & A. Bharath Kumar

practice. Cardiovascular disease is noted to be one of the leading causes of mortality worldwide and results in 18 million deaths every year. Previous literature works stated that 80 percent of all deaths occurring worldwide are due to cardiovascular diseases. The advancement of age can cause the progression of cardiovascular diseases. A greater burden of cardiovascular disease deaths occurs at younger ages in low-middle income countries was high as compared to high-income countries.

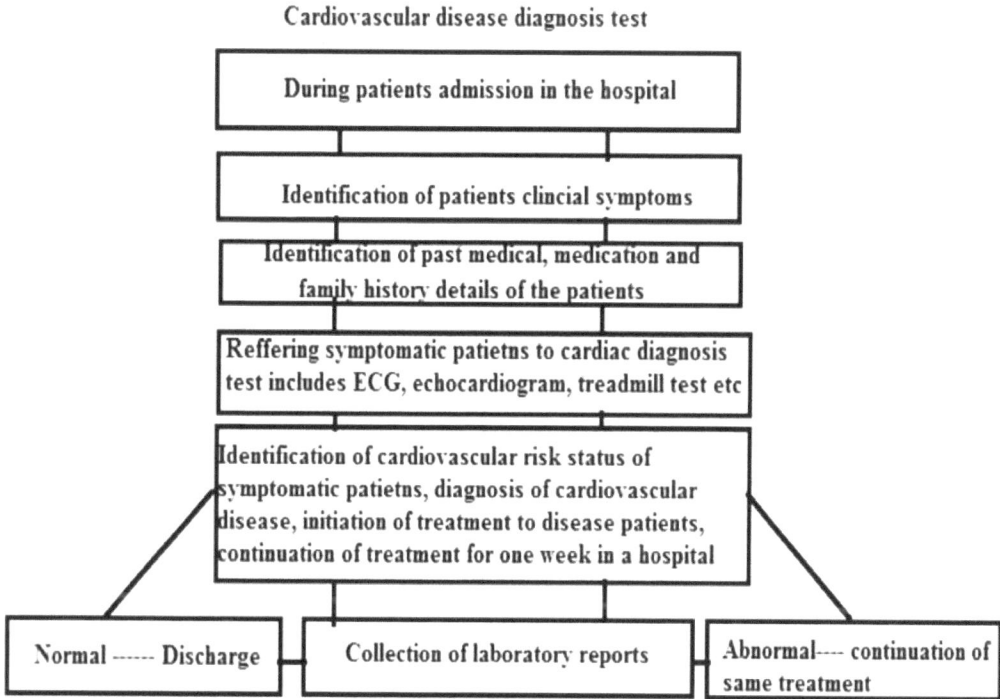

Cardiovascular disease diagnosis test

During patients admission in the hospital

Identification of patients clincial symptoms

Identification of past medical, medication and family history details of the patients

Reffering symptomatic patietns to cardiac diagnosis test includes ECG, echocardiogram, treadmill test etc

Identification of cardiovascular risk status of symptomatic patietns, diagnosis of cardiovascular disease, initiation of treatment to disease patients, continuation of treatment for one week in a hospital

Normal ----- Discharge

Collection of laboratory reports

Abnormal---- continuation of same treatment

Fig. (1). Cardiovascular disease diagnosis test flow chart.

The number of adults with raised blood pressure increased from 594 million in 1975 to 1.13 billion in 2015, with the increase largely in low- and middle-income countries. High blood pressure is the leading risk factor for the progression of cardiovascular disease. The prevalence was found to 24.1% in men and 20.1% in women.

Coronary artery disease diagnostic investigations

```
┌─────────────────────────────────────────────────────┐
│  Patient admitted with coronary artery disease in a   │
│  hospital, identification of clinical history of patient │
└─────────────────────────────────────────────────────┘
                          │
┌─────────────────────────────────────────────────────┐
│  Identification of past medical, medication and family │
│  history details of the patient                       │
└─────────────────────────────────────────────────────┘
                          │
┌─────────────────────────────────────────────────────┐
│  Reffering symptomatic patient  to cardiovascular disease │
│  diagnosis test include ECG, echocardiogram, treadmill │
│  test, stress test, MRI scan, doppler test etc.       │
└─────────────────────────────────────────────────────┘
                          │
┌─────────────────────────────────────────────────────┐
│  Observation of abnormal clinical reports of the patient, │
│  sugesting for one week admission in a hospital, initiation of │
│  treatment, continuation of treatment for one week    │
└─────────────────────────────────────────────────────┘

┌──────────────────┐  ┌──────────────────────────┐  ┌──────────────────────────┐
│ Normal: Discharge │  │ Collection of clinical reports │  │ Abnormal: Continuation of │
│                  │  │                          │  │ same treatment            │
└──────────────────┘  └──────────────────────────┘  └──────────────────────────┘
```

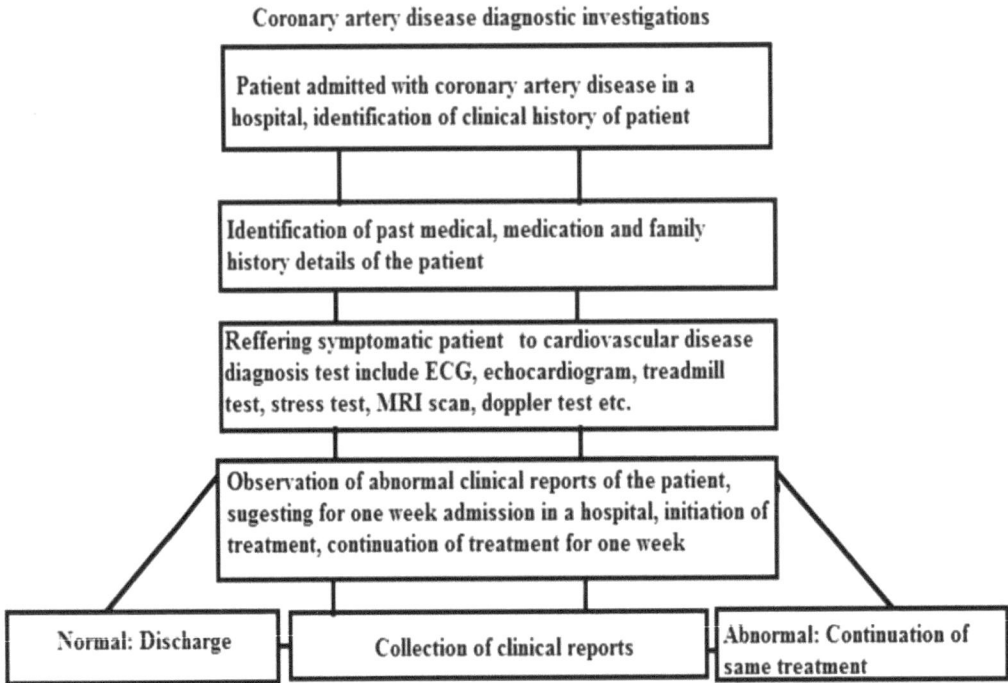

Fig. (2). Coronary artery disease diagnostic investigations flow chart.

The prevention of cardiovascular diseases needs knowledge on cardiovascular risk factors, newer advance treatment strategies and continuous support from the health care team may identify to effective for successful management and prevention of cardiovascular complications. The reduction of cardiovascular

complications can be achieved through addressing the risk factors and early initiation of screening and diagnostic techniques could lower the progression of cardiovascular complications. The cardiovascular disease diagnosis test was shown in Figs. (**1** & **2**). Cardiovascular disease prevention through meeting with a healthier lifestyle and cardiovascular risk factors reduction practices can helpful for the prevention of cardiovascular disease burden in the community. The low-middle income countries do not have sophisticated health care facilities and disease detection devices for the identification of chronic diseases so therefore the disease progression rate was very high [1 - 6]. The reduction of incidences of hypertension by approaching lifestyle modification practices such as smoking and alcohol cessation, reduction in salt intake. Reducing the incidence of hypertension by implementing population-wide policies to reduce behavioral risk factors, including harmful use of alcohol, physical inactivity, overweight, obesity, and high salt intake, is essential to attaining this target.

CARDIOVASCULAR DISEASES: A GROUP OF DISORDERS OF THE HEART AND BLOOD VESSELS

Coronary Heart Disease

It is a disease of the blood vessels that causes a lack of blood supply to the cardiac muscles leads to the development of coronary artery disease.

Cerebrovascular Disease

It causes a low level of blood supply to the brain can cause an ischemic condition which leads to the development of stroke.

Peripheral Arterial Disease

The low level of blood supply to the arms and legs can cause the development of peripheral artery disease.

Rheumatic Heart Disease

The damage to the heart muscles and heart valves from rheumatic fever which is caused by the presence of streptococcal bacteria.

Congenital Heart Disease

The malformations of heart structure can cause the formation of the abnormal limbs which leads to the development of congenital heart disease.

Deep Vein Thrombosis and Pulmonary Embolism

The clotting of blood in the leg veins and also lowers the blood flow to the heart and lungs.

RISK FACTORS FOR CARDIOVASCULAR DISEASE

Congestive heart failure is usually caused by blockage of coronary arteries which can prevent the flow of blood to the coronary arteries. The deposition of fatty materials in the walls of blood vessels can cause heart disease problems. The development of cardiovascular diseases is associated with complex risk factors such as smoking, alcohol, obesity, unhealthy diet, physical inactivity, hypertension and diabetes mellitus can increase the risk of cardiovascular disease complications. The smoking cessation, reduction of salt in the diet, consuming fruits and vegetables, regular physical activity and stress management can reduce the further progression of cardiovascular disease complications [7, 8]. The early initiation of treatment steps for cardiovascular risk prevention and management could reduce the progression of cardiovascular disease complications.

DIAGNOSTIC INVESTIGATIONS FOR CARDIOVASCULAR DISEASES

Blood Analysis

The blood test plays an essential role in the identification of infectious status and cardiovascular risk conditions of individual patients.

Biomarkers for Detection of Cardiovascular Disease

B-type Natriuretic Peptides

It is produced by the heart and the high levels of BNP can damage the heart muscle which leads to the development of heart failure.

Blood Urea Nitrogen

This test is used for the detection of heart failure. The abnormal level of blood urea nitrogen is a sign of kidney failure.

C-reactive Protein

It is produced by the liver in response to inflammatory conditions. The high levels of C-reactive protein can cause atherosclerosis.

Enzymes

The elevated conditions of the enzyme levels which may indicate the cardiovascular risk.

Fibrinogen

it is a protein that helps for blood clotting. The high levels of fibrinogen can indicate the risk of a blood clot which results in the development of a heart attack.

Blood Sugar Test

Abnormal glucose levels can cause diabetes mellitus, which is a major risk factor for the development of coronary artery disease.

Homocysteine

It is a protein and elevated levels of homocysteine increase the risk of coronary artery disease.

Lipid

It refers deposition of more lipids in the bloodstream. Elevated lipid levels can increase the risk of cardiovascular diseases.

OTHER CARDIOVASCULAR DISEASE DIAGNOSTIC INVESTIGATIONS

CT Scan

The computed tomography scans are used to produce high-resolution images of the heart and surrounding arteries. This test is used to detect plaque formation in the arteries.

Cardiac Catheterization

A flexible tube is inserted through an artery to the heart to detect blood pressure, blood oxygen capacity. A contrast dye may inject into the blood vessels to see the blockage in the coronary arteries.

Echocardiography

An echocardiogram is a noninvasive ultrasound of the heart. The test enables the information about size, structure, and function of the heart, valve abnormality, and calculation of cardiac output [9 - 12].

Ejection Fraction Testing

It is used to measures how much blood remains in the heart's pumping chambers after each heartbeat.

Electrocardiogram

It is used to record the electrical activity of the heart. An ECG measures the heart's electrical activity through electrodes placed in the chest, arms, and legs. An ECG can help to detect the heart rhythm,

Electrophysiology Study

An EP study investigates the electrical patterns of the heart and can help in determining the cause of an abnormal rhythm of the heart. In this method, a catheter is used to identify the blood pumping to the heart. At the end of the catheter, tiny electrodes are placed and it will transmit electrical impulses to the heart muscle to identify an abnormal heart rhythm.

Cardiac Stress Test

It is used to record an electrocardiogram while the patient reaching increased levels of physical strain at specific conditions. The test can be performed on a treadmill which increases the speed and resistance progressively. This will provide information about heart activity after scheduled exercise which is used to detect cardiac abnormalities [13 - 17].

Cardiac CT Scan Angiography

The CCTA is a noninvasive test that allows for detecting the important blood vessels in the heart muscle. The contrast dye solution is injected during the scan which shows blood flow in the coronary arteries. This comprehensive test shows that the narrowing in the arteries, heart chamber size, valves working status, pressures within the heart chambers and arteries and veins. The patient lies on a table that enters into a tomography scanner and produces images of the heart which is used to determine the degree of obstruction in the coronary arteries and risk of cardiovascular diseases [18 - 21].

Coronary Angiogram

It is a diagnostic tool that detects plaques in the bloodstream. These plaques are responsible for sudden cardiac deaths, strokes and cardiac failure.

Magnetic Resonance Imaging

It is a noninvasive and painless test that is used to evaluate the function of cardiac valves. A combination of large magnets with designed radio frequencies which are connected to a computer to record the images of the organs and structures in the body. It can also detect cardiac abnormality and blood vessels functioning status can help for the identification of cardiac diseases.

Transesophageal Echocardiogram

This method an ultrasound waves can produce images of the heart and blood vessels. The ultrasound device is placed on the esophagus to identify the images of heart valves, chambers, ribs, and lungs *etc*. It is used to record the blood clots in the heart filling chambers during atrial fibrillation. The small probe is inserted into the esophagus, which lies directly behind the heart and sends the images of heart function.

Ultrasound Examination

It uses high-frequency ultra sound waves to create graphic images of the heart and blood vessels. This ultrasound can create the images of the heart and direction of blood flow to the arteries and body organs. It is a leading test for the identification of peripheral vascular disease which is a major risk factor for the development of cardiovascular diseases.

Chest X-rays

It can help for the detection of congestive heart failure, heart infections, and inflammation, enlargement, and calcified heart valves lead to the progression of cardiovascular diseases.

Nuclear Perfusion Imaging

The radioactive agents are called radioisotopes are injected into the bloodstream to identify the blood flow to the heart. It can be performed at the resting stage to assess the adequacy of blood flow to the heart in a non-exertional state. A PET scan can detect the extent of heart muscle damage and helps to improve blood flow to the area of the affected area of the heart muscle.

Myocardial Perfusion Imaging

It is a nuclear medicine procedure shows the function of the heart muscle to identify cardiovascular diseases such as coronary artery disease, cardiomyopathy, and abnormalities associated with heart wall motion.

Holter and Event Monitoring Test

This test can progressively monitor heart beating capacity. It is placed around the waist for scheduled durations and continuously records the heart activity. The test can be performed during the patients suffering from cardiac symptoms to assess the burden of cardiovascular diseases [22 - 25].

CONCLUSION

Cardiovascular disease is a leading cause of mortality worldwide and results in 18 million deaths every year. Previous research studies stated that 80 percent of all deaths occurring in the worldwide is due to cardiovascular diseases. The prevention of cardiovascular diseases needs knowledge on cardiovascular risk factors, newer advance treatment strategies and continuous support from the health care team may identify to effective for successful management and prevention of cardiovascular complications. The lifestyle modifications for the prevention of cardiovascular diseases include termination of smoking and alcohol habits, eating healthy foods, DASH diet, scheduled exercise, weight control, and stress management can reduce the individual risk burden. Initiation of regular treatment with aspirin, cholesterol lowering drugs, hypertensive medications, and instigation of novel diagnostic tests and patient follow-up care services are needed to control the future attack of cardiovascular disease events in clinical practice.

REFERENCES

[1]   Deaton C, Froelicher ES, Wu LH, Ho C, Shishani K, Jaarsma T. The global burden of cardiovascular disease. Eur J Cardiovasc Nurs 2011; 10(2): 5-13.

[2]   Baroncini LAV, Borsoi R, Vidal MEB, Valente NJ, Veloso J, Pecoits Filho R. Assessment of dipyridamole stress echocardiography for risk stratification of diabetic patients. Cardiovasc Ultrasound 2015; 13: 35.
[http://dx.doi.org/10.1186/s12947-015-0030-7] [PMID: 26209102]

[3]   de Azevedo CF, Hadlich MS, Bezerra SG, *et al.* Prognostic value of CT angiography in patients with inconclusive functional stress tests. JACC Cardiovasc Imaging 2011; 4(7): 740-51.
[http://dx.doi.org/10.1016/j.jcmg.2011.02.017] [PMID: 21757164]

[4]   de Andrade L, Lynch C, Carvalho E, *et al.* System dynamics modeling in the evaluation of delays of care in ST-segment elevation myocardial infarction patients within a tiered health system. PLoS One 2014; 9(7): e103577.
[http://dx.doi.org/10.1371/journal.pone.0103577] [PMID: 25079362]

[5]   de Paula JA, Moreira OC, da Silva CD, Silva DS, dos Santos Amorim PR. Metabolic syndrome prevalence in elderly of urban and rural communities participants in the HIPERDIA in the city of Coimbra/MG, Brazil. Invest Educ Enferm 2015; 33(2): 325-33.
[PMID: 26535853]

[6]   Machado JP, Martins M, Leite ID. Quality of hospital databases in Brazil: some elements. Revista brasileira de epidemiologia = Brazilian journal of epidemiology 2016; 19(3): 81-567.

[7]   Stone NJ, Robinson JG, Lichtenstein AH, *et al.* 2013 ACC/AHA guideline on the treatment of blood cholesterol to reduce atherosclerotic cardiovascular risk in adults: a report of the American College of Cardiology/American Heart Association Task Force on Practice Guidelines Circulation 2014; 25(2): 1-45.

[8]   Ngui AN, Apparicio P. Optimizing the two-step floating catchment area method for measuring spatial accessibility to medical clinics in Montreal. BMC Health Serv Res 2011; 11: 166.
[http://dx.doi.org/10.1186/1472-6963-11-166] [PMID: 21745402]

[9]   Lucas FL, DeLorenzo MA, Siewers AE, Wennberg DE. Temporal trends in the utilization of diagnostic testing and treatments for cardiovascular disease in the United States, 1993-2001. Circulation 2006; 113(3): 374-9.
[http://dx.doi.org/10.1161/CIRCULATIONAHA.105.560433] [PMID: 16432068]

[10]   de Fatima Marinho de Souza M, Gawryszewski VP, Orduñez P, Sanhueza A, Espinal MA. Cardiovascular disease mortality in the Americas: current trends and disparities. Heart 2012; 98(16): 1207-12.
[http://dx.doi.org/10.1136/heartjnl-2012-301828] [PMID: 22826558]

[11]   Badano LP, Muraru D, Rigo F, *et al.* High volume-rate three-dimensional stress echocardiography to assess inducible myocardial ischemia: a feasibility study. J Am Soc Echocardiogr 2010; 23(6): 628-35.
[http://dx.doi.org/10.1016/j.echo.2010.03.020] [PMID: 20434877]

[12]   Mordi I, Tzemos N. Incremental value of CT perfusion in the diagnosis of coronary artery disease. Eur Heart J Cardiovasc Imaging 2013; 14(5): 504.
[http://dx.doi.org/10.1093/ehjci/jes237] [PMID: 23148081]

[13]   Banerjee A, Newman DR, Van den Bruel A, Heneghan C. Diagnostic accuracy of exercise stress testing for coronary artery disease: a systematic review and meta-analysis of prospective studies. Int J Clin Pract 2012; 66(5): 477-92.

[http://dx.doi.org/10.1111/j.1742-1241.2012.02900.x] [PMID: 22512607]

[14]   Roger VL, Jacobsen SJ, Pellikka PA, Miller TD, Bailey KR, Gersh BJ. Prognostic value of treadmill exercise testing: a population-based study in Olmsted County, Minnesota. Circulation 1998; 98(25): 2836-41.
[http://dx.doi.org/10.1161/01.CIR.98.25.2836] [PMID: 9860784]

[15]   Mark DB, Shaw L, Harrell FE Jr, *et al.* Prognostic value of a treadmill exercise score in outpatients with suspected coronary artery disease. N Engl J Med 1991; 325(12): 849-53.
[http://dx.doi.org/10.1056/NEJM199109193251204] [PMID: 1875969]

[16]   Pflugi S, Roujol S, Akçakaya M, *et al.* Accelerated cardiac MR stress perfusion with radial sampling after physical exercise with an MR-compatible supine bicycle ergometer. Magn Reson Med 2015; 74(2): 384-95.
[http://dx.doi.org/10.1002/mrm.25405] [PMID: 25105469]

[17]   Foster EL, Arnold JW, Jekic M, *et al.* MR-compatible treadmill for exercise stress cardiac magnetic resonance imaging. Magn Reson Med 2012; 67(3): 880-9.
[http://dx.doi.org/10.1002/mrm.23059] [PMID: 22190228]

[18]   Agatston AS, Janowitz WR, Hildner FJ, Zusmer NR, Viamonte M Jr, Detrano R. Quantification of coronary artery calcium using ultrafast computed tomography. J Am Coll Cardiol 1990; 15(4): 827-32.
[http://dx.doi.org/10.1016/0735-1097(90)90282-T] [PMID: 2407762]

[19]   Einstein AJ. Radiation dose reduction in coronary CT angiography: time to buckle down. JACC Cardiovasc Imaging 2015; 8(8): 897-9.
[http://dx.doi.org/10.1016/j.jcmg.2015.02.021] [PMID: 26271086]

[20]   Douglas PS, Hoffmann U, Patel MR, *et al.* Outcomes of anatomical*versus* functional testing for coronary artery disease. N Engl J Med 2015; 372(14): 1291-300.
[http://dx.doi.org/10.1056/NEJMoa1415516] [PMID: 25773919]

[21]   Andreini D, Pontone G, Mushtaq S, *et al.* A long-term prognostic value of coronary CT angiography in suspected coronary artery disease. JACC Cardiovasc Imaging 2012; 5(7): 690-701.
[http://dx.doi.org/10.1016/j.jcmg.2012.03.009] [PMID: 22789937]

[22]   Liew GY, Feneley MP, Worthley SG. Appropriate indications for computed tomography coronary angiography. Med J Aust 2012; 196(4): 246-9.
[http://dx.doi.org/10.5694/mja11.10130] [PMID: 22409689]

[23]   Doris M, Newby DE. Coronary CT angiography as a diagnostic and prognostic tool: perspectives from the SCOT-HEART trial. Curr Cardiol Rep 2016; 18(2): 18.
[http://dx.doi.org/10.1007/s11886-015-0695-4] [PMID: 26782999]

[24]   Carpeggiani C, Picano E, Brambilla M, *et al.* Variability of radiation doses of cardiac diagnostic imaging tests: the RADIO-EVINCI study (RADIationdOse subproject of the EVINCI study). BMC Cardiovasc Disord 2017; 17(1): 63.
[http://dx.doi.org/10.1186/s12872-017-0474-9] [PMID: 28202051]

[25]   Lebtahi NE, Stauffer JC, Delaloye AB. Left bundle branch block and coronary artery disease: accuracy of dipyridamole thallium-201 single-photon emission computed tomography in patients with exercise anteroseptal perfusion defects. J Nucl Cardiol 1997; 4(4): 266-73.
[http://dx.doi.org/10.1016/S1071-3581(97)90103-3] [PMID: 9278872]

CHAPTER 4

Heart Valve Disease

Abstract: Valvular heart disease occurs by the defects in tricuspid, aortic, mitral, pulmonary artery leads to develop heart valve abnormalities. Gender, age, hypertension, diabetes mellitus, alcohol, smoking and hypercholesterolemia can contribute to the progression of valvular heart disease. Previous research studies stated that one-third of elderly patients echocardiographic examination showed that the evidence of calcific aortic valve sclerosis. Patients with age more than 60 years suffer from the calcific aortic stenosis. It is more prevalent in western countries as compared with other cardiovascular diseases such as coronary artery disease, angina pectoris, myocardial infarction, and hypertension. Previous research studies demonstrated that 40 million people are affected by the age group of 65 years in the 2010 year and expected to rise 55 million in 2020 and 72 million in 2030. Patients with clinical signs of aortic stenosis during the physical examination should undergo various other examinations like chest x-ray, electrocardiogram, and echocardiogram useful for the detection of valvular heart disease risk at the early stages. Aortic valve replacement is used to lower the progression of aortic stenosis among high-risk patients.

Keywords: Diabetes Mellitus, Electrocardiogram, Hypercholesterolemia, Myocardial Infarction, Valvular Heart Disease.

INTRODUCTION

Aortic stenosis affects people of older age being 65 years. The presence of left ventricular hypertrophy and atrial augmentation of preload compensate for the increase in after-load caused by aortic stenosis. The worsening of heart valve disease condition leads to the development of various cardiovascular diseases such as coronary artery disease, heart failure, and angina pectoris. Aortic valve replacement is strongly recommended for most symptomatic patients diagnosed with aortic stenosis. Surgical valve replacement is the standard treatment for patients at low to moderate surgical risk. Trans catheter aortic valve replacement may beneficial for patients having high surgical risk. Regular health care visit is recommended for patients with symptomatic having moderate to severe aortic stenosis. Medical management of concurrent hypertension, atrial fibrillation, and coronary artery disease can improve the health related quality of life of individual patients. The progression of aortic stenosis occurs earlier in patients with congenital bicuspid aortic valves, and renal failure can increase the risk developing aortic valve disease. valvular heart disease is defined as a defect in one of the four heart valves: the mitral, aortic, tricuspid or pulmonary. The mitral and tricuspid valves direct the blood flow between the atria and the ventricles [1 - 5]. The pulmonary valve monitors the blood flow from the heart to the lungs, and aortic valve controls the blood flow between the heart and the aorta. The mitral and aortic valves are commonly affected by valvular heart disease. Heart valves monitor the blood flows with appropriate direction to the heart. In valvular heart disease condition the valves become too narrow and unable to close completely leads to the development of valvular defects in the heart. The heart valves are shown in Fig. (1). The improper circulation of blood to the heart muscles leads to losing its efficiency and increases the risk of the pulmonary embolism. The ineffective treatment of valvular heart may increase the risk of developing cardiovascular complications.

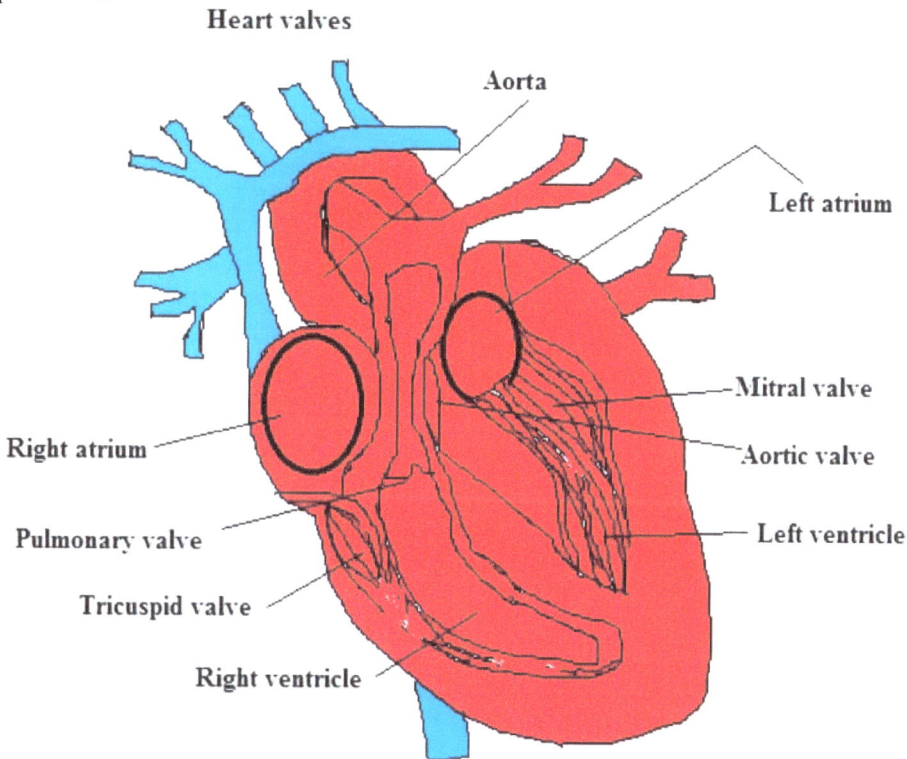

Fig. (1). Heart valves.

PREVALENCE

It is estimated from the previous research studies demonstrated that the 40 million people are affected with age group of 65 years in the year 2010 and expected to rise 55 million in 2020 and 72 million in 2030.

TYPES OF HEART VALVE DISEASE

Valvular Stenosis

It occurs when the defect in the heart valve and narrowing of valves reduce the blood flow to the heart which leads to the development of valvular stenosis.

Valvular Insufficiency

It occurs due to the improper close of valves leads to blockage of valves and causes leakage of blood from the valves. The heart will depend on more energy to pump the blood to all the organs in the body. The damage of the valves is called aortic regurgitation [6 - 8]. The leakage of the valves leads to a low level of blood flow to the body. The damage of the valve is known as pulmonary regurgitation, mitral regurgitation and tricuspid regurgitation.

RISK FACTORS FOR HEART VALVE DISEASE

- Heart attack
- Infection
- Aging
- Congenital birth defect
- Syphilis
- History of rheumatic fever

CAUSES OF HEART VALVE DISEASE

- Normal aging process
- Damage from a previous heart attack
- Damage by rheumatic fever
- A buildup of calcium on the valve
- Infection in the lining of the heart walls and valves
- Heart attack
- Atherosclerosis
- High blood pressure
- Autoimmune disorders
- Metabolic disorders

SYMPTOMS [9, 10]

- Swelling of ankles and feet
- Dizziness
- Fainting
- Irregular heartbeat

- Chest pain
- Abnormal heart sounds
- Fatigue
- Shortness of breath
- Fever
- Weight gain

DIAGNOSTIC INVESTIGATIONS

- Transesophageal echocardiogram
- Electrocardiogram
- Chest X-ray
- Cardiac ultrasound
- Electrocardiogram
- A stress test
- Cardiac magnetic resonance image
- Cardiac catheterization

PATHOPHYSIOLOGY

The progression of the aortic valve starts from sclerosis to stenosis. In this condition, the presence of high resistance on the left ventricle reduces the blood ejection from the heart. The ventricles must produce high systolic pressure compared with the contrasting force produced by the calcified aortic valve. The high resistance pressure during the time of blood ejection from systole known as after load. The thickening of the left ventricular wall is called hypertrophy and maintaining and improves cardiac output. The presence of high left ventricular after load reduces the cardiac function. The left ventricular pressure is greater in the aortic pressure at the time of ejection of the blood from the left ventricle. The pressure across the aortic valve is much greater during the stenosis and increases the resistance of aortic valve leads to create turbulence on the valve. The pressure gradient is calculated by the severity of stenosis and the flow of blood across the valve. The impediment of the left ventricular outflow increases the pressure thereby activation of compensatory mechanisms to maintain the normal systolic function. Narrowing of aortic valve causes shrinkage of the left ventricular outflow results in the development of left ventricular hypertrophy. The continuous progression of the left ventricular hypertrophy leads to reduce blood to the coronary arteries [11 - 16]. The presence of high after load in the ventricles reduces the left ventricular ejection fraction and cardiac output leads to the development of congestive heart failure in aortic valve sclerosis patients. Effects of high left ventricular after load include decreased left ventricular myocardial elasticity and coronary blood flow and increased myocardial workload, oxygen consumption, and mortality. The inveterate of blood increases the risk of developing causes the development of angina pectoris.

PHARMACOTHERAPEUTIC MANAGEMENT

- Diuretics
- Anti-arrhythmic drugs
- Vasodilators
- ACE inhibitors
- Beta blockers
- Anticoagulants

SURGERY OPTIONS

Heart Valve Repair

It is used to improve heart function. During the valve repairing process the partition of valve cups and removal of higher valve tissue leads to valve cups that may close properly. The replacement of a valve ring can be performed with embedding an artificial ring around the valve. To repair a valve, surgeons may separate valve flaps (leaflets or cusps) that have fused, replace the cords that support the valve, remove excess valve tissue so that the leaflets or cusps can close tightly or patch holes in a valve [17 - 19]. Surgeons may often tighten or reinforce the ring around a valve by implant an artificial ring.

Biological Valve Replacement

The biological tissue valves can degeneration process may require prolonged time. Patients treated with mechanical valves need anti coagulant medications for the prevention of blood clot.

Biological tissue valves degenerate over time, and often eventually need to be replaced. People with mechanical valves will need to take blood-thinning medications for life to prevent blood clots.

Surgery and other Procedures

Surgical options include heart valve repair or replacement. Valves can be repaired or replaced with traditional heart valve surgery or a minimally invasive heart valve surgical procedure. Heart valves may also be repaired by other procedures such as percutaneous balloon valvotomy. The surgical treatment for aortic valve disease includes heart valve replacement and percutaneous balloon valvotomy.

Aortic Stenosis

Aortic stenosis (AS) is the most common VHD in adults, increasing in prevalence with age. AS presents a mechanical problem, when hemodynamically severe and adversely affects the myocardium and aortic valve replacement is used to reduce the valvular complications. The clinical manifestations in aortic stenosis result from the combined mechanical effects of the structural valve abnormality and the myocardial response to the resulting mechanical stresses. Consequently, several studies have evaluated the role of statins, angiotensin-converting enzyme inhibitors (ACEIs), angiotensin receptor blockers (ARBs), and bisphosphonates to slow AS progression [20 - 22].

Lipid-Lowering Therapy

Statins

The potential of statins to retard valvular calcification initially was inferred from the similarities in risk factors and histological findings in calcific aortic stenosis and coronary artery disease. Subsequent demonstration of the similarity of cellular pathways leading to valve calcification and atherosclerotic plaque formation gave credence to the statin hypothesis. It is used to prevent the progression of valvular calcification. The various classes of statins include Atorvastatin, lovastatin, simvastatin, pitavastatin, fluvastatin, rosuvastatin and pravastatin is the commonly prescribed drugs in the current medical practice.

Angiotensin-Converting Enzyme Inhibitors/Angiotensin Receptor Blockers

Histopathological studies demonstrated that up regulation of angiotensin II in sclerotic aortic valves may cause aortic stenosis. ACE inhibitors generate angiotensin II, facilitates the degradation of anti fibrotic bradykinin causes atrio-ventricular fibrosis. The renin-angiotensin system is believed to modulate adverse left ventricular remodeling and myocardial fibrosis and produces angiotensin II which can initiate the inflammation process and promotes the degradation of bradykinins. The ACE inhibitor drugs include Captopril, Benazepril, Enalapril, Fosinopril, Lisinopril, Perindopril, Quinapril, Ramipril and Trandolapril.

Vasodilator Therapy

Vasodilator therapy is a cornerstone in the management of patients with left ventricular dysfunction but was historically contraindicated in patients with severe aortic stenosis. It was previously believed that cardiac output across a fixed stenotic aortic valve and vasodilatation from vasodilator therapy would reduce the systemic vascular resistance without compensatory increase in the cardiac output that will result in severe hypotension. Vasodilator therapy could lower the systemic vascular resistance and to increase the cardiac output. The previous research studies suggested the usefulness of this therapy as a bridge in patients who present with severe aortic stenosis and severe congestive heart failure, indicating that after load reduction may be used to stabilize the patient before valve replacement or switching to oral vasodilators in patients who choose not to undergo surgery. Previous research studies demonstrated that improving the prescribing pattern of vasodilators can reduce the after load and to alleviate the normal heart function [23].

Beta Blockers

Beta blockers improve the contraction of the heart muscles and reduce the preload and after load results in normalizing the valvular functions. The commonly prescribed beta-blockers include

- Acebutolol
- Atenolol
- Betaxolol
- Bisoprolol
- Carteolol
- Carvedilol
- Labetalol
- Metoprolol
- Nadolol
- Nebivolol
- Penbutolol
- Pindolol
- Propanolol
- Sotalol
- Timolol

Aortic Valve Replacement

Aortic valve replacement is the only effective treatment for symptomatic, hemodynamically severe aortic stenosis. It is recommended for symptomatic patients with severe aortic stenosis with left ventricular ejection fraction is less than 50 percent. Surgical replacement leads to significant improvement in survival, usually accompanied by symptom improvement. Surgical replacement can improve the quality of life and also improve the left ventricular function. Aortic valve replacement is also recommended for asymptomatic patients with severe stenosis accompanied by LV systolic dysfunction (EF less than 50%).

When severe stenosis is found to be the primary pathology in this setting, aortic valve replacement is a lifesaving therapy and improves LV function. Aortic valve replacement is also indicated in asymptomatic patients with severe or even moderate stenosis who are undergoing cardiac surgery for other indications; this avoids the need for repeat surgery once the valve disease inevitably progresses. It is indicated in asymptomatic patients with moderate stenosis with patients undergoing cardiac surgery for the previous history of coronary artery disease problems.

Surgical and Transcatheter Aortic Valve Replacement

Surgical aortic valve replacement is the standard of care in patients with low or intermediate surgical risk. Transcatheter aortic valve replacement is recommended for patients who have an indication for valve replacement. Surgical aortic valve replacement is effective care in patients diagnosed with intermediate surgical risk [24, 25]. Transcatheter aortic valve replacement is suggested for patients who are diagnosed with valve replacement having high surgical risk. Transcatheter valve replacement is also a reasonable alternative to surgical valve replacement in high-risk patients. Surgical risk should be assessed by a multidisciplinary team composed at minimum of a clinical cardiologist and a cardiac surgeon, and usually including subspecialists in interventional cardiology, cardiovascular imaging, anesthesiology, and heart failure management. Transcatheter valve replacement is another alternative method for surgical valve replacement in high-risk patients.

Aortic Balloon Valvuloplasty

Percutaneous aortic balloon valvoplasty is essentially balloon inflation across the aortic valve to reduce the severity of AS. Aortic balloon valvoplasty is fixed across the aortic valve to lower the risk of Aortic stenosis. The mechanism by which reduction in aortic valve gradient and improvement in symptoms with valvuloplasty occurs is yet unknown, but fracture of the calcific deposits, and separation of commissures, or stretching of the aortic annulus may play a part. Its current role is mainly as a part of the Trans catheter aortic valve replacement (TAVR) procedure or sometimes as a bridge to more definitive therapy.

HEALTHY LIFESTYLE CHANGES TO TREAT OTHER RELATED HEART CONDITIONS

• Eating a heart-healthy diet
• Maintaining a healthy weight
• Regular physical activity

- Managing stress
- Quitting smoking and alcohol
- Regular medication adhernece

CONCLUSION

Valvular heart diseases are reaching high prevalence in developed and developing countries. There is a need for an effective prescribing pattern of drugs and an understanding of molecular mechanisms associated with the pathogenesis of valvular heart disease guides for reducing the disease complications in primary care areas. The degenerative valve disorders are likely to rise at the population ages. Effective diagnosis, an early stage of screening, risk factors detection and better treatment options can lower the chronic mortality in health care settings. The improper circulation of blood to the heart muscles lead to losing its efficiency results in the occurrence of pulmonary embolism.

A better understanding of the patient's clinical history, previous medication history, and advanced diagnostic imaging tools, and surgical approaches could direct for appropriate selection of individual drug regimen. The ineffective treatment of valvular heart may increase the risk of developing cardiovascular complications. Regular health care visit is recommended for patients who are diagnosed with severe aortic stenosis. Medical management of complex diseases such as atrial fibrillation, hypertension, and coronary artery disease can improve the health-related quality of life of individual patients.

REFERENCES

[1]   Nkomo VT, Gardin JM, Skelton TN, Gottdiener JS, Scott CG, Enriquez-Sarano M. Burden of valvular heart diseases: a population-based study. Lancet 2006; 368(9540): 1005-11.
       [http://dx.doi.org/10.1016/S0140-6736(06)69208-8] [PMID: 16980116]

[2]   Berry C, Lloyd SM, Wang Y, Macdonald A, Ford I. The changing course of aortic valve disease in Scotland: temporal trends in hospitalizations and mortality and prognostic importance of aortic stenosis. Eur Heart J 2013; 34(21): 1538-47.
       [http://dx.doi.org/10.1093/eurheartj/ehs339] [PMID: 23111418]

[3]   Gaede L, Di Bartolomeo R, van der Kley F, Elsässer A, Iung B, Möllmann H. Aortic valve stenosis: what do people know? A heart valve disease awareness survey of over 8,800 people aged 60 or over. EuroIntervention 2016; 12(7): 883-9.
       [http://dx.doi.org/10.4244/EIJY16M06_02] [PMID: 27283409]

[4]   Pawade TA, Newby DE. Treating aortic stenosis: arresting the snowball effect. Expert Rev Cardiovasc Ther 2015; 13(5): 461-3.
       [http://dx.doi.org/10.1586/14779072.2015.1037284] [PMID: 25882205]

[5]   Lindroos M, Kupari M, Heikkilä J, Tilvis R. Prevalence of aortic valve abnormalities in the elderly: an echocardiographic study of a random population sample. J Am Coll Cardiol 1993; 21(5): 1220-5.
       [http://dx.doi.org/10.1016/0735-1097(93)90249-Z] [PMID: 8459080]

[6]   Roberts WC, Janning KG, Ko JM, Filardo G, Matter GJ. Frequency of congenitally bicuspid aortic valves in patients ≥80 years of age undergoing aortic valve replacement for aortic stenosis (with or

without aortic regurgitation) and implications for transcatheter aortic valve implantation. Am J Cardiol 2012; 109(11): 1632-6.
[http://dx.doi.org/10.1016/j.amjcard.2012.01.390] [PMID: 22459301]

[7]   Otto CM, Kuusisto J, Reichenbach DD, Gown AM, O'Brien KD. Characterization of the early lesion of 'degenerative' valvular aortic stenosis. Histological and immunohistochemical studies. Circulation 1994; 90(2): 844-53.
[http://dx.doi.org/10.1161/01.CIR.90.2.844] [PMID: 7519131]

[8]   Mick SL, Keshavamurthy S, Gillinov AM. Mitral valve repair *versus* replacement. Ann Cardiothorac Surg 2015; 4(3): 230-7.
[PMID: 26309824]

[9]   Zhuge RQ, Hou XP, Qi XL, Wu YJ, Zhang MZ. Clinical features and treatment options for mitral regurgitation in elderly inpatients. J Geriatr Cardiol 2018; 15(6): 428-33.
[PMID: 30108615]

[10]   Iung B, Baron G, Butchart EG, *et al.* A prospective survey of patients with valvular heart disease in Europe: The Euro Heart Survey on Valvular Heart Disease. Eur Heart J 2003; 24(13): 1231-43.
[http://dx.doi.org/10.1016/S0195-668X(03)00201-X] [PMID: 12831818]

[11]   Dweck MR, Boon NA, Newby DE. Calcific aortic stenosis: a disease of the valve and the myocardium. J Am Coll Cardiol 2012; 60(19): 1854-63.
[http://dx.doi.org/10.1016/j.jacc.2012.02.093] [PMID: 23062541]

[12]   Towler DA. Molecular and cellular aspects of calcific aortic valve disease. Circ Res 2013; 113(2): 198-208.
[http://dx.doi.org/10.1161/CIRCRESAHA.113.300155] [PMID: 23833294]

[13]   Hoffman JI, Kaplan S. The incidence of congenital heart disease. J Am Coll Cardiol 2002; 39(12): 1890-900.
[http://dx.doi.org/10.1016/S0735-1097(02)01886-7] [PMID: 12084585]

[14]   Larson EW, Edwards WD. Risk factors for aortic dissection: a necropsy study of 161 cases. Am J Cardiol 1984; 53(6): 849-55.
[http://dx.doi.org/10.1016/0002-9149(84)90418-1] [PMID: 6702637]

[15]   Siu SC, Silversides CK. Bicuspid aortic valve disease. J Am Coll Cardiol 2010; 55(25): 2789-800.
[http://dx.doi.org/10.1016/j.jacc.2009.12.068] [PMID: 20579534]

[16]   Otto CM, Burwash IG, Legget ME, *et al.* Prospective study of asymptomatic valvular aortic stenosis. Clinical, echocardiographic, and exercise predictors of outcome. Circulation 1997; 95(9): 2262-70.
[http://dx.doi.org/10.1161/01.CIR.95.9.2262] [PMID: 9142003]

[17]   Lancellotti P, Donal E, Magne J, *et al.* Risk stratification in asymptomatic moderate to severe aortic stenosis: the importance of the valvular, arterial and ventricular interplay. Heart 2010; 96(17): 1364-71.
[http://dx.doi.org/10.1136/hrt.2009.190942] [PMID: 20483891]

[18]   Goel SS, Ige M, Tuzcu EM, *et al.* Severe aortic stenosis and coronary artery disease--implications for management in the transcatheter aortic valve replacement era: a comprehensive review. J Am Coll Cardiol 2013; 62(1): 1-10.
[http://dx.doi.org/10.1016/j.jacc.2013.01.096] [PMID: 23644089]

[19]   Dhoble A, Enriquez-Sarano M, Kopecky SL, *et al.* Cardiopulmonary responses to exercise and its utility in patients with aortic stenosis. Am J Cardiol 2014; 113(10): 1711-6.
[http://dx.doi.org/10.1016/j.amjcard.2014.02.027] [PMID: 24698467]

[20]   Domanski O, Richardson M, Coisne A, *et al.* Cardiopulmonary exercise testing is a better outcome predictor than exercise echocardiography in asymptomatic aortic stenosis. Int J Cardiol 2017; 227: 908-14.
[http://dx.doi.org/10.1016/j.ijcard.2016.10.070] [PMID: 27916346]

[21]   Leskelä HV, Satta J, Oiva J, *et al.* Calcification and cellularity in human aortic heart valve tissue determine the differentiation of bone-marrow-derived cells. J Mol Cell Cardiol 2006; 41(4): 642-9.
[http://dx.doi.org/10.1016/j.yjmcc.2006.07.014] [PMID: 16938307]

[22]   Aikawa E, Nahrendorf M, Sosnovik D, *et al.* Multimodality molecular imaging identifies proteolytic and osteogenic activities in early aortic valve disease. Circulation 2007; 115(3): 377-86.
[http://dx.doi.org/10.1161/CIRCULATIONAHA.106.654913] [PMID: 17224478]

[23]   Garcia D, Pibarot P, Kadem L, Durand LG. Respective impacts of aortic stenosis and systemic hypertension on left ventricular hypertrophy. J Biomech 2007; 40(5): 972-80.
[http://dx.doi.org/10.1016/j.jbiomech.2006.03.020] [PMID: 16750211]

[24]   Lewin MB, Otto CM. The bicuspid aortic valve: adverse outcomes from infancy to old age. Circulation 2005; 111(7): 832-4.
[http://dx.doi.org/10.1161/01.CIR.0000157137.59691.0B] [PMID: 15723989]

[25]   Grimard BH, Larson JM. Aortic stenosis: diagnosis and treatment. Am Fam Physician 2008; 78(6): 717-24.
[PMID: 18819236]

CHAPTER 5

Dyslipidemia

Abstract: Hyperlipidemia is one of the major risk factors for developing cardiovascular complications. The cardiovascular diseases connected with complex risk factors include diabetes, smoking, alcohol, physical inactivity, dyslipidemia, hypertension, and obesity. Cardiovascular disease is causing more deaths in developed and developing countries. Hyperlipidemia associated with high levels of fatty materials deposition in systemic circulation. Cholesterol is a waxy fat protein produced naturally in the liver, present in bloodstream as proteins called lipoproteins. Cholesterol is a fatty substance found in several fatty foods such as eggs, red meat, and cheese. The large amounts of low-density lipoprotein cholesterol deposits in the arterial walls cause narrowing of blood vessels that can increase the risk of serious cardiovascular complications. Dyslipidemia is categorized into primary and secondary types. It includes primary and secondary dyslipidemia. The primary dyslipidemia is noted to be inherited. Secondary dyslipidemia is an acquired condition and develops from obesity and diabetes. Patients diagnosed with dyslipidemia may have xanthomas which are deposits of cholesterol under the skin and also under the eyes. The commonly prescribed medications for the management of dyslipidemia include fibric acid derivatives, bile acid drugs, statins, nicotinic acid, and reduce the progression of dyslipidemia complications in health practice. Early identification of risk factors, diagnosis and cholesterol screening programmes can prevent the progression of the dyslipidemic burden among high cholesterol risk patients.

Keywords: Cholesterol, Hyperlipidemia, Hypertension, Lipoproteins, Xanthomas.

INTRODUCTION

Dyslipidemia is characterized by the deposition of a high amount of fatty materials in the blood. Low density level cholesterol is a "bad" type of cholesterol. It can deposit in the blood vessels leads to the formation of plaques in the arteries. The excessive deposition of cholesterol in the blood can cause the progression of cardiovascular problems. HDL is the good cholesterol and it helps to eliminate the LDL from blood. Triglycerides are stored in adipose tissue cells. The high levels of LDL and triglycerides can increase the risk of cardiac problems. Low level of HDL cholesterol is associated with the development of higher heart disease risks. Cholesterol is one type of lipid, waxy white substance and an essential element for body growth.

M.S. Umashankar & A. Bharath Kumar

Cholesterol having several functions such as secretion of bile, sex hormones, vitamin D and present in the outer layer of the body cells. It comes from animal food sources and diet leads to produce the cholesterol in the body. These fatty substances will adhere to the arterial walls and form plaques in the blood vessels [1 - 4]. High cholesterol increases the risk of cardiovascular disease and stroke. The risk factors for cardiovascular disease include high in saturated fats and cholesterol, obesity, and physical inactivity. The other medical conditions such as hypothyroidism, kidney disease, diabetes mellitus, liver disease and alcoholism can elevate the higher lipid levels.

MAIN TYPES OF LIPIDS

• High-Density Lipoprotein
• Low-Density Lipoprotein
• Triglycerides

MOST COMMON GOALS FOR CHOLESTEROL

• Total cholesterol Below 200 mg/dL
• HDL cholesterol Men - above 40 mg/dL; Women - above 50 mg/dL
• LDL cholesterol Below 100 mg/dL; Below 70 mg/dL
• Triglycerides Below 150 mg/dL

Lipids are naturally occurring molecules that contain hydrocarbons that build the structure and makes functioning of the cells in the body. The lipids are undergoing the oxidation process during the metabolism and release energy is needed for living creatures. Lipids are the non-polar molecules and which are not soluble in water and soluble in non-polar solutions such as ether, chloroform and other lipids. Lipids are composed of phospholipids, fats, waxes and steroids.

Dyslipdiemia consists of various lipoproteins. Low density level lipoproteins transfer the diverse lipid substances into the bloodstream. The High density lipoprotein carries the cholesterol from the tissue of the body to hepatic cells. The bad cholesterol has a role in developing high cardiovascular risk. High density lipoprotein is identified as good cholesterol that eliminates the bad cholesterol from arteries and sends back to the hepatic cells for elimination. The incidence of dyslipidemia affects the health burden to the individuals which leads to developing narrowing of coronary arteries (atheroscleoris) and manifests the clinical symptoms of cardiovascular diseases [5 - 8].

TYPES OF DYSLIPIDEMIAS

Dyslipidemia is categorized into primary and secondary types. It includes primary and secondary dyslipidemia. The primary dyslipidemia is noted to be inherited.

Secondary dyslipidemia is an acquired condition and develops from obesity and diabetes.

SPECIFIC TYPES OF PRIMARY DYSLIPIDEMIA

Familial Combined Hyperlipidemia

It is the most common inherited cause of both high LDL cholesterol levels and high triglycerides. These abnormal cholesterol levels can increase the risk of developing cardiovascular diseases.

Familial Hypercholesterolemia

It is characterized by abnormal levels of cholesterol in the blood. A total cholesterol level is exceeding more than 200 milligrams per deciliter (mg/dL) in the blood.

Familial hyperapobetalipoproteinemia

These high levels of apolipoprotein B and high LDL levels are deposited in the blood leads to an increase in the risk of cardiovascular complications.

PREVALENCE

According to the world health organization estimated that every year 7.4. million deaths are occurring in the worldwide. The dyslipdemia complications are still developing from low- and middle-income countries. Dyslipidemia is one of the risk factors for developing chronic diseases and is estimated to raise 2.6 million deaths are occurring in the worldwide. Previous research studies showed that the cholesterol complications were seen in adults 9.7 percent, 8.5 percent in males and 10.7% in females. Jamaica health and lifestyle survey in the 2008 year demonstrated that a high prevalence of total cholesterol 11.7% is noted in the age group ranges from 15-74 years and 17.7% among an aged group of 65–74 years. The prevalence ranged from 7% among females aged 15–24 years to 32% among those aged 55–64 years [9 - 11].

CAUSES

There are many factors are associated with the development of dyslipidemia include primary and secondary factors. Primary dyslipidemia is linked with abnormal lipid levels are present in the blood which is caused due to genetic mutations. The defective gene mutations may cause abnormal clearance of lipids from the body. Primary dyslipidemia increases LDL levels in the blood which results in increases in the risk of developing cardiovascular diseases. Secondary dyslipidemia is connected with various lifestyle risk factors and chronic diseases [12, 13].

Secondary Hyperlipidemia Causes

- High fat diet
- Lack of exercise
- Certain medications such as beta blockers and oral contraceptives
- Liver disease
- Cigarette smoking and alcohol
- Hypothyroidism
- Uncontrolled diabetes
- Smoking
- Being overweight
- A diet high in total fat, saturated fat, and cholesterol such as cheese, egg yolks, red meat, fried and processed foods
- Physical inactivity
- Excessive alcohol consumption
- Steroids

CLINICAL SYMPTOMS OF DYSLIPIDEMIA

It includes:

- Chest pain
- Xanthomas in skin and eyes
- Shortness of breath
- Pain, tightness, and pressure in the neck, jaw, shoulders, and back
- Indigestion and heartburn
- Sleep problems
- Dizziness
- Heart palpitations
- Vomiting and nausea
- swelling in the legs, ankles, feet, stomach, and veins of the neck
- Fainting

DIAGNOSIS

It includes:

- Blood test
- Liver test

- Renal function test
- Lipid test

COMPLICATIONS OF HYPERLIPIDEMIA

Atherosclerosis

Hyperlipidemia is one of the risk factor for developing atherosclerotic cardiovascular diseases. Atherosclerosis is a pathological condition that is characterized by an accumulation of lipids that forms fibrous plaques in the arteries [14, 15].

Coronary Artery Disease

Atherosclerosis is the major cause for the development of cardiovascular diseases. It is characterized by the deposition of fatty materials within the walls of arteries which will narrow the arteries leads to reduce blood to cardiac protective layers which is strongly associated with the development of coronary artery disease [16 - 18].

Myocardial Infarction

It is associated with a low level of blood flow and oxygen supply to the coronary arteries which result in occlusion of coronary arteries. It results in the development of atherosclerotic plaque formation.

Ischemic Stroke

Stroke is the fourth leading cause of death in the world. The blockage of arteries by a bit of atherosclerotic plaque and lipid particles can damage the blood vessels present in brain and increases the risk of developing ischemic stroke.

PREVENTION OF DYSLIPIDEMIA

It includes

- Maintaining a healthy weight
- Quit smoking and alcohol
- Physical exercise for at least 30 minutes per day
- Stress management
- Reducing the consumption of unhealthy fats
- Maintaining a healthy body weight

Mechanism of action of dyslipidemia drugs

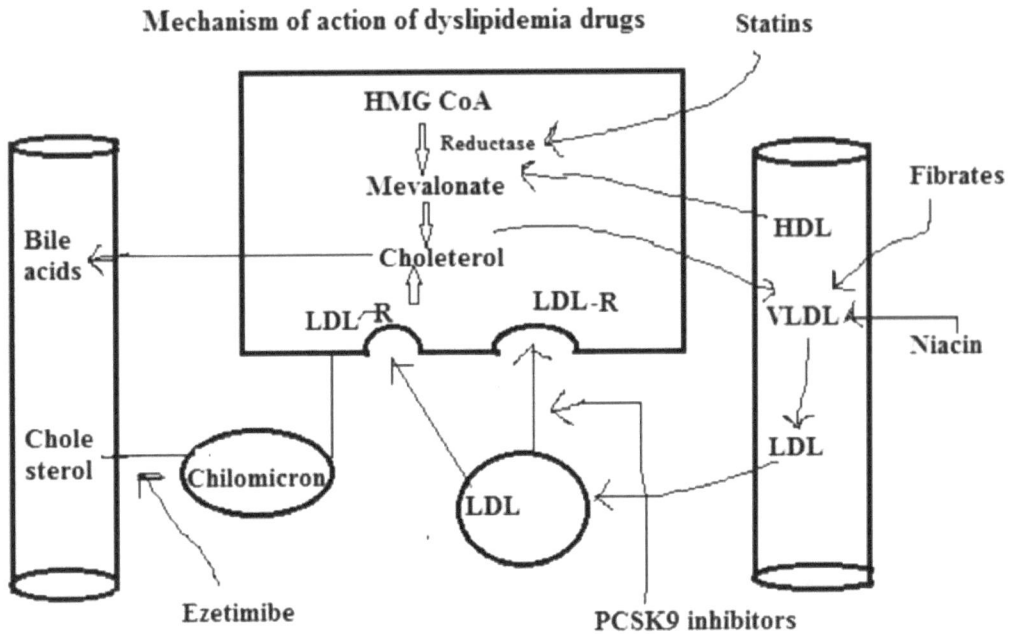

Fig. (1). Mechanism of action of dyslipidemia drugs.

HYPERLIPIDMIA MANAGEMENT

Dyslipidemia Medications

There are several medications used to treat dyslipidemias. The mechanism of action of dylipidemia drugs was shown in Fig. (**1**).

Statins

Statins are a class of medications that will inhibit HMG CoA reductase the enzyme which is needed for cholesterol synthesis in the body. It will reduce LDL cholesterol and increases HDL and modest decreases in triglycerides. The statin drugs include lovastatin, pravastatin, simvastatin, fluvastatin and atorvastatin. It works by lowering total cholesterol and LDL cholesterol and which results in the reduction of cardiovascular morbidity and mortality.

Side Effects

It includes nausea, vomiting, diarrhea, headache, myalgia and dizziness.

Bile Acid Sequestrants

It is marketed as colestipol and colesevelam, this class of drugs works by preventing bile acids from being reabsorbed by the gut. Bile acids are produced from cholesterol and aid in the digestion and absorption of lipids. These drugs force our liver to produce more bile acids from cholesterol, thereby reducing cholesterol levels in the body. These medications are appropriate for elevated cholesterol levels and not hypertriglyceridemia. The bile acid sequesterants drugs include cholestyramine, colestipol, colestimide and colesevelam [19 - 22].

Side Effects

It includes constipation, nausea, indigestion, bloating and flatulence.

Cholesterol Absorption Inhibitors

It will inhibit NPC1L1 in the gut, which reduces the amount of cholesterol is absorbed from our guts. It is a major transporter in the gut for absorption of the fatty materials. The low level of cholesterol coming from gut pushes into liver to synthesize the cholesterol and reduces the LDL particles in the blood.

Side Effects

It includes headache, diarrhea and abdominal pain and diarrhea *etc.*

Niacin

It works by interacting with NIACR receptors located on the adipose tissue cells and inhibit the triglycerides and converted into VLDL in the liver. The conversion can reduce the VLDL, tri glycerides, and LDL levels and increases HDL cholesterol in the blood.

Side Effects

The most common side effects include itching, headache, nausea and abdominal discomfort.

Fibrates

The fibrate medications activate gene transcription of PPAR alpha can control the expression of the gene in lipoprotein metabolism. The fibrate drugs can lower the triglycerides levels and increases the HDL level. The fibrates medications include Bezafibrate, ciprofibrate, gemfibrozil and fenofibrate [23].

Side Effects

It includes arrhythmia, myopathy, skin rashes and gallstones.

PCSK9 Monoclonal Antibodies

These drugs are bind to the PCSK9 receptors which are connected to the LDL receptors. It can regulate the plasma concentration of LDL by interacting with LDL receptors present in the liver cells. It will degrade the lysosomes and inhibits the recycling of the hepatocytes and delays the catabolism of LDL particles. It will inhibit the proprotein convertase subtilisin/kexin type 9 (PCSK9) enzymes which will act on the LDL receptor and lowers the cholesterol levels. Omega-3 fatty acids consist of eicosapentaenoic acid [EPA] and docosahexaenoic acid [DHA]) are present in marine fish which can effectively reduce the tri gllycerides. It will inhibit the thromboxane, release of inflammatory mediators and cytokine production which could reduce the vascular inflammation.

NEW POTENTIAL TARGETS AND TREATMENTS [24, 25]

Cholesteryl Ester Transfer Protein (CETP) Inhibitors

Cholesteryl ester transfer protein present in liver promotes the distribution of cholesteryl esters from anti-atherogenic cholesterol to atherogenic apolipoprotein B containing lipoproteins such as LDL and VLDL. Previous studies stated that the CETP involved in the proatherogenic process which involves inhibition of CETP can reduce the progression of atheroslcerosis.

Antisense Oligonucleotides

Mipomersen is an antisense oligonucleotide that is connected to messenger RNA to prevent translation and forms the apolipoprotein-B. It can reduce the formation of apoB-containing lipoproteins such as VLDL, LDL, TG *etc.* in the blood which leads to preventing the development of dyslipidemic complications.

Microsomal Triglyceride Transfer Protein (MTP) Inhibitors

It is a USFDA approved drug for the treatment of homozygous familial hypercholsterolemia. Lomitapide is the microsomal triglyceride transfer protein inhibitor. These agents will inhibit the transfer of triglyceride to apoB-48, apoB-100 in intestinal and liver cells. It will reduce the formation of chylomicrons and very-low-density lipoprotein (VLDL) in liver.

Microsomal triglyceride transfer protein transfers the neutral lipids between membrane vesicles. It can participate in bio synthesis of CD1 and antigen-presenting molecules and also regulates the cholesterol biosynthesis. Therefore inhibition of Microsomal triglyceride transfer protein cause reduction of triglycerides, VLDL, total cholesterol and LDL can lower the progression of hyperlipidemic complications.

Acyl-CoA Cholesterol Acyl Transferase Inhibitors (ACAT)

Acyl-CoA cholesterol acyl transferase is the enzyme has a significant role in switching of intracellular cholesterol into cholesteryl esters. It consists of two isomers which include ACAT1 and ACAT2. These drugs will inhibit the ACAT-1 and ACAT-2 which results in the reduction of cholesterol absorption in the intestine.

ATP Citrate Lyase Inhibitors

*ATP citrate lyase is the enzyme responsible for the synthesis of cytosolicacetyl-*CoA and oxaloacetate. It will inhibit the synthesis the cytosolicacetyl-CoA and oxalo acetate thereby reduces the synthesis of cholesterol. Therefore it is widely used in the treatment of hyperlipidemia.

Squalene Epoxidase Inhibitors

It is an enzyme that inhibits the squalene epoxidase is responsible for sterol biosynthesis. NF-598 *is* a potent competitive inhibitor of *squalene* epoxidase and inhibits the cholesterol synthesis.

Lanosterol Synthase Inhibitors

Lanosterol synthase catalyzes the conversion of oxidosqualene to lanosterol. It is the primary step in the cholesterol biosynthesis pathway. LSS inhibitors include U18666A and Ro 48-8071 have a vital role in the reduction of plasma low-density level lipoproteins.

Acyl Coenzyme A Diacyl Glycerol Acyltransferase (DGAT)

It is a microsomal enzyme having a vital role in tri glyceride bio synthesis. It is available in two forms, which include DGAT-1 and DGAT-2. Previous research studies proved that the DGAT-1 had used in the treatment of hyperlipidemia.

Squalene Synthase Inhibitors

Squalene synthase catalyzes the conversion of farnesyl pyrophosphate to squalene and it having a significant role in cholesterol biosynthesis. Squalene synthase inhibitors are identified to lead compounds in the development of hypelipidemic drugs.

CONCLUSION

Dyslipidemia is a disorder of lipoprotein metabolism and that is manifested by elevated total cholesterol, low-density lipoproteins, triglycerides, and low level of high density level cholesterol that can increase the risk of dyslipidemic complications. The incidence of dyslipidemia affects the health burden to the individuals which leads to develop narrowing of coronary arteries and manifests the clinical symptoms of cardiovascular diseases. The global incidence of dyslipidemia is caused by eating high fatty foods, obesity, stress and physical inactivity can aggravate the risk of various complications.

Early screening of cholesterol levels, diagnosis and newer therapeutic options can reduce the progression of dyslipidemia burden in health care. Strict implementation of cholesterol guidelines for effective prescribing of lipid medications and rapid implementation of the clinical pharmacist intervened services on risk screening, advanced patient counseling on diet, disease, lifestyle modification, medication adherence, regular patient follow-up care can help for improving the health-related quality of life and also reduces the risk of progression of cardiovascular disease in health care.

REFERENCES

[1]   Robinson JG, Smith B, Maheshwari N, Schrott H. Pleiotropic effects of statins: benefit beyond cholesterol reduction? A meta-regression analysis. J Am Coll Cardiol 2005; 46(10): 1855-62.
[http://dx.doi.org/10.1016/j.jacc.2005.05.085] [PMID: 16286171]

[2]   Ference BA, Yoo W, Alesh I, *et al.* Effect of long-term exposure to lower low-density lipoprotein cholesterol beginning early in life on the risk of coronary heart disease: a Mendelian randomization analysis. J Am Coll Cardiol 2012; 60(25): 2631-9.
[http://dx.doi.org/10.1016/j.jacc.2012.09.017] [PMID: 23083789]

[3]   Strong JP, Malcom GT, McMahan CA, *et al.* Prevalence and extent of atherosclerosis in adolescents and young adults: implications for prevention from the Pathobiological Determinants of Atherosclerosis in Youth Study. JAMA 1999; 281(8): 727-35.
[http://dx.doi.org/10.1001/jama.281.8.727] [PMID: 10052443]

[4]   Cohen JC, Boerwinkle E, Mosley TH Jr, Hobbs HH. Sequence variations in PCSK9, low LDL, and protection against coronary heart disease. N Engl J Med 2006; 354(12): 1264-72.
[http://dx.doi.org/10.1056/NEJMoa054013] [PMID: 16554528]

[5]   Zhao Z, Tuakli-Wosornu Y, Lagace TA, *et al.* Molecular characterization of loss-of-function mutations in PCSK9 and identification of a compound heterozygote. Am J Hum Genet 2006; 79(3): 514-23.
[http://dx.doi.org/10.1086/507488] [PMID: 16909389]

[6]   Simopoulos AP. Evolutionary aspects of diet, the omega-6/omega-3 ratio and genetic variation: nutritional implications for chronic diseases Biomed Pharmacother 2006 2006; 60: 7-502.

[7]   Connor WE, DeFrancesco CA, Connor SL. N-3 fatty acids from fish oil. Effects on plasma lipoproteins and hypertriglyceridemic patients. Ann N Y Acad Sci 1993; 683: 16-34.
[http://dx.doi.org/10.1111/j.1749-6632.1993.tb35689.x] [PMID: 8352438]

[8]   Studer M, Briel M, Leimenstoll B, Glass TR, Bucher HC. Effect of different antilipidemic agents and diets on mortality: a systematic review. Arch Intern Med 2005; 165(7): 725-30.
[http://dx.doi.org/10.1001/archinte.165.7.725] [PMID: 15824290]

[9]   Nordestgaard BG, Langsted A. Lipoprotein (a) as a cause of cardiovascular disease: insights from epidemiology, genetics, and biology. J Lipid Res 2016; 57(11): 1953-75.
[http://dx.doi.org/10.1194/jlr.R071233] [PMID: 27677946]

[10]   Ebrahimi M, Ghayour-Mobarhan M, Rezaiean S, *et al*. Omega-3 fatty acid supplements improve the cardiovascular risk profile of subjects with metabolic syndrome, including markers of inflammation and auto-immunity. Acta Cardiol 2009; 64(3): 321-7.
[http://dx.doi.org/10.2143/AC.64.3.2038016] [PMID: 19593941]

[11]   Eslick GD, Howe PR, Smith C, Priest R, Bensoussan A. Benefits of fish oil supplementation in hyperlipidemia: a systematic review and meta-analysis. Int J Cardiol 2009; 136(1): 4-16.
[http://dx.doi.org/10.1016/j.ijcard.2008.03.092] [PMID: 18774613]

[12]   Mattar M, Obeid O. Fish oil and the management of hypertriglyceridemia. Nutr Health 2009; 20(1): 41-9.
[http://dx.doi.org/10.1177/026010600902000105] [PMID: 19326719]

[13]   Heber D, Yip I, Ashley JM, Elashoff DA, Elashoff RM, Go VL. Cholesterol-lowering effects of a proprietary Chinese red-yeast-rice dietary supplement. Am J Clin Nutr 1999; 69(2): 231-6.
[http://dx.doi.org/10.1093/ajcn/69.2.231] [PMID: 9989685]

[14]   Joshi SR, Anjana RM, Deepa M, *et al*. Prevalence of dyslipidemia in urban and rural India: the ICMR-INDIAB study. PLoS One 2014; 9(5): e96808.
[http://dx.doi.org/10.1371/journal.pone.0096808] [PMID: 24817067]

[15]   Raal FJ, Pilcher GJ, Panz VR, *et al*. Reduction in mortality in subjects with homozygous familial hypercholesterolemia associated with advances in lipid-lowering therapy. Circulation 2011; 124(20): 2202-7.
[http://dx.doi.org/10.1161/CIRCULATIONAHA.111.042523] [PMID: 21986285]

[16]   Brouwers MC, van Greevenbroek MM, Stehouwer CD, de Graaf J, Stalenhoef AF. The genetics of familial combined hyperlipidaemia. Nat Rev Endocrinol 2012; 8(6): 352-62.
[http://dx.doi.org/10.1038/nrendo.2012.15] [PMID: 22330738]

[17]   Jain KS, Kathiravan MK, Somani RS, Shishoo CJ. The biology and chemistry of hyperlipidemia. Bioorg Med Chem 2007; 15(14): 4674-99.
[http://dx.doi.org/10.1016/j.bmc.2007.04.031] [PMID: 17521912]

[18]   Pattis P, Wiedermann CJ. Ezetimibe-associated immune thrombocytopenia. Ann Pharmacother 2008; 42(3): 430-3.
[http://dx.doi.org/10.1345/aph.1K614] [PMID: 18252832]

[19]   Arnold MA, Swanson BJ, Crowder CD, *et al*. Colesevelam and colestipol: novel medication resins in the gastrointestinal tract. Am J Surg Pathol 2014; 38(11): 1530-7.
[http://dx.doi.org/10.1097/PAS.0000000000000260] [PMID: 24921636]

[20]   Hussain MM, Rava P, Walsh M, Rana M, Iqbal J. Multiple functions of microsomal triglyceride transfer protein. Nutr Metab (Lond) 2012; 9(9): 14-30.
[http://dx.doi.org/10.1186/1743-7075-9-14] [PMID: 22353470]

[21]   Chang TY, Li BL, Chang CC, Urano Y. Acyl-coenzyme A:cholesterol acyltransferases. Am J Physiol Endocrinol Metab 2009; 297(1): E1-9.
[http://dx.doi.org/10.1152/ajpendo.90926.2008] [PMID: 19141679]

[22]   McLaren JE, Michael DR, Ashlin TG, Ramji DP. Cytokines, macrophage lipid metabolism and foam cells: implications for cardiovascular disease therapy. Prog Lipid Res 2011; 50(4): 331-47.
[http://dx.doi.org/10.1016/j.plipres.2011.04.002] [PMID: 21601592]

[23]   Hegele RA. Plasma lipoproteins: genetic influences and clinical implications. Nat Rev Genet 2009; 10(2): 109-21.
[http://dx.doi.org/10.1038/nrg2481] [PMID: 19139765]

[24]   Wang H, Eckel RH. Lipoprotein lipase: from gene to obesity. Am J Physiol Endocrinol Metab 2009; 297(2): E271-88.
[http://dx.doi.org/10.1152/ajpendo.90920.2008] [PMID: 19318514]

[25]   Amarenco P, Labreuche J. Lipid management in the prevention of stroke: review and updated meta-analysis of statins for stroke prevention. Lancet Neurol 2009; 8(5): 453-63.
[http://dx.doi.org/10.1016/S1474-4422(09)70058-4] [PMID: 19375663]

CHAPTER 6

Hypertension

Abstract: Hypertension is a major health problem and its incidence was rapidly growing from urban and rural communities. The narrowed arteries can reduce the blood flow in the arteries due to this condition the development of pressure can increase the blood flowing capacity in the arteries is called arterial blood pressure. Patients who are diagnosed with more than 140/90 mmHg reading is known as hypertension. Uncontrolled blood pressure can damage the various vital organs which include cardiac, retinal, renal, neurological diseases. The reduction of systolic and diastolic blood pressure can lower the occurrence of cardiovascular disease. Various pharmacological classes of drugs are available for the treatment of high blood pressure includes beta blockers, diuretics, angiotensin receptor blockers, calcium channel blockers, central sympatholytics, alpha blockers, angiotensin converting enzyme inhibitors, vasodilator drugs can lower the progression of hypertensive complications in the health care.

Keywords: Angiotensin Receptor Blockers, Cardiovascular Disease, Diuretics, Hertension, Hypertension.

INTRODUCTION

The narrowed arteries can reduce the blood flow in the arteries due to this condition the development of pressure can increase the blood flowing capacity in the arteries is called arterial blood pressure. The blood pressure is defined as the systolic blood pressure reading is more than 140 mm hg and diastolic blood pressure is more than 90 mm hg is called diastolic blood pressure. The systolic pressure is connected with cardiac output and diastolic pressure is caused due to peripheral resistance. The cardiac output, heart rate and venous return can increase the systolic pressure. Total peripheral resistance results from constriction of arteries which is due to diastolic blood pressure. Hypertension is one of the causative factors for the development of cardiovascular diseases [1 - 3].

The blood pressure is recorded as 120/80 mm hg. 120 mm hg indicates systolic pressure and 80 mm hg indicate diastolic pressure.

Blood pressure is demonstrated by the product of cardiac output and total peripheral vascular resistance *i.e.,*

M.S. Umashankar & A. Bharath Kumar

Blood pressure = Cardiac output × total peripheral resistance

CLASSIFICATION

The normal physiological conditions the blood pressure is normal. During the abnormal emotional conditions and more stress leads to cause high blood pressure. The presence of uncontrolled hypertension leads to the development of various cardiovascular diseases such as angina, stroke, myocardial infarction and renal failure and previous history of cardiovascular disease. The pressure difference between systolic and diastolic blood pressure is called pulse pressure. The classification of blood pressure is shown in Table **1**.

Table 1. JNC 7 Classification of blood pressure.

Blood Pressure Classification	SBP (mm Hg)	DBP (mm Hg)
Normal	<120	<80
Pre hypertension	120–139	80–89
Stage 1	140–159	90–99
Stage 2	≥160	≥100
Hypertensive crisis	≥180	≥120

CAUSES OF HYPERTENSION

The Causes of Hypertension are Classified into Two Types

Primary hypertension

Secondary hypertension

Primary Hypertension

There is no specific identifiable cause for the development of high blood pressure. This type of blood pressure is called essential hypertension.

Secondary Hypertension

Various conditions and medications can lead to secondary hypertension, including [4, 5]:

- Obstructive sleep apnea
- Kidney problems

- Adrenal gland tumors
- Thyroid problems
- Diabetes mellitus
- Defects in blood vessels
- Certain medications, such as decongestants, birth control pills, cold remedies, over-the-counter medications
- Illegal drugs, such as cocaine and amphetamines

RISK FACTORS

There are various factors significantly linked with increasing the risk of developing hypertension.

It includes

Age

Hypertension is more common in people who are more than 60 years of age. Blood pressure can increase steadily with age as the arteries stiffen and narrow due to plaque buildup.

Ethnicity

African Americans have a higher risk than other ethnic groups.

Alcohol and Tobacco Use

Regular habitat of consuming large quantities of alcohol or tobacco can increase blood pressure.

Sex

The males have a higher risk of developing hypertension than females.

Existing Health Conditions

Cardiovascular disease, diabetes, renal disease, and obesity can lead to hypertension.

PATHOPHYSIOLOGY

Neural Mechanisms

Central and autonomic nervous systems are associated with controlling of blood pressure. Activation of alpha receptors present in the nervous system lowers the blood pressure by inhibiting the vasomotor center. Activation of pre synaptic receptors releases the norepinephrine causes vasoconstriction. Activation of β 1 receptors present in the heart raises the heart rate and stimulation of β 2 receptors present in the arterials causes vasodilation. The synaptic nervous system controls the baro receptor reflexes pathway. These nerve endings connected to the carotial and aortic arch located in baro receptor. The minute elevation of arterial blood pressure increases the activity of the baro receptor discharges. These results in vasodilatation and reduces the contraction of the heart.

Pathogenesis of Hypertension

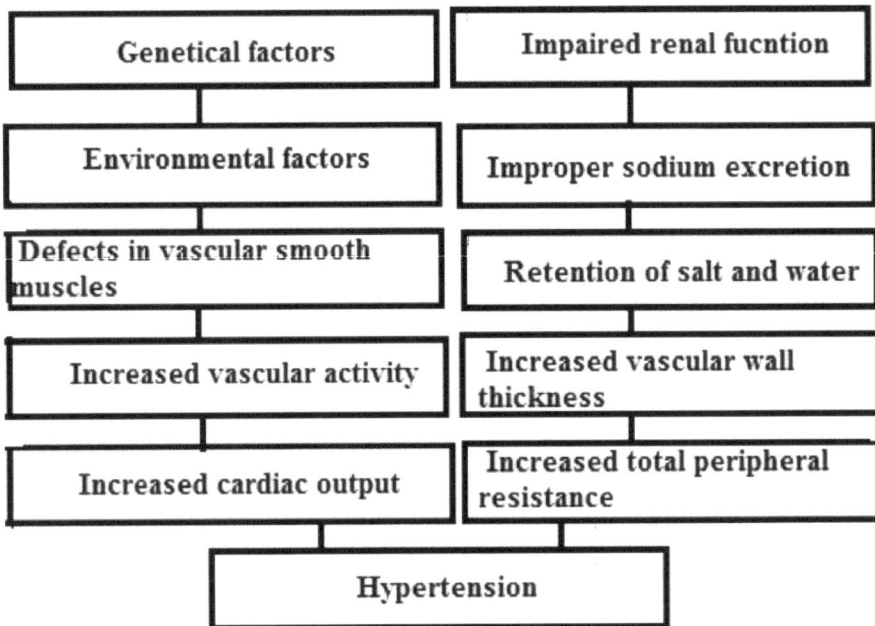

Fig. (1). Pathogenesis of Hypertension.

Peripheral Auto Regulatory Components

The defects in auto regulatory mechanisms cause the development of hypertension. The lowering of blood pressure causes retaining sodium and water results in the expansion of plasma volume and increases blood pressure. The abnormal function of the renal protective mechanism may impair the blood pressure regulatory mechanism which leads to elevating the blood pressure. Cells can control oxygen transportation to the peripheral tissues. The elevated metabolic demand causes arteries vasodilation. It can lower the peripheral resistance and increase the oxygen demands for metabolic functions. These metabolic defects lead to an increase in the plasma volume and blood flow to the peripheral tissues

[6 - 8]. The initial defect in the adaptive mechanism can lead to plasma volume expansion and increased blood flow to peripheral tissues and enhance the peripheral resistance ultimately raise the blood pressure. The pathogenesis of hypertension is shown in Fig. (**1**).

Hormonal Mechanism

The hormonal mechanism was controlled by renin angiotensionogen aldosterone system (RAAS). The matriuritic hormone and hyperinsulincmia are involved in the progression of hypertension. The RAAS system controls the sodium potassium and fluid balance during the development of hypertension. The rennin is secreted and stored in juxtra glomerular cells present in the kidney. The rennin released in blood catalyzes the conversion of catalyzes the conversion of angiotensinogen to angiotensin I. The angiotensin I is converted to angiotensin II by ACE enzyme. The activation of catecholamine releases aldosterone from the adrenal gland which retains both sodium and fluid and elevates the blood pressure. The second humoral factor is the nutrimetric hormone inhibits the Na^+,K^+ ATPase causes an increase of sodium retention, extra cellular fluid and ultimately elevates the blood pressure. Hyperinsulinemia may raise sodium on retention and increases the sympathetic nervous system activity causes the elevation of blood pressure [9 - 13].

Vascular Endothelial Mechanism

Vascular endothelial cells release the various inflammatory mediators such as prostaglandins, bradykinins and endothelium factors that can cause vasoconstriction. Deficient of synthesizing vasodialting substances causes the development of hypertension.

SIGNS AND SYMPTOMS

Uncontrolled blood pressure can damage the various vital organs which include cardiac, retinal, renal, neurological diseases. Patients with primary secondary hypertension are initially normal and elevation of blood pressure may progress the manifestation of hypertension.

- Nausea and vomiting
- Dizziness
- Fatigue
- Chest pain
- Shortness of the breath
- Irregular heart beats

- Blood in urine
- Blurred vision
- Nose bleeding
- Heart palpitations
- Breathlessness

COMPLICATIONS

Improper treatment of blood pressure leads to damage of blood vessels and causes the progression of hypertensive complications.

The possible complications of blood pressure include

- Stroke
- Heart failure
- Blood clots
- Aneurysm
- Kidney disease
- Metabolic syndrome
- Cognitive defects
- Pharmacotherapy

The First-line therapy for the management of hypertension includes diuretics, angiotensin-converting enzyme inhibitors, angiotensin receptor blockers, beta-blockers, and calcium channel blockers [14 - 20].

LIFESTYLE CHANGES FOR PREVENTION OF HYPERTENSION [21]

- Eating a healthy diet with less salt
- Getting regular physical activity
- Smoking cessation
- Alcohol cessation
- Stress management
- Regular physical exercise
- Maintaining a healthy weight

TREATMENT

Anti-hypertensive Drugs [22 - 25]

The commonly prescribed anti-hypertensive drugs were shown in Table **2**.

Table 2. Commonly prescribed anti-hypertensive drugs.

Drug		
Diuretics	**Dose**	**Adverse effects**
Furosemide	20-40 mg	GI disturbances, dizziness, weakness, muscle cramps
Hydrochlorothiazide	12.5–50 mg	electrolyte abnormalities, hypercalcemia, dizziness, weakness, muscle
Amiloride	5–10 mg	Hyperkalemia, GI disturbances, muscle cramps, weakness
Spironolactone	25–50 mg	Hyperkalemia, menstrual irregularities, gynecomastia
ACE inhibitors	**Dose**	**Adverse effects**
Benazepril	10–40 mg	Hypotension, cough, hyperkalemia, dizziness, headache, diarrhea loss of taste perception
Captopril	25–100 mg	
Enalapril	2.5–40 mg	
Fosinopril	10–40 mg	
Perindopri	4–16 mg	
Ramipril	1.25–20 mg	
Angiotensin II receptor antagonists	**Dose**	**Adverse effects**
Candesartan	8–32 mg	Hypotension, hyperkalemia, dizziness, fatigue, diarrhea
Losartan	25–100 mg	
Olmesartan	20–40 mg	
Telmisartan	20–80 mg	
Valsartan	80–320 mg	
Beta-blockers	**Dose**	**Adverse effects**
Atenolol	25–100 mg	Bradycardia, hypotension, GI disturbances, dizziness, fatigue, insomnia, heart failure, reduced peripheral circulation
Bisoprolol	2.5–10 mg	
Carvedilol	12.5–50 mg	
Metoprolol tartrate	50–100 mg	
Propranolol	40–160 mg	
Calcium channel blockers	**Dose**	**Adverse effects**
Amlodipine	2.5–10 mg	Peripheral edema, palpitations, headache, dizziness, fatigue, dizziness, bradycardia, hypotension, constipation, nausea, weakness
Felodipine	2.5–20 mg	
Nicardipine	60–120 mg	
Nifedipine	30–60 mg	
Verapamil	120–480	
Diltiazem	120–420	

Drug		
Alpha₁-blockers	**Dose**	**Adverse effects**
Doxazosin	1–16 mg	Dizziness, headache, lack of energy, nausea, palpitations, orthostatic hypotension
Prazosin	2–20 mg	
Terazosin (Hytrin)	1–20 mg	
Alpha₂-agonists	**Dose**	**Adverse effects**
Clonidine	0.1–0.8 mg	Dry mouth, dizziness, drowsiness, constipation
Methyldopa	250–1000 mg	Drowsiness, orthostatic hypotension, nasal congestion, bradycardia
Renin inhibitor	**Dose**	**Adverse effects**
Aliskiren	150–300 mg	Diarrhea, headache, dizziness, fatigue, cough
Vasodilators	**Dose**	**Adverse effects**
Hydralazine	25–100 mg	Tachycardia, palpitations, GI disturbances, headache
Minoxidil	2.5–80 mg	

Diuretics

It includes thiazide diuretics, loop diuretics, and potassium-sparing diuretics.

Thiazides: It acts by inhibiting the absorption of sodium and chloride in the distal convoluted tubule.

Loop diuretics: It will act on the ascending loop of henle and inhibit the luminal Na+/K+/2Cl– symporter, therefore reducing NaCl reabsorption. These medications are prescribed single or in combination for the management of hypertension. It is mostly prescribed in the treatment of congestive heart failure, acute pulmonary edema, or renal disease.

Potassium-Sparing Diuretics

It acts on the distal and cortical collecting tubules to reduce sodium reabsorption by inhibiting Na+ influx through epithelium sodium ion channels in the collecting tubule. These are effective in the treatment of hypertensive patients.

ACE inhibitors: It will inhibit the conversion of the inactive angiotensin I to the active angiotensin II and increases bradykinins and subsequently prostaglandins which lead to lower blood pressure. It is prescribed in the treatment of heart failure, post myocardial infarction, high risk of CAD, diabetes, chronic kidney disease, and stroke.

Angiotensin receptor: blockers It blocks the angiotensin II receptor, thereby prevents the vasoconstriction and reduces blood pressure.

Renin inhibitors : It will inhibit the conversion of angiotensinogen to angiotensin I by inhibition of rennin enzyme.

Calcium channel blockers: It will prevent the entry of calcium into vascular smooth muscles, causes vasodilation and reduces vascular contractility.

Beta-blockers: it will inhibit the beta-1 adrenergic receptors and results in slower heart rate, decreased cardiac contractility, and reduced cardiac output. It will also inhibit renin release and subsequently angiotensin II production and lowers the blood pressure.

Alpha and beta blockers: It will reduce the nerve impulses to blood vessels and slow the heartbeat to reduce the amount of blood that must be pumped through the vessels and lowers the blood pressure.

Alpha-blockers: It will block the alpha-1 adrenoreceptors on vascular smooth muscles and inhibits the vasoconstriction and lower the blood pressure.

Direct vasodilators: These drugs relax vascular smooth muscle, primarily arterioles, and inhibit the vasoconstriction thereby lowers the blood pressure.

CONCLUSION

Hypertension is a leading risk factor for developing various cardiovascular disease complications. Low income and middle income countries are in the front of high incidence of hypertension which causes a huge health care expenditure to the affected population. The improper sedentary life style contributes to the progression of the high incidence of hypertension. The non-pharmacological intervention for management of hypertension includes reducing the salt intake, termination of smoking and alcohol, regular physical exercise for 30 minutes, weight reduction, and stress management can reduce the hypertensive complications in health care.

Regular implementation of clinical pharmacist services with the health care team on risk factors screening and control, diagnosis, patient follow-up care services, medication adherence, and effective implementation of anti-hypertensive therapy guidelines to improve the prescribing pattern of drugs can helpful for controlling blood pressure.

REFERENCES

[1]   Chobanian AV, Bakris GL, Black HR, *et al.* Seventh report of the Joint National Committee on

Prevention, Detection, Evaluation, and Treatment of High Blood Pressure. Hypertension 2003; 42(6): 1206-52.
[http://dx.doi.org/10.1161/01.HYP.0000107251.49515.c2] [PMID: 14656957]

[2]   Huai P, Xun H, Reilly KH, Wang Y, Ma W, Xi B. Physical activity and risk of hypertension: a meta-analysis of prospective cohort studies. Hypertension 2013; 62(6): 1021-6.
[http://dx.doi.org/10.1161/HYPERTENSIONAHA.113.01965] [PMID: 24082054]

[3]   Lloyd-Jones D, Adams R, Carnethon M, *et al.* Heart Disease and Stroke Statistics 2009 Update: a Report from the American Heart Association Staistics Committee and Stroke Statistics Subcommittee. Circulation 2009; 119: 21-181.

[4]   Alcocer L, Cueto L. Hypertension, a health economics perspective. Ther Adv Cardiovasc Dis 2008; 2(3): 147-55.
[http://dx.doi.org/10.1177/1753944708090572] [PMID: 19124418]

[5]   Psaty BM, Lumley T, Furberg CD, *et al.* Health outcomes associated with various antihypertensive therapies used as first-line agents: a network meta-analysis. JAMA 2003; 289(19): 2534-44.
[http://dx.doi.org/10.1001/jama.289.19.2534] [PMID: 12759325]

[6]   Lewington S, Clarke R, Qizilbash N, Peto R, Collins R. Age-specific relevance of usual blood pressure to vascular mortality: a meta-analysis of individual data for one million adults in 61 prospective studies. Lancet 2002; 360(9349): 1903-13.
[http://dx.doi.org/10.1016/S0140-6736(02)11911-8] [PMID: 12493255]

[7]   Spurgeon D. NIH promotes use of lower cost drugs for hypertension. BMJ 2004; 328(7439): 539.
[http://dx.doi.org/10.1136/bmj.328.7439.539] [PMID: 15001483]

[8]   Vasan RS, Beiser A, Seshadri S, *et al.* Residual lifetime risk for developing hypertension in middle-aged women and men: The Framingham Heart Study. JAMA 2002; 287(8): 1003-10.
[http://dx.doi.org/10.1001/jama.287.8.1003] [PMID: 11866648]

[9]   Screening for high blood pressure: U.S. Preventive Services Task Force reaffirmation recommendation statement. Ann Intern Med 2007; 147(11): 783-6.
[http://dx.doi.org/10.7326/0003-4819-147-11-200712040-00009] [PMID: 18056662]

[10]   The sixth report of the Joint National Committee on prevention, detection, evaluation, and treatment of high blood pressure. Arch Intern Med 1997; 157(21): 2413-46.
[http://dx.doi.org/10.1001/archinte.1997.00440420033005] [PMID: 9385294]

[11]   Forman JP, Brenner BM. 'Hypertension' and 'microalbuminuria': the bell tolls for thee. Kidney Int 2006; 69(1): 22-8.
[http://dx.doi.org/10.1038/sj.ki.5000056] [PMID: 16374419]

[12]   Appel LJ, Champagne CM, Harsha DW, *et al.* Effects of comprehensive lifestyle modification on blood pressure control: main results of the PREMIER clinical trial. JAMA 2003; 289(16): 2083-93.
[PMID: 12709466]

[13]   Effects of treatment on morbidity in hypertension. Results in patients with diastolic blood pressures averaging 115 through 129 mm Hg. JAMA 1967; 202(11): 1028-34.
[http://dx.doi.org/10.1001/jama.1967.03130240070013] [PMID: 4862069]

[14]   Prevention of stroke by antihypertensive drug treatment in older persons with isolated systolic hypertension. Final results of the Systolic Hypertension in the Elderly Program (SHEP). JAMA 1991; 265(24): 3255-64.
[http://dx.doi.org/10.1001/jama.1991.03460240051027] [PMID: 2046107]

[15]   Jamerson K, Weber MA, Bakris GL, *et al.* Benazepril plus amlodipine or hydrochlorothiazide for hypertension in high-risk patients. N Engl J Med 2008; 359(23): 2417-28.
[http://dx.doi.org/10.1056/NEJMoa0806182] [PMID: 19052124]

[16]   Saklayen MG. Which diuretic should be used for the treatment of hypertension? Am Fam Physician 2008; 78(4): 444-446, 446.

[PMID: 18756650]

[17]   Ernst ME, Carter BL, Basile JN. All thiazide-like diuretics are not chlorthalidone: putting the ACCOMPLISH study into perspective. J Clin Hypertens (Greenwich) 2009; 11(1): 5-10.
[http://dx.doi.org/10.1111/j.1751-7176.2008.00009.x] [PMID: 19125852]

[18]   Pitt B, Zannad F, Remme WJ, *et al.* The effect of spironolactone on morbidity and mortality in patients with severe heart failure. N Engl J Med 1999; 341(10): 709-17.
[http://dx.doi.org/10.1056/NEJM199909023411001] [PMID: 10471456]

[19]   Pitt B, Remme W, Zannad F, *et al.* Eplerenone, a selective aldosterone blocker, in patients with left ventricular dysfunction after myocardial infarction. N Engl J Med 2003; 348(14): 1309-21.
[http://dx.doi.org/10.1056/NEJMoa030207] [PMID: 12668699]

[20]   Dimeo F, Pagonas N, Seibert F, Arndt R, Zidek W, Westhoff TH. Aerobic exercise reduces blood pressure in resistant hypertension. Hypertension 2012; 60(3): 653-8.
[http://dx.doi.org/10.1161/HYPERTENSIONAHA.112.197780] [PMID: 22802220]

[21]   Geleijnse JM, Kok FJ, Grobbee DE. Blood pressure response to changes in sodium and potassium intake: a metaregression analysis of randomised trials. J Hum Hypertens 2003; 17(7): 471-80.
[http://dx.doi.org/10.1038/sj.jhh.1001575] [PMID: 12821954]

[22]   de la Sierra A, Lluch MM, Coca A, *et al.* Assessment of salt sensitivity in essential hypertension by 24-h ambulatory blood pressure monitoring. Am J Hypertens 1995; 8(10 Pt 1): 970-7.
[http://dx.doi.org/10.1016/0895-7061(95)00225-1] [PMID: 8845078]

[23]   Langford HG, Blaufox MD, Oberman A, *et al.* Dietary therapy slows the return of hypertension after stopping prolonged medication. JAMA 1985; 253(5): 657-64.
[http://dx.doi.org/10.1001/jama.1985.03350290063027] [PMID: 3881608]

[24]   Fleming S, Atherton H, McCartney D, *et al.* Self-screening and non-physician screening for hypertension in communities: a systematic review. Am J Hypertens 2015; 28(11): 1316-24.
[http://dx.doi.org/10.1093/ajh/hpv029] [PMID: 25801901]

[25]   Stojanova A, Koceski S, Koceska N. Continuous blood pressure monitoring as a basis for ambient assisted living (AAL) review of methodologies and devices. J Med Syst 2019; 43(2): 24.
[http://dx.doi.org/10.1007/s10916-018-1138-8] [PMID: 30603777]

CHAPTER 7

Atherosclerosis

Abstract: Atherosclerosis is a long-lasting inflammatory disease that is caused by the more accumulation of fatty materials in the arteries leads to create plaques in blood vessels. The risk factors for atherosclerosis include diabetes mellitus, alcohol, smoking, hypertension, dyslipidemia, and genetic abnormalities can increase the risk of atherosclerotic cardiovascular complications. The incidence of atherosclerotic cardiovascular disease per 1,000 patients was 98.25 in 2014 and 101.11 in 2015. Atherosclerosis major clinical manifestations include ischemic stroke, ischemic heart disease, and peripheral arterial disease. The consumption of cholesterol free diet, regular health care visit, weight control, medication adherence, physical exercises, stress management and maintaining the controlled levels of the lipid, blood pressure, and glycemic levels could reduce the progression of cardiovascular events in the health care.

Keywords: Atherosclerosis, Dyslipidemia, Hypertension, Ischemic Heart Disease, Stroke.

INTRODUCTION

Vascular problems such as thrombosis and embolism may suddenly affect the health of individual people at any age and leads to an increase in the future risk of developing cardiovascular diseases.

Atherosclerosis is a disease affecting the arterial blood vessel. It is a chronic inflammatory response in the walls of arteries due to the formation of plaques which in turn is promoted by low density lipoproteins. Simply it is a disease in which plaque builds up on the inside of the arteries. A plaque is made up of fat, cholesterol, calcium and other substances found in the blood as macrophages. Over time the plaque may harden and narrow the arteries. Atherosclerosis is a general term describing any hardening with loss of elasticity of medium or large arteries.

Atherosclerosis is hardening with loss of elasticity of arterioles. Atherosclerosis mainly involves the media of the blood vessel. Atherosclerosis also refers to the hardening of any artery especially due to atheromatous plaque. Therefore atheros-

M.S. Umashankar & A. Bharath Kumar

clerosis with marked cholesterol lipid calcium deposits forming a swollen area in arterial linings called atheromatous plaque. Large and medium sized are usually narrowed by fibro-lipid atherosclerotic lesions where small arteries and arterioles show proliferative or hyaline changes of arteriolosclerosis. The lesion of atherosclerosis includes the arterial chances of atheromatous plaque, fatty streaks and cushion lesions [1, 2].

Atherosclerosis

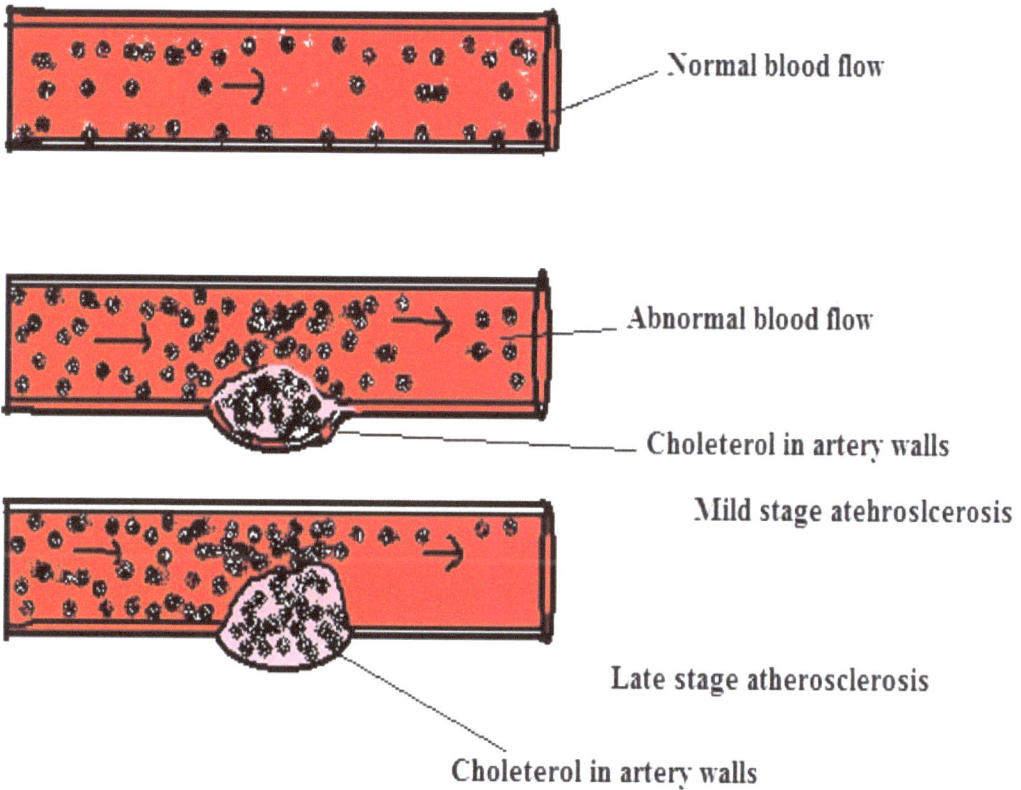

Normal blood flow

Abnormal blood flow

Choleterol in artery walls

Mild stage atehroslcerosis

Late stage atherosclerosis

Choleterol in artery walls

Fig. (1). Atherosclerosis.

Atheromatous Plaque

Atheromatous plaque is also called as fibrous or fibro lipid plaque is a raised, swollen area the surface surrounding the intima and it produces into the lumen of the vessel. It is usually whitish yellow in colour, and it may grow in size if adjacent plaques coalesce. The plaque may contain a soft yellow gruel like lipid center covered by a fibrous cap. The lipid center includes the mass of lipid cellular debris, cholesterol clefts, plasma proteins, and lipid loaded cells are derived from the macrophases and smooth muscle cells.

The fibrous cap is composed of smooth muscle cells, collagen, elasitn and proteoglycans. In between this fibrous cap and lipid center, there is a more cellular region of macrophases, smooth muscles. Plauques are common in the aorta, femoral, central and coronary arteries. The plaques may cause complete occlusion, thrombosis, and embolism. Plaques may be stable or unstable. Stable plaques may have a large lipid pool with a thin fibrous cap. Unstable plaques are liable to cause problems, when ruptured. Plaques are general are not elastic lesions but can change gradually. The changes may be influenced by other layers of the vessel wall. These results which increase permeability to proteins, lipids lead to aggregation of platelets and monocytes. These leukocytes migrate into the sub endothelial layers from the blood and there they become macrophases and ingest the lipid. This eventually develops into an atheromatous plaque may not be involved in producing any clinical effect. However these problems may occur due to the rupture of plaque promotes local thrombosis. The atherosclerosis is shown in Fig. (**1**).

Fatty Streaks

A fatty streak occurs on the endothelial surface of the aorta and coronary artery arteries. Initially, it appears as tiny, round or oval flat yellow dots composed of lipids, and presence of macrophages and T cells in the intima. They then become arranged in rows and finally coalesce to form a streak. The earliest streaks do not have any smooth muscle proliferation of these blood vessel or extracellular lipid. Through they do not affect blood flow. It could represent a precursor lesion or atheroamtous plaque depends on hemodynamic forces such as hypertension and the plasma levels of atherogenic lipoproteins.

Intimal Cushion Lesions

It refers to thickening at a branching point, a small opening in the artery as a result of increases in the extra cellular matrix and smooth muscles. It is suggested that this may be a precursor lesion for fibro lipid plaques.

RISK FACTORS FOR ATHEROSCLEROSIS [3 - 6]

The risk factors involved in causing atherosclerosis are important and hence it is necessary to consider them.

Age

Atheroma offers different vessels at different ages. Generally, small aortic lesions appear in the first decade, coronary artery in the second decade and cerebral arterial lesion in the third decade.

Gender

Males are more affected than females. The incidence is more or less similar in both males and females after the age of 75. In pre menopausal women myocardial infarction due to atherosclerosis is extreme rare.

Genes

Genetic influences such as changes in cholesterol levels through changes to LDL .receptor, apolipoproteinB, apolipirpotein C, variation in angiotensinogen, predisposition to type 2 diabetes mellitus, altered in activation of nicotine and ion channel proteins leads to cause cardiovascular disease.

Smoking

It is likely that smoking promotes artheroma and also causes occlusion of vessels. This may due to increasing a local clotting tendency as a result of altered platelet function. Smoking increases the risk of coronary artery disease. The damage to vessels caused by smoking has been suggested to increased free radical activity and raised carbon monoxide levels.

Hypertension

It may increase the risk of ischemic heart disease and strokes diastolic blood pressure level more than 95 mm hg is deemed harmful. Patients with congenital heart disease, narrowing of aorta develop atheroma in the proximal hypertensive segment but not in the distal region where the pressure in lower. The coronary artery, linked to the aorta develops the atheromatous changes with age where as artery linked to the pulmonary supply is not affected.

Diabetes

The risk of developing the myocardial infarction in diabetics is twice that in non diabetics a possible mechanism may be a rise in LDL and a decrease in HDL in diabetics as a result of a reduction in receptor mediated catabolism.

Hyperlipidemia

In families with a genetic disorder that causes that hypercholesterolemia or is persons with acquired hyper-cholesterolemia can increase the risk of atherosclerosis.

Low density level lipoproteins rich in cholesterol appear most harmful and the high density lipoproteins appear cardio protective.

Pathogenesis of Atherosclerosis

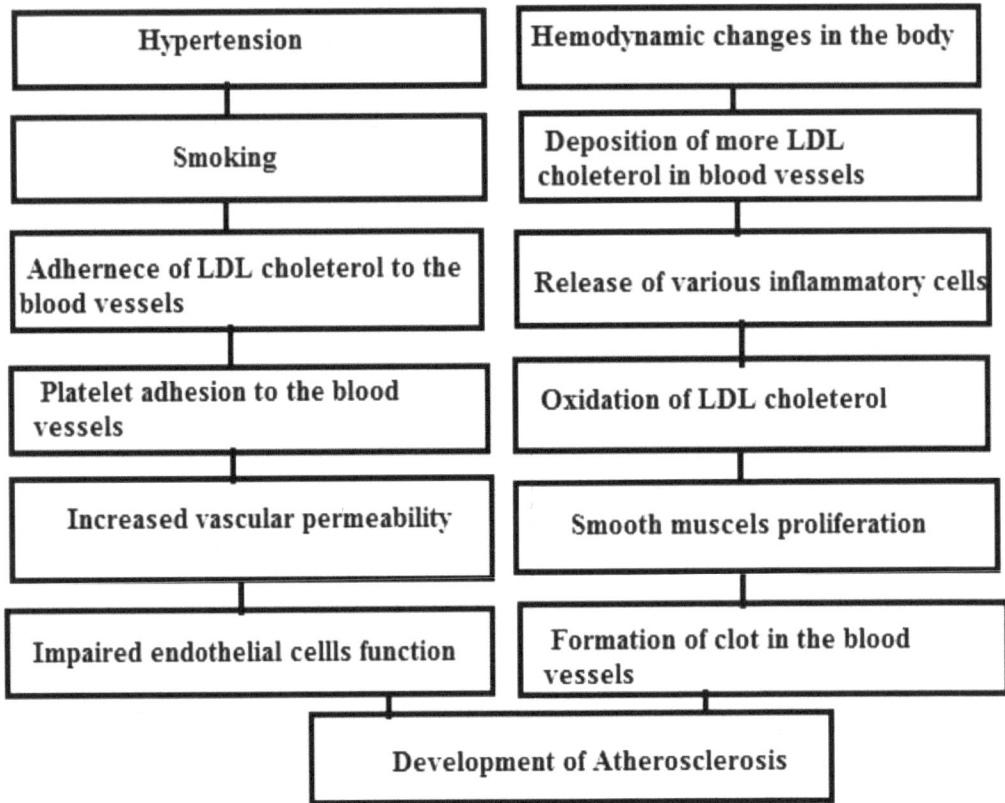

Hypertension	Hemodynamic changes in the body
Smoking	Deposition of more LDL choleterol in blood vessels
Adhernece of LDL choleterol to the blood vessels	Release of various inflammatory cells
Platelet adhesion to the blood vessels	Oxidation of LDL choleterol
Increased vascular permeability	Smooth muscels proliferation
Impaired endothelial cellls function	Formation of clot in the blood vessels

Development of Atherosclerosis

Fig. (2). Pathogenesis of Atherosclerosis.

Arteriosclerosis

Arteriosclerosis may be hyaline Arteriosclerosis or hyperplatic arteriosclerosis. These are very different atheromatous damage. They only affect small vessel and not have increased in lipids. They primarily affect the media of the vessel and are strongly associated with hypertension.

Hyaline arteriosclerosis occurs in elderly and diabetic patients. It involves the deposition of homogenous glassy pink material that thickens the media and hence the walls. Calcium accumulates in the fatty material causing hardening or arteries leading to the condition atherosclerosis. The pathogenesis of atherosclerosis is shown in Fig. (2). Hyperplastic arteriosclerosis may develop in a patient who has rather sudden or severe prolonged increase in blood pressure. The media of the arteriole wall is thickened by a concentrate proliferation of smooth muscle cells. There may also be an increase in basement material.

Causes

Arteriosclerosis causes two main problems.1.Atheromatous plaque eventually ends in rupture. Stenosis of artery results in insufficient blood supply to the organ if feeds. If the compensatory enlargement is exclusive, it leads to development of aneurysm.

Aneurysm

There may bleed in the space below the outer most layers. Berry aneurysms look like a cherry struck on the side of vessel. It usually develops due to a defect in the media of the blood vessels at the sites at bifurcation. Patients with berry aneurysm may have a sudden severe headache. The patient may lose consciousness when aneurysms leaks. Micro aneurysms affect cerebral vessels. They present as multiple small aneurysms on small arteries within cerebral hemispheres. This occurs in hypertensive patients and is common cause of intra cerebral hemorrhage, a form of stroke. Atherosclerotic aneurysms are the most commonly found in the abdominal potion of the aorta [7 - 9]. They occur in individuals with risk factors for atheroma and develop as a result of an exacerbation of the media by hypertension. Aneurysm secondary to inflammation includes those due to syphilis, arthritis and infection. Aneurysm secondary to infection is called mycotic aneurysm.

DIAGNOSIS TEST [10 - 14]

Blood Tests Blood tests check the levels of certain fats, cholesterol, sugar, and proteins in the blood and abnormal levels may indicate risk factors for atherosclerosis.

Chest X ray A chest x ray takes a picture of the organs and structures inside the chest, including the heart, lungs, and blood vessels - a chest x ray can also reveal signs of heart failure.

Ankle brachial index This test compares the blood pressure in ankle with the blood pressure in arms to see how well blood is flowing.

Echocardiography This test uses sound waves to create a moving picture of heart and provides information about the size and shape of heart and how well heart chambers and valves are working.

Computed tomography scan It creates a computer generated image of the heart, brain, and other parts of the body and helpful for detection of abnormality of the affected organ.

Stress Testing During stress testing, exercise is used to make the heart work hard and beat fast while heart tests are performed - if a person is unable to exercise, medicines are given to speed up the heart rate.

Angiography Angiography is a test that uses dye and special x -rays to show the insides of arteries and can reveal whether plaque is blocking the arteries and how severe the plaque is.

CLINICAL MANIFESTATIONS

- Chest Pain
- Pain in leg, arm
- Shortness of breath
- Fatigue
- Confusion
- Muscle weakness in legs

THE PREVENTION OF ATHEROSCLEROSIS

It includes

- Eating just a little or moderate amount of fat
- Eating just a moderate amount of sugar
- Eating much fish and just a little red meat
- Eating a good amount of fruit and vegetables each day
- Supply of enough vitamins, minerals and anti-oxidants
- Only consuming moderate amount of salt
- Stop smoking
- Getting high blood pressure treated if lifestyle measures do not bring blood pressure down
- Daily exercise for 20 minutes
- Stress management
- Stressing down and getting enough rest.

PHARAMACOTHERAPY FOR TREATING ATHEROSCLEROSIS

Cholesterol Lowering Drugs

Cholesterol lowering medications include [15 - 19]

Statins

These drugs act by inhibiting HMG-CoA reductase enzyme and inhibit the cholesterol biosynthetic pathway and shows anti atherosclerotic effect in the blood vessels.

- Atorvastatin
- Fluvastatin
- Lovastatin
- Pitavastatin
- Pravastatin
- Rosuvastatin
- Simvastatin

Adverse effects Headache, dizziness, insomnia, flushing of the skin, drowsiness and myalgia.

Niacin

In prescription form, niacin is sometimes used to lower LDL cholesterol. It can be more effective in raising HDL cholesterol than other medications.

Side effects Redness, stomach upset, headache, dizziness, blurred vision, and liver damage.

Bile Acid Sequestrates

These are used to treat high levels of LDL. Common side effects include bloating, constipation, heartburn, and elevated triglycerides. People who have high levels of triglycerides should not take bile acid sequestrants.

The drugs include

- Cholestyramine
- Colestipol
- Colesevelam

Cholesterol Absorption Inhibitors

The medication ezetimibe limits how much LDL cholesterol can be absorbed in the small intestine.

Side effects Headaches, nausea, muscle weakness.

Fibric Acid Derivatives

These medicines are effective at lowering triglyceride levels, and moderately effective at lowering LDL. They are used to treat high triglycerides and low HDL in people who cannot take niacin.

It includes

- Gemfibrozil
- Fenofibrate

Side effects Myositis, stomach upset, sun sensitivity, gallstones, irregular heartbeat, and liver damage.

Blood Pressure Lowering Drugs

Beta Blockers

It reduces the work load on the heart and reduces stress and hormones levels in the body which leads to vasodilatation in the blood vessels.

Commonly prescribed beta blockers include

- Atenolol
- Bisoprolol
- Nadolol
- Nebivolol
- Carvedilol
- Labetalol
- Nebivolol
- Pindolol
- Propranolol
- Timolol
- Metoprolol

Adverse effects Dry mouth, dry skin, feelings of coldness, diarrhea, shortness of breath and insomnia.

Angiotensin Converting Enzyme (ACE) Inhibitors

ACEs block the conversion of angiotensin I to angiotensin II by the action of angiotensinogen in the body and help to lower the vasoconstriction and promote vasodilation.

It includes

- Captopril
- Lisinopril
- Fosinopril
- Ramipril
- Benazepril
- Enalapril
- Perindopril
- Quinapril
- Moexipril
- Trandolapril

Adverse effects Dry cough, hyperkalemia, fatigue, headaches and loss of taste.

Angiotensin II Receptor Blockers

It blocks the conversion of angiotensin II from its binding to angiotensin II receptors located on the blood vessels and produces vasodialtion in the blood vessels.

These drugs include

- Candesartan
- Telmisartan
- Valsartan
- Eprosartan
- Irbesartan
- Losartan

Adverse effects Hyperkalemia, dizziness, headache, cough, diarrhea, hypotension and angioedema.

Calcium Channel Blockers

This drug blocks the entry of calcium ions into the calcium channels and lowers the work load on the heart and dilates the arteries leads to vasodilatation [20 - 23].

These drugs include

- Diltiazem
- Verapamil
- Isradipine
- Nifedipine
- Nicardipine

- Nimopidine
- Amlodipine
- Nisoldipine
- Bepridil
- Felodipine

Adverse effects Rashes, headache, constipation, flushing, edema, drowsiness

Thrombolytic Drugs

Thrombolytic drugs are prescribed to reduce the formation of blood clot in the blood vessels and also lower the severity of stroke. These drugs will act by conversion of plasminogen which forms plasmin and activates the fibrin bound plasminogen. Fibrin molecules are inhibited by plasmin which leads to breakdown of clot in the blood vessels and reduces the occurrence of stroke complications.

It includes

- Anistreplase
- Reteplase
- Streptokinase
- T-pa
- Tenecteplase
- Alteplase
- Urokinase

Adverse drug reactions Internal bleeding, damage to the blood vessels, renal damage.

Anti Platelet Drugs

These drugs are help to prevent the platelet aggregation and reduce the clot in the blood vessels [24].

Types of Antiplatelet Agents

- Aspirin
- Dipyridamole
- Clopidogrel
- Ticagrelor

Clinical Uses of Antiplatelet Agents

It is used to treat the following disease conditions which include

- Coronary artery disease
- Heart attack
- Angina (chest pain)
- Stroke and transient ischemic attacks
- Peripheral artery disease

Side Effects Nausea, gastric problems, diarrhea, rashes, itching,

Diuretics

Loop Diuretics

These drugs will inhibit the sodium potassium co transport mechanism in the ascending loop of henle it leads to increase the distal tubular concentration of sodium and reduced levels of hyprertonicity of the sodium levels in the intestine cause's diueresis [25].

Loop diuretics include

- Bumetanide
- Furosemide
- Ethacrynate
- Torsemide

Adverse effects Hypokalemia, alkalosis, hypomagnesemia, hyperuricemia, dehydration, ototoxicity.

Thiazides Diuretics

These drugs inhibit the sodium-chloride transporter in the distal tubule and reabsorption of sodium ions causes elimination of more water from the body.

- Chlorothiazide
- Chlorthalidone
- Indapamide
- Hydrochlorothiazide
- Methyclothiazide

Adverse effects Hyponatremia, hyperglycemia, dehydration, hypokalemia, hypertriglyceridemia, hyperuricemia, azotemia.

Carbonic Anhydrase Inhibitors

These drugs will inhibit the transport of bicarbonate ions from the proximal convulted tubule which leads to loss of sodium, hydrogen and bicarbonate ions in the urine.

The drugs include

- Acetazolamide
- Methazolamide

Adverse effects Metabolic acidosis and hypokalemia

Potassium Sparing Diuretics

It acts on the distal segment of the distal tubules and causes more water to enter inside the collecting tubule. It will inhibit the aldosterone-sensitive sodium reabsorption thereby loss of potassium and hydrogen from the urine.

- Amiloride
- spironolactone
- Triamterene

Adverse effects Metabolic acidosis, gynecomastia, hyperkalemia, gastric ulcers.

CONCLUSION

Atherosclerosis is a potential cause of mortality and morbidity in all countries. Atherosclerosis is a metabolic disorder in which the deposition of more fatty materials in the arteries can form the plaques. Atherosclerosis is a vascular process that occurs in the third decade of life. Diabetes, hypertension, smoking, alcohol and hyperlipidemia can enhance atherosclerotic risk. Early diagnosis and identification of plaques severity in the vascular stream may create new opportunities for treating atherosclerosis. The atherosclerotic therapy based on lipid lowering therapy in combined with anti-inflammatory therapeutic options can lower atherosclerosis events. Currently, many medications are available to treat atherosclerosis that includes statins, fibrates, niacin, ezetimibe, and bile acid sequestrants are greatly implicated to treat the lipid abnormalities. Regular implementation of clinical pharmacist services with health care team on detection of risk factors, regular health care visit, medications use, patient referral services, patient counseling on diet, disease and lifestyle modifications and maintaining controlled levels of risk factors can improve the health related quality of life among high atherosclerosis risk profile patients.

REFERENCES

[1]   Davies MJ. The pathophysiology of acute coronary syndromes. Heart 2000; 83(3): 361-6.
[http://dx.doi.org/10.1136/heart.83.3.361] [PMID: 10677422]

[2]   W van Lammeren G, L Moll F, Borst GJ, de Kleijn DP, P M de Vries JP, Pasterkamp G. Atherosclerotic plaque biomarkers: beyond the horizon of the vulnerable plaque. Curr Cardiol Rev 2011; 7(1): 22-7.
[http://dx.doi.org/10.2174/157340311795677680] [PMID: 22294971]

[3]   Sakakura K, Nakano M, Otsuka F, Ladich E, Kolodgie FD, Virmani R. Pathophysiology of atherosclerosis plaque progression. Heart Lung Circ 2013; 22(6): 399-411.
[http://dx.doi.org/10.1016/j.hlc.2013.03.001] [PMID: 23541627]

[4]   Ylä-Herttuala S, Bentzon JF, Daemen M, *et al.* Stabilization of atherosclerotic plaques: an update. Eur Heart J 2013; 34(42): 3251-8.
[http://dx.doi.org/10.1093/eurheartj/eht301] [PMID: 23966311]

[5]   Kronenberg F, Utermann G. Lipoprotein(a): resurrected by genetics. J Intern Med 2013; 273(1): 6-30.
[http://dx.doi.org/10.1111/j.1365-2796.2012.02592.x] [PMID: 22998429]

[6]   Cannon CP, Braunwald E, McCabe CH, *et al.* Intensive*versus* moderate lipid lowering with statins after acute coronary syndromes. N Engl J Med 2004; 350(15): 1495-504.
[http://dx.doi.org/10.1056/NEJMoa040583] [PMID: 15007110]

[7]   Bruckert E, Hayem G, Dejager S, Yau C, Bégaud B. Mild to moderate muscular symptoms with high-dosage statin therapy in hyperlipidemic patients--the PRIMO study. Cardiovasc Drugs Ther 2005; 19(6): 403-14.
[http://dx.doi.org/10.1007/s10557-005-5686-z] [PMID: 16453090]

[8]   Ross R. Atherosclerosis--an inflammatory disease. N Engl J Med 1999; 340(2): 115-26.
[http://dx.doi.org/10.1056/NEJM199901143400207] [PMID: 9887164]

[9]   Weber C, Noels H. Atherosclerosis: current pathogenesis and therapeutic options. Nat Med 2011; 17(11): 1410-22.
[http://dx.doi.org/10.1038/nm.2538] [PMID: 22064431]

[10]   McCrindle BW. Cardiovascular risk factors in adolescents: relevance, detection, and intervention. Adolesc Med 2001; 12(1): 147-62.
[PMID: 11224028]

[11]   Liao JK, Laufs U. Pleiotropic effects of statins. Annu Rev Pharmacol Toxicol 2005; 45: 89-118.
[http://dx.doi.org/10.1146/annurev.pharmtox.45.120403.095748] [PMID: 15822172]

[12]   Stoll G, Bendszus M. Inflammation and atherosclerosis: novel insights into plaque formation and destabilization. Stroke 2006; 37(7): 1923-32.
[http://dx.doi.org/10.1161/01.STR.0000226901.34927.10] [PMID: 16741184]

[13]   Nissen SE, Nicholls SJ, Sipahi I, *et al.* Effect of very high-intensity statin therapy on regression of coronary atherosclerosis: the ASTEROID trial. JAMA 2006; 295(13): 1556-65.
[http://dx.doi.org/10.1001/jama.295.13.jpc60002] [PMID: 16533939]

[14]   Blankenhorn DH, Johnson RL, Nessim SA, Azen SP, Sanmarco ME, Selzer RH. The Cholesterol Lowering Atherosclerosis Study (CLAS): design, methods, and baseline results. Control Clin Trials 1987; 8(4): 356-87.
[http://dx.doi.org/10.1016/0197-2456(87)90156-5] [PMID: 3327654]

[15]   Brown G, Albers JJ, Fisher LD, *et al.* Regression of coronary artery disease as a result of intensive lipid-lowering therapy in men with high levels of apolipoprotein B. N Engl J Med 1990; 323(19): 1289-98.
[http://dx.doi.org/10.1056/NEJM199011083231901] [PMID: 2215615]

[16]   Prasad K, Lee P. Suppression of hypercholesterolemic atherosclerosis by pentoxifylline and its

mechanism. Atherosclerosis 2007; 192(2): 313-22.
[http://dx.doi.org/10.1016/j.atherosclerosis.2006.07.034] [PMID: 16963055]

[17]   Hsia J, MacFadyen JG, Monyak J, Ridker PM. Cardiovascular event reduction and adverse events among subjects attaining low-density lipoprotein cholesterol <50 mg/dl with rosuvastatin. The JUPITER trial (Justification for the Use of Statins in Prevention: an Intervention Trial Evaluating Rosuvastatin). J Am Coll Cardiol 2011; 57(16): 1666-75.
[http://dx.doi.org/10.1016/j.jacc.2010.09.082] [PMID: 21492764]

[18]   Whayne TF Jr, Zielke JC, Dickson LG, Winters JL. State of the art treatment of the most difficult low density lipoprotein (LDL) cholesterol problems: LDL apheresis. J Ky Med Assoc 2002; 100(12): 535-8.
[PMID: 12522946]

[19]   Gimbrone MA Jr, Topper JN, Nagel T, Anderson KR, Garcia-Cardeña G. Endothelial dysfunction, hemodynamic forces, and atherogenesis. Ann N Y Acad Sci 2000; 902: 230-9.
[http://dx.doi.org/10.1111/j.1749-6632.2000.tb06318.x] [PMID: 10865843]

[20]   Berliner JA, Territo MC, Sevanian A, *et al.* Minimally modified low density lipoprotein stimulates monocyte endothelial interactions. J Clin Invest 1990; 85(4): 1260-6.
[http://dx.doi.org/10.1172/JCI114562] [PMID: 2318980]

[21]   Després JP. Body fat distribution and risk of cardiovascular disease: an update. Circulation 2012; 126(10): 1301-13.
[http://dx.doi.org/10.1161/CIRCULATIONAHA.111.067264] [PMID: 22949540]

[22]   Law MR, Morris JK, Wald NJ. Use of blood pressure lowering drugs in the prevention of cardiovascular disease: meta-analysis of 147 randomised trials in the context of expectations from prospective epidemiological studies. BMJ 2009; 338: b1665-5.
[http://dx.doi.org/10.1136/bmj.b1665] [PMID: 19454737]

[23]   Nissen SE. Effect of intensive lipid lowering on progression of coronary atherosclerosis: evidence for an early benefit from the Reversal of Atherosclerosis with Aggressive Lipid Lowering (REVERSAL) trial. Am J Cardiol 2005; 96(5A): 61F-8F.
[http://dx.doi.org/10.1016/j.amjcard.2005.07.013] [PMID: 16126025]

[24]   Okazaki S, Yokoyama T, Miyauchi K, *et al.* Early statin treatment in patients with acute coronary syndrome: demonstration of the beneficial effect on atherosclerotic lesions by serial volumetric intravascular ultrasound analysis during half a year after coronary event: the ESTABLISH Study. Circulation 2004; 110(9): 1061-8.
[http://dx.doi.org/10.1161/01.CIR.0000140261.58966.A4] [PMID: 15326073]

[25]   Riccioni G. Integrated control of hypertension, dyslipidemia and carotid atherosclerosis in the reduction of cardiovascular risk. Expert Rev Cardiovasc Ther 2007; 5(3): 371-4.
[http://dx.doi.org/10.1586/14779072.5.3.371] [PMID: 17489661]

CHAPTER 8

Deep Vein Thrombosis

Abstract: Deep vein thrombosis is a serious health problem due to thrombosis in the systemic circulation. Ineffective treatment of deep vein thrombosis increases the risk of pulmonary embolism. Venous thrombosis condition decreases the blood flow to the veins in the legs. Valves help to promote the blood flow to the veins, during the hypoxia condition the low level of the blood flow to the veins can manifest the symptoms of venous thrombosis. The incidence of deep vein thrombosis is estimated to one patient per 1000 cases annually. The clinical manifestations of venous thromboembolism include swelling; redness can increase the progression of venous thromboembolism. The blood test, doppler ultra sound, venogram and magnetic resonance imaging test are helpful for the detection of deep vein thrombosis. The pharmacological and non-pharmacological treatment modalities are encouraged in the inpatient and outpatient wards could useful for reducing the progression of disease complications.

Keywords: Hypoxia, Pulmonary Embolism, Venous Thromboembolism, Venous Circulation, Veins.

INTRODUCTION

The development of blood clot in the veins of the body particularly in the leg is known as deep vein thrombosis. It usually occurs in deep leg veins and calf and thigh muscles. The swelling in the legs may lead to the progression of pulmonary embolism. Deep vein thrombosis causes pain, swelling in the legs. It is a serious clinical condition that develops during the formation of a blood clot in the legs and blocks the blood vessels leads to thrombosis in the blood vessels. Venous thromboembolism is a medical disorder which includes deep vein thrombosis and pulmonary embolism. A pulmonary embolism occurs when the blood clot that travels through the blood stream to the lungs. Patients with heart failure, cancer and previous history of surgery can increase the risk of developing venous thromboembolism. The venous thromboembolism is shown in Fig. (**1**). The clinical manifestations of venous thromboembolism include swelling; redness can increase the progression of venous thromboembolism. Effective treatment options can reduce the formation of blockages in the blood vessels [1 - 3].

M.S. Umashankar & A. Bharath Kumar

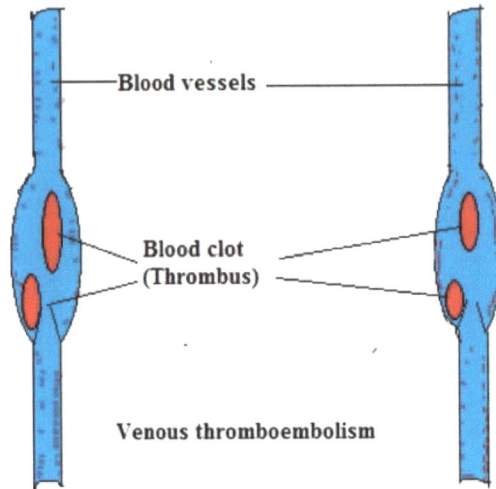

Fig. (1). Venous thromboembolism.

TYPES OF THROMBOSIS
Deep Vein Thrombosis (DVT)

It is a clot that occurs in deep veins usually in the legs. The deep vein thrombosis is shown in Fig. (**2**).

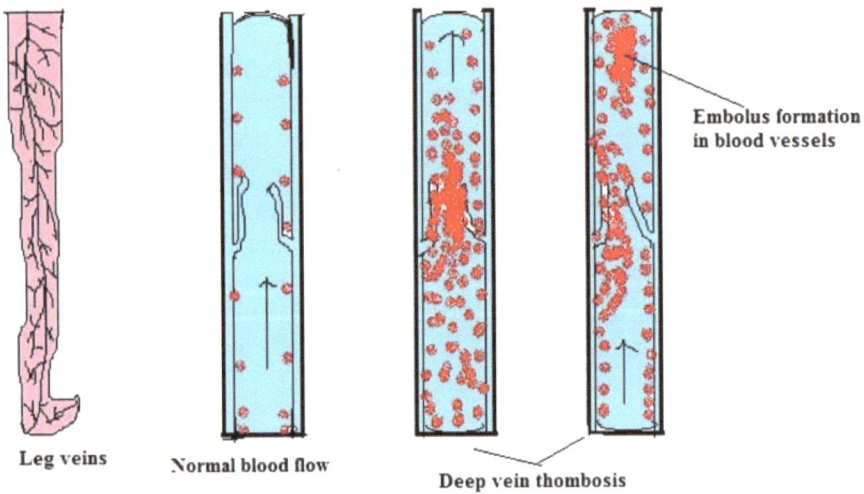

Fig. (2). Deep vein thrombosis.

Pulmonary Embolism (PE)

It occurs when a blood clot breaks in veins and transport to the lungs and blocks the blood flow in the blood vessels.

PREVALENCE OF DEEP VEIN THROMBOSIS

The annual incidence of venous thrombosis was 1 per 1000 in adult patients. The incidence rate was high in males as compared with females. Post-thrombotic syndrome can impair the quality of life of post-thrombotic patients. It occurs due to aging and higher incidence was seen in after age 45 years, and five to six percent of cases were occurring per 1000 patients annually at the age of 80 years. Recent research studies demonstrated that the disease severity was low in the United States, in Asians pacific countries and high in African countries.

RISK FACTORS [4 - 8]

Many factors can increase the risk of developing deep vein thrombosis which includes

Inheriting Blood Clotting Defects

The inherited blood clotting disorder can increase blood clotting defects easily.

Neuronal Paralysis

Prolong nerve defects decrease the blood supply to the calf muscles which leads to an increase in the risk of blood clot.

Injury

Injury to the veins and previous history of surgery can increase the risk of blood clots.

Pregnancy

Pregnancy increases the pressure in the pelvis and legs. Female patients with an inherited clotting disorder can increase the risk of clotting defects.

Hormone replacement therapy

Patients who are under current medications therapy can increase the risk of blood clotting.

Obesity

Patients with overweight increase the pressure in the veins which can increase the blood clotting problems.

Smoking

Smoking affects the blood circulation and increases the risk of DVT.

Cancer

The presence of tumors in the body can increase the risk of a blood clot.

Inflammatory Bowel Disease

Inflammatory bowel diseases such as crohn's disease or ulcerative colitis and increase the risk of progression of DVT.

Family History of Deep Vein Thrombosis

Family history of DVT van increases the higher risk of developing DVT.

Age

Patients with older age more than 60 years increase the risk burden to the individuals.

CLINICAL SYMPTOMS

Symptoms of DVT occur in the leg affected by the blood clot and include

- Swelling
- Pain in legs
- Distended veins
- Red or discolored skin
- Shortness of breath
- Sudden onset of chest pain
- Cough
- Vomiting blood
- Feeling lightheaded
- Rapid pulse

DIAGNOSIS [9 - 11]
Blood Tests

It is used to identify blood disorders and also to predict the risk of DVT.

Doppler Ultrasound

A Doppler device is kept in veins which use the sound waves to measure the blood flow. The pressure is applied to see if the vein responds normally. The sound waves signal is captured by the visual monitoring device and produces the images of the blood clot. This test is most often used to confirm the DVT in the legs.

Magnetic Resonance Imaging

It is used to detect the images of blood clots present in the veins.

Ventilation Scan

This is an image based examination that measures the pattern of air and blood move through the lungs.

Pulse Oximetry

It is used to identify the level of oxygen absorption present in the blood.

Chest X-ray

This test is used to identify the images of pneumonia in the lungs and other cardiac abnormalities.

Spiral Computed Tomography

This test is used to identify the cross sectional images of the lungs.

Pulmonary Angiogram

This is an invasive test, a catheter placed into a vein and to identify clots in veins and arteries located in the lungs and heart.

Echocardiogram

It is used to identify the blood flow pattern to the heart and also to detect cardiovascular abnormalities.

COMPLICATIONS
Pulmonary Embolism

It occurs when the damage of blood vessels present in the lungs due to blood clot. It is a life-threatening condition and regular treatment is needed for the prevention of pulmonary embolism risk among affected patients.

Signs and symptoms of pulmonary embolism include

- Shortness of breath
- Chest pain
- Cough
- Headache
- Dizziness
- Rapid pulse rate

Postphlebitic Syndrome

It is one of the complications of deep vein thrombosis. The formation of a blood clot in the veins lowers the blood flow to the damaged area which leads to cause the development of post phlebitic syndrome.

Signs and symptoms of post phlebitic syndrome include

- Legs swelling
- Edema
- Leg pain
- Skin discoloration
- Skin sores
- Pathogenesis

Venous thrombosis condition decreases the blood flow to the valves and veins of the legs. Valves help to promote the blood flow to the venous circulation but during the conditions of hypoxia condition, the low level of the blood flow to the veins can manifest the symptoms of venous thrombosis. The low level of blood flow can alter the oxygen binding capacity with hemoglobin and raise the hematocrit cells count. The hyper-coagulable micro-environment conditions in the blood vessels can slow down the working nature of the antithrombotic proteins which is binding to the endothelial protein C receptor. The P-selectin adhesion molecules send the immunological tissue factors to the endothelium which leads to forming the thrombus in the blood vessels. The blood clotting factors such as factor VII, factor VIII, von wille brand factor and pro thrombin can strongly influence the formation of clotting in the blood vessels. Fibrin and extracellular DNA attached with histone proteins to form the outer scaffold which is an essential factor in the thrombus formation. The thrombus formation is strongly influenced by several anticoagulant pathways which include heparin-antithrombin pathway, tissue factor inhibitor pathway and protein C anticoagulant pathway. The defects in the clotting mechanisms can increase the risk of thrombus formation [12 - 14].

PROGRESSION OF THE VENOUS THROMBOEMBOLISMS

It includes

- Endothelial injury
- Abnormal blood flow
- Hypercoagulability

Endothelial Injury

The injury of the endothelial cells is caused by bacterial endotoxins, vasculitis and cigarette smoke which lead to changes in the platelet adherence in the blood vessels.

Abnormal Blood Flow

The presence of aneurism condition cause turbulence in the atrium and dilation of atrial cells may aggravate thrombus formation. Several clinical hematological diseases such as polycythemia and sickle cell anemia can increase the risk of thrombus formation in the blood vessels.

Hypercoagulability

The alteration in the coagulation pathways in the systemic stream can increase the risk of thrombus formation. The hypercoagulability disorders include primary and secondary disorder. The primary hypercoagulability disorders are genetically inherited which is caused due to elevation of prothrombin levels and factor V genetic mutations [15 - 18]. Secondary hypercoagulability disorders are acquired type which is caused by burns, fractures, cancer *etc.*

PREVENTION [19 - 22]

- Avoiding prolong sitting

- Wight management

- Quit smoking.

- Regular physical exercise

- Drinking plenty of fluids

- Regular leg and ankle exercises

- Wearing loose-fitting clothes.

• Walk and stretch at regular intervals

• Regular physical active

TREATMENT GOALS FOR DEEP VEIN THROMBOSIS

It includes

• Prevent the clot from breaking off and traveling to the lungs where it could lead to pulmonary embolism

• Reduce the chance of developing another clot

• Minimize the risk of developing other complications

• Avoiding the patients exposure to the risk factors

• Preventing the development of deep vein thrombosis complications

• Minimizing the risk of a blood clot in the veins

Anticoagulation Therapy

The prescribing pattern of anticoagulation therapy to the high risk patients can reduce the extensive risk of venous thromboembolism. Low molecular weight heparin therapy was widely used for the treatment of venous thromboembolism complications [23 - 25].

Initial Choice of Anticoagulation

The primary therapy for the management of venous thromboembolism includes Low molecular weight heparin. It is prescribed once daily for 5-7 days as a starting treatment. Fondaparinux a new drug is used for the treatment of venous thromboembolism. It is a safety drug molecule similar as low molecular weight heparin.

Long-term Treatment

A Vitamin K antagonist such as warfarin is effective for long-term prevention of recurrent incidences of thrombosis. The long term therapy can differ depending upon the risk status of the affected population.

Medications

Anticoagulants

It will prevent blood clot and reduces the risk of venous thromboembolsim. Anticoagulants include injectables drugs such as heparin or low molecular weight heparin, and oral medications such as edoxaban and warfarin. apixaban, dabigatran and rivaroxaban. Thrombolytic therapy can initiate with prescribing of tissue plasminogen activator (tPA) which is a clot dissolving enzyme and administered through vein.

Thrombolytic Agents

These drugs are given through intravenous injection and help to dissolve the clot. The thrombolytic drugs such as anistreplase, reteplase, streptokinase, t-PA (class of drugs that includes activase, tenecteplase and rokinase.

Compression Stockings

It will protect the lower legs and improves the blood flow to the heart and lowers the leg swelling.

Surgery

Patients with high risk group the surgery is recommended. In this procedure a small filter may be inserted into the veins which are connected to the heart. After the surgical procedures it will prevent the clot formation in the heart and lungs.

IVC Filters

Filters are the mechanical devices that dissolve the clot formation in the veins and reduce the further progression of complications. The failure of the anticoagulation therapy in the venous thromboembolism patients IVC filters is recommended. IVC filters are positioned in the vein of the abdomen especially inferior vena cava which receives blood from the lungs and heart. It can be used to treat pulmonary embolism complications.

CONCLUSION

Deep vein thrombosis is a severe condition that is associated with many risk factors. Deep vein thrombosis mostly occurs in less than 45years of age patients. Venous thromboembolism mainly occurs in the veins of the arm, and cerebral sinus. American heart association stated that patients affected with deep vein thrombosis were more as compared with other heart diseases annually. The prevalence was 80-100 per 1, 00,000 in western countries and 4 per in the south-asian population. The chest x-ray, echo studies, doppler examinations, electrocardiogram, D-dimer test, pulmonary angiography examinations are useful for better investigation of vein abnormalities. The prescribing pattern of thrombolytic and anticoagulation medications can reduce the recurrence of disease burden. Non pharmacological treatment options include suction, embolectomy, and catheter-directed therapies colud lower the development of venous thromboembolism risk in veins.

REFERENCES

[1]   Hirsh J, Hoak J. Management of deep vein thrombosis and pulmonary embolism. A statement for healthcare professionals. Council on Thrombosis (in consultation with the Council on Cardiovascular Radiology), American Heart Association. Circulation 1996; 93(12): 2212-45.
[http://dx.doi.org/10.1161/01.CIR.93.12.2212] [PMID: 8925592]

[2]   Silverstein MD, Heit JA, Mohr DN, Petterson TM, O'Fallon WM, Melton LJ III. Trends in the incidence of deep vein thrombosis and pulmonary embolism: a 25-year population-based study. Arch Intern Med 1998; 158(6): 585-93.
[http://dx.doi.org/10.1001/archinte.158.6.585] [PMID: 9521222]

[3]   Naess IA, Christiansen SC, Romundstad P, Cannegieter SC, Rosendaal FR, Hammerstrøm J. Incidence and mortality of venous thrombosis: a population-based study. J Thromb Haemost 2007; 5(4): 692-9.
[http://dx.doi.org/10.1111/j.1538-7836.2007.02450.x] [PMID: 17367492]

[4]   Rosendaal FR. Risk factors for venous thrombosis: prevalence, risk, and interaction. Semin Hematol 1997; 34(3): 171-87.
[PMID: 9241704]

[5]   Anderson FA Jr, Spencer FA. Risk factors for venous thromboembolism. Circulation 2003; 107(23) (Suppl. 1): I9-I16.
[PMID: 12814980]

[6]   Gerotziafas GT. Risk factors for venous thromboembolism in children. Int Angiol 2004; 23(3): 195-205.
[PMID: 15765033]

[7]   Rosendaal FR, Reitsma PH. Genetics of venous thrombosis. J Thromb Haemost 2009; 7(1) (Suppl. 1): 301-4.
[http://dx.doi.org/10.1111/j.1538-7836.2009.03394.x] [PMID: 19630821]

[8]   Kyrle PA, Minar E, Bialonczyk C, Hirschl M, Weltermann A, Eichinger S. The risk of recurrent venous thromboembolism in men and women. N Engl J Med 2004; 350(25): 2558-63.
[http://dx.doi.org/10.1056/NEJMoa032959] [PMID: 15201412]

[9]   Keenan CR, White RH. The effects of race/ethnicity and sex on the risk of venous thromboembolism. Curr Opin Pulm Med 2007; 13(5): 377-83.
[http://dx.doi.org/10.1097/MCP.0b013e3281eb8ef0] [PMID: 17940480]

[10]   Andrew M, David M, Adams M, *et al.* Venous thromboembolic complications (VTE) in children: first analyses of the Canadian Registry of VTE. Blood 1994; 83(5): 1251-7.
[http://dx.doi.org/10.1182/blood.V83.5.1251.1251] [PMID: 8118029]

[11]   Tapson VF, Carroll BA, Davidson BL, *et al.* The diagnostic approach to acute venous thromboembolism. Clinical practice guideline. Am J Respir Crit Care Med 1999; 160(3): 1043-66.
[http://dx.doi.org/10.1164/ajrccm.160.3.16030] [PMID: 10471639]

[12]   Kahn SR. The clinical diagnosis of deep venous thrombosis: integrating incidence, risk factors, and

symptoms and signs. Arch Intern Med 1998; 158(21): 2315-23.
[http://dx.doi.org/10.1001/archinte.158.21.2315] [PMID: 9827782]

[13]   Wells PS, Anderson DR, Bormanis J, *et al.* Value of assessment of pretest probability of deep-vein thrombosis in clinical management. Lancet 1997; 350(9094): 1795-8.
[http://dx.doi.org/10.1016/S0140-6736(97)08140-3] [PMID: 9428249]

[14]   Anderson DR, *et al.* Evaluation of D-dimer in the diagnosis of suspected deep-vein thrombosis N Engl J Med 2003; 349: 1227-35.

[15]   Aguilar C, del Villar V. Combined D-dimer and clinical probability are useful for exclusion of recurrent deep venous thrombosis. Am J Hematol 2007; 82(1): 41-4.
[http://dx.doi.org/10.1002/ajh.20754] [PMID: 16947316]

[16]   Brotman DJ, Segal JB, Jani JT, Petty BG, Kickler TS. Limitations of D-dimer testing in unselected inpatients with suspected venous thromboembolism. Am J Med 2003; 114(4): 276-82.
[http://dx.doi.org/10.1016/S0002-9343(02)01520-6] [PMID: 12681454]

[17]   Curry N, Keeling D. Venous thromboembolism: the role of the clinician. J R Coll Phys Edinb 2009; 39: 243-6.

[18]   Hirsh J, Lee AY. How we diagnose and treat deep vein thrombosis. Blood 2002; 99(9): 3102-10.
[http://dx.doi.org/10.1182/blood.V99.9.3102] [PMID: 11964271]

[19]   Tovey C, Wyatt S. Diagnosis, investigation, and management of deep vein thrombosis. BMJ 2003; 326(7400): 1180-4.
[http://dx.doi.org/10.1136/bmj.326.7400.1180] [PMID: 12775619]

[20]   Zierler BK. Ultrasonography and diagnosis of venous thromboembolism. Circulation 2004; 109(12) (Suppl. 1): I9-I14.
[http://dx.doi.org/10.1161/01.CIR.0000122870.22669.4a] [PMID: 15051663]

[21]   Kearon C, Julian JA, Newman TE, Ginsberg JS. Noninvasive diagnosis of deep venous thrombosis. McMaster Diagnostic Imaging Practice Guidelines Initiative. Ann Intern Med 1998; 128(8): 663-77.
[http://dx.doi.org/10.7326/0003-4819-128-8-199804150-00011] [PMID: 9537941]

[22]   Tapson VF, Carroll BA, Davidson BL, *et al.* The diagnostic approach to acute venous thromboembolism. Clinical practice guideline. Am J Respir Crit Care Med 1999; 160(3): 1043-66.
[http://dx.doi.org/10.1164/ajrccm.160.3.16030] [PMID: 10471639]

[23]   Bates SM, Ginsberg JS. How we manage venous thromboembolism during pregnancy. Blood 2002; 100(10): 3470-8.
[http://dx.doi.org/10.1182/blood-2002-03-0965] [PMID: 12393666]

[24]   Hovens MM, Snoep JD, Tamsma JT, Huisman MV. Aspirin in the prevention and treatment of venous thromboembolism. J Thromb Haemost 2006; 4(7): 1470-5.
[http://dx.doi.org/10.1111/j.1538-7836.2006.01928.x] [PMID: 16839339]

[25]   Segal JB, Streiff MB, Hofmann LV, Thornton K, Bass EB. Management of venous thromboembolism: a systematic review for a practice guideline. Ann Intern Med 2007; 146(3): 211-22.
[http://dx.doi.org/10.7326/0003-4819-146-3-200702060-00150] [PMID: 17261856]

Aortic Aneurysm

Abstract: The weakening of the artery causes abnormal bulging and rupture of the artery with bleeding results in the development of an aneurysm. An aneurysm occurs in the various vital organs in the body which include the brain, aorta, legs, and spleen. Patients with age more than 60 years, hypertension, smoking, can drastically increase the risk of the aortic aneurysm. The development of aneurysm rupture is influenced by the aneurysm size, expansion rate, and uncontrolled hypertension increases the risk of more bleeding in the arteries. The arteries of brain cells and heart are the most common sites of developing serious aneurysm complications. The incidence of abdominal aortic aneurysms has been increasing from the past few decades. The aortic aneurysm has an incidence of 5-10 cases per 100,000 was seen in more than the age of 60 years. An aneurysm is detected with a computed tomography scan, magnetic resonance image scan, ultrasonography, angiography examinations helpful for detecting the abnormalities in the arteries. The prevention and management of aneurysm through lifestyle modification practices, eating a healthy diet, stress management, regular medication adherence and maintaining controlled levels of risk factors could minimize the future complications of an aneurysm in primary care settings.

Keywords: Aneurysm, Bleeding, Hypertension, Legs, Spleen, Ultrasonography.

INTRODUCTION

An aneurysm is the bulge of artery cause wakening of arterial wall results in rupture of arterial cells develops fatal complications. Aorta is the main arteries that supply the blood to the heart and all the organs present in the body. The severe condition of an aneurysm increases the risk of internal bleeding in blood vessels. The development of the aortic aneurysm is the abdominal cavity. The rupture of the aortic aneurysms can cause bleeding and clot in the blood vessels. A brain aneurysm can cause bleeding in the cerebral cells. During this condition, the permanent damage of the covering layers of the brain may occur which is called a hemorrhagic stroke. Therefore rapid screening programmes and prompt medical therapy can help for reducing the burden of an aneurysm.

The Aortic aneurysm is represented with the location, size and morphology of the cells. It occurs in the aortic cells which are strong and low levels of blood supply may weaken the aortic walls resulting in the progression of the aneurysm. An aortic aneurysm develops in the aortic root and the presence of inflammation damages the aortic valves and appears balloon-like shape. An aortic aneurysm can occur in the various places of the body which includes abdominal area; thoracic area leads to develops aortic complications in the blood vessels [1 - 4].

CLASSIFICATION OF THE AORTIC ANEURYSMS BULGING

Aneurysms are categorized according to their location in the body. The arteries of the brain cells and heart are the most common sites of developing serious aneurysm complications.

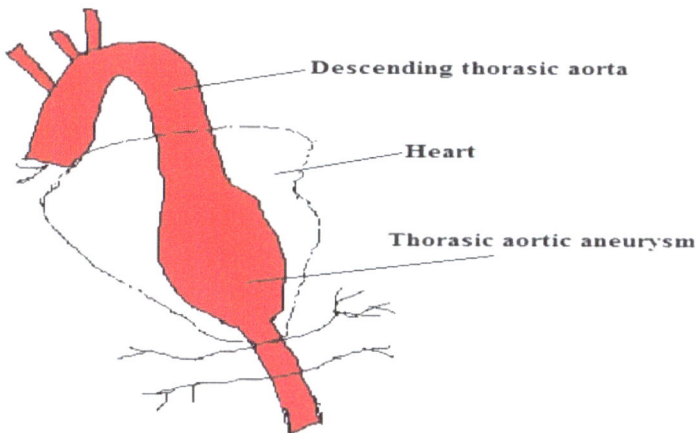

Fig. (1). Thorasic aortic aneurysm.

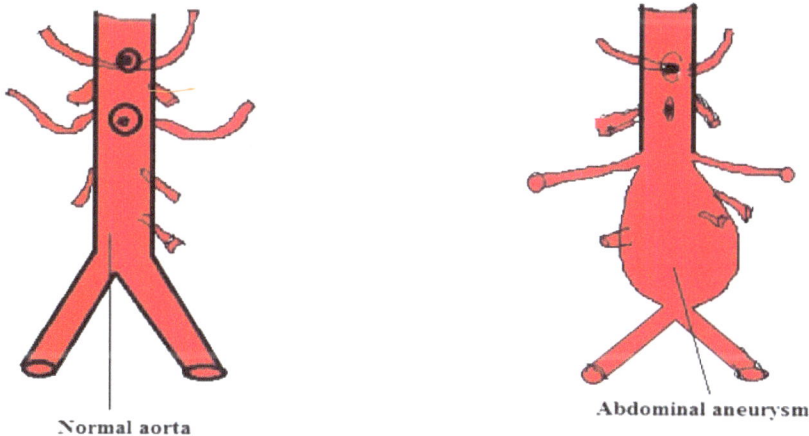

Fig. (2). Abdominal aneurysm.

The bulge can take two main shapes

• Fusiform aneurysms bulge all sides of a blood vessel

• Saccular aneurysms bulge only on one side

Aorta is the large artery that originates from the left ventricle and passes through the chest and abdominal region. The normal diameter of the aorta is ranging from 2 and 3 centimeters but more than 5cm of arterial swelling leads to the development of an aneurysm. The common aneurysm of the aorta is the abdominal aortic aneurysm.

TYPES OF AORTIC ANEURYSMS [5 - 9]

Abdominal Aortic Aneurysm

It occurs in the aorta that passes through the abdominal region. It is shown in Fig. **(2)**.

Thoracic Aortic Aneurysm

It occurs in the aorta that passes through the chest cavity. It is shown in Fig. **(1)**.

THORACIC AORTIC ANEURYSM

• The clinical symptoms may include

• Chest tightness

• Chest pain

• Back pain

• Shortness of breath

• Abdominal aortic aneurysm

• The clinical symptoms may include

• Back pain in the mid to lower part of the back

• Abdominal pain

• Abdominal discomfort

• Pulsating sensation in the abdomen

RUPTURED AORTIC ANEURYSM

The clinical symptoms may include:

• Loss of consciousness

• Light headedness

• Blurred vision

• Dizziness

• Severe weakness

• Chest pain

• Abdominal pain

• Back pain

Aortic Aneurysm Affecting other Organs

The blood clot travels to the body and damages the vital organs in the body which leads to damage the heart failure, renal failure and stroke.

Clinical symptoms

It includes

• Difficult or painful swallowing

• Difficulty breathing

• Hoarseness

• Pain

• Pulsating or throbbing

• Shortness of breath

• Swelling of the face, neck, or arms

• Back or chest pain

• Light-headedness

• Rapid heart rate

• Severe pain in abdomen

• Changes in thinking ability, confusion, disorientation

• Clammy skin, sweating

• Dizziness, fainting, nausea, and vomiting

• Dry skin Excessive yawning

• High blood pressure

• Intense anxiety

• Pallor

• Rapid pulse or weak/absent pulse

• Shortness of breath

PREVALENCE

The incidence of abdominal aortic aneurysms has been increasing from the past few decades. The aging, presence of risk factors, ineffective screening programmes and in effective diagnostic tools can increase the risk of aneurysm complications. An aneurysm is more common to male patients than female patients and the incidence was 1.3–8.9% in males and 1.0–2.2% in females. The thoracic aortic aneurysms incidence was estimated that 5-10 percent 100,000 person-years. The aortic aneurysm has an incidence of 5-10 cases per 100,000 was seen in more than the age of 60 years. The aortic aneurysms are do not cause death to the patients but the improper treatment of aneurysm causes various disease complications [10 - 12].

PATHOPHYSIOLOGY

Aneurysms are characterized by localized dilation of the arterial segment greater than its normal diameter. It occurs in the infra renal segment. The normal size for thoracoabdominal aorta is larger than infra renal aorta. The development of aneurysm involves hemodynamic factors. The medial layer of the aorta has effective tensile strength and elastic nature. The structural proteins include collagen and elastin is essential for protecting aorta. The infiltration of the arterial vessel by the action of lymphocytes and macrophage cells damage and destruction of the elastin and collagen in the cell matrix results in the progression of inflammatory conditions in the aorta. The elastin content was high in ascending aorta as compared with descending aorta. The infra renal aorta has a paucity of elastin and most of the aneurysms are occurred in the infra renal aorta. The enzymatic action in the infra renal portion leads to degrading the structural proteins. The fragmentation of the elastic fibers causes the weakening of aortic walls and dilation of the blood vessels causes the development of an aneurysm. The hemodynamic factors have a major role in the formation of aortic aneurysms. The aorta has a low resistance and path for the circulation of blood to all the vital organs present in the body. The lower extremities have a greater arterial resistance and repeated injury to the arterial walls cause aneurysmal degeneration. The elevated levels of pressure in the arterial walls can accelerate the formation of an aneurysm. According to the law of laplace aneurysmal dilation states that the wall tension is proportional to the pressure and radius of the artery. The diameter of the artery and wall tension increases, which contributes to the development of systemic hypertension thereby increase the risk of wall rupture and leads to the development of aneurysm [13 - 15].

CAUSES OF AORTIC ANEURYSM

There are several causes to develop aortic aneurysms which include

• Hypertension

• High cholesterol

• Injury to the chest

• Atherosclerosis

• Inflammation

• Endocarditis

• Smoking

• Genes associated with aortic aneurysms include ACTA2, FBN1 *etc.*

COMPLICATIONS [16 - 18]

The bleeding can cause damage to cerebral cells and increases the pressure in the brain which leads to raising the risk of a aneurysm. Complications that can develop after the rupture of an aneurysm include

Re bleeding: It may increase the risk of brain cells rupture thereby progression of an aneurysm in the cerebrum.

Vasospasm The rupture of an aneurysm may cause narrow the blood flow to the brain cells which causes the development of stroke.

Hydrocephalus: The deposition of fluid in the ventricle of the brain cavities causes the progression of Hydrocephalus.

Hyponatremia Subarachnoid hemorrhage from a ruptured brain aneurysm can disrupt the balance of sodium in the blood. This may occur from damage to the hypothalamus, an area near the base of the brain.

Aortic rupture: It causes severe bleeding inside the tissue cells which leads to the development of shock and reduced levels of oxygen results in the development of **aortic rupture.**

DIAGNOSIS

It includes

CT scan This test is used to identify the images of muscles, fat, and organs present in the body.

MRI: Radio waves are used to create detailed images of organs and structures in the body.

Echocardiogram This test can detect the functioning of the heart valves and associated cardiac defects.

Arteriogram Angiogram studies are used to evaluate blockages in the blood vessels.

Ultrasound An ultrasound and high-frequency sound waves are used to identify the abnormal nature of blood vessels, tissues, and organs.

Chest X-ray A chest X-ray is used to detect the inflammatory conditions of the chest.

SCREENING

• People who have Turner syndrome

• First-degree relatives of people who have a thoracic aortic aneurysm

• Patients with age of 65 to 75 years old

• Patients with smoking habit

• Family history of abdominal aortic aneurysms

PREVENTION STRATEGIES

• Smoking cessation

• Healthy eating

• Regular physical exercises

• Stress management

• Maintaining controlled levels of blood pressure

• Maintaining controlled levels of blood cholesterol levels

• Regular medication adherence

TREATMENT [19 - 22]

The aortic aneurysms can be managed through prescribing beta blockers, calcium channel blockers, angiotensin-converting-enzyme inhibitors, angiotensin receptor blockers and statins, can reduce the progression of aortic aneurysm complications.

Calcium Channel Blockers This drug blocks the entry of calcium ions into the calcium channels and lowers the work load on the heart and dilates the arteries leads to vasodilatation.

These drugs include

• Diltiazem

• Verapamil

• Isradipine

• Nifedipine

• Nicardipine

• Nimopidine

• Amlodipine

• Nisoldipine

• Bepridil

• Felodipine

Adverse effects Rashes, headache, constipation, flushing, edema, drowsiness

Cholesterol Lowering Medications
Statins

These drugs act by inhibiting HMG-CoA reductase enzyme and inhibit the cholesterol biosynthetic pathway and show anti atherosclerotic effect in the blood vessels.

• Atorvastatin

• Fluvastatin

• Lovastatin

• Pitavastatin

• Pravastatin

• Rosuvastatin

• Simvastatin

Adverse effects Headache, dizziness, insomnia, flushing of the skin, drowsiness and myalgia.

Beta Blockers

It reduces the work load on the heart and reduces stress and hormones levels in the body which leads to vasodilatation in the blood vessels. Some commonly prescribed beta blockers include

• Atenolol

• Bisoprolol

• Nadolol

• Nebivolol

• Carvedilol

• Labetalol

- Nebivolol

- Pindolol

- Propranolol

- Timolol

- Metoprolol

Adverse effects Dry mouth, dry skin, feelings of coldness, diarrhea, shortness of breath and insomnia.

Angiotensin Converting Enzyme Inhibitors [23 - 25]

ACEs block the conversion of angiotensin I to angiotensin II by the action of angiotensinogen in the body and help to lower the vasoconstriction and promote vasodilation.

It includes

- Captopril

- Lisinopril

- Fosinopril

- Ramipril

- Benazepril

- Enalapril

- Perindopril

- Quinapril

- Moexipril

- Trandolapril

Adverse effects Dry cough, hyperkalemia, fatigue, headaches and loss of taste.

Angiotensin II Receptor Blockers

It blocks the conversion of angiotensin II from its binding to angiotensin II receptors located on the blood vessels and produce vasodialtion in the blood vessels. These drugs include

• Candesartan

• Telmisartan

• Valsartan

• Eprosartan

• Irbesartan

• Losartan

Adverse effects Hyperkalemia, dizziness, headache, cough, diarrhea, hypotension and angioedema.

CONCLUSION

The incidence of abdominal aortic aneurysms has been increasing from the past few decades. The aging, presence of risk factors, ineffective risk screening programmes and in effective diagnostic tools can increase the risk of aneurysm complications. The implication of clinical pharmacist services with the health care team on diet counseling, disease counseling, lifestyle modification counseling, stress management, physical exercise, weight management, cessation of smoking, and alcohol practices could lower the risk severity among high risk profile patients. The surgical invention is suggested for symptomatic aneurysms cases in clinical settings. Regular prescribing of beta blockers, calcium channel blockers and statins, and maintaining controlled levels of risk factors can helpful for effective management of aneurysm complications in health care.

REFERENCES

[1]   Lederle FA, Johnson GR, Wilson SE, *et al.* The aneurysm detection and management study screening program: validation cohort and final results. Arch Intern Med 2000; 160(10): 1425-30.
[http://dx.doi.org/10.1001/archinte.160.10.1425] [PMID: 10826454]

[2]   Kuzmik GA, Sang AX, Elefteriades JA. Natural history of thoracic aortic aneurysms. J Vasc Surg 2012; 56(2): 565-71.
[http://dx.doi.org/10.1016/j.jvs.2012.04.053] [PMID: 22840907]

[3]   Johansen K, Koepsell T. Familial tendency for abdominal aortic aneurysms. JAMA 1986; 256(14): 1934-6.
[http://dx.doi.org/10.1001/jama.1986.03380140104031] [PMID: 3761500]

[4]   Lederle FA, Johnson GR, Wilson SE, *et al.* Prevalence and associations of abdominal aortic aneurysm detected through screening. Ann Intern Med 1997; 126(6): 441-9.
[http://dx.doi.org/10.7326/0003-4819-126-6-199703150-00004] [PMID: 9072929]

[5]   Helgadottir A, Thorleifsson G, Magnusson KP, *et al.* The same sequence variant on 9p21 associates

with myocardial infarction, abdominal aortic aneurysm and intracranial aneurysm. Nat Genet 2008; 40(2): 217-24.
[http://dx.doi.org/10.1038/ng.72] [PMID: 18176561]

[6]   Ailawadi G, Eliason JL, Upchurch GR Jr. Current concepts in the pathogenesis of abdominal aortic aneurysm. J Vasc Surg 2003; 38(3): 584-8.
[http://dx.doi.org/10.1016/S0741-5214(03)00324-0] [PMID: 12947280]

[7]   Doyle JJ, Gerber EE, Dietz HC. Matrix-dependent perturbation of TGFβ signaling and disease. FEBS Lett 2012; 586(14): 2003-15.
[http://dx.doi.org/10.1016/j.febslet.2012.05.027] [PMID: 22641039]

[8]   Davies RR, Gallo A, Coady MA, *et al.* Novel measurement of relative aortic size predicts rupture of thoracic aortic aneurysms. Ann Thorac Surg 2006; 81(1): 169-77.
[http://dx.doi.org/10.1016/j.athoracsur.2005.06.026] [PMID: 16368358]

[9]   Conway KP, Byrne J, Townsend M, Lane IF. Prognosis of patients turned down for conventional abdominal aortic aneurysm repair in the endovascular and sonographic era: Szilagyi revisited? J Vasc Surg 2001; 33(4): 752-7.
[http://dx.doi.org/10.1067/mva.2001.112800] [PMID: 11296328]

[10]   Lindholt JS, Ashton HA, Scott RA. Indicators of infection with Chlamydia pneumoniae are associated with expansion of abdominal aortic aneurysms. J Vasc Surg 2001; 34(2): 212-5.
[http://dx.doi.org/10.1067/mva.2001.115816] [PMID: 11496270]

[11]   Elefteriades JA. Indications for aortic replacement. J Thorac Cardiovasc Surg 2010; 140(6) (Suppl.): S5-9.
[http://dx.doi.org/10.1016/j.jtcvs.2010.10.001] [PMID: 21092797]

[12]   Fleming C, Whitlock EP, Beil TL, Lederle FA. Screening for abdominal aortic aneurysm: a best-evidence systematic review for the U.S. Preventive Services Task Force. Ann Intern Med 2005; 142(3): 203-11.
[http://dx.doi.org/10.7326/0003-4819-142-3-200502010-00012] [PMID: 15684209]

[13]   Moll FL, Powell JT, Fraedrich G, *et al.* Management of abdominal aortic aneurysms clinical practice guidelines of the European society for vascular surgery. Eur J Vasc Endovasc Surg 2011; 41 (Suppl. 1): S1-S58.
[http://dx.doi.org/10.1016/j.ejvs.2010.09.011] [PMID: 21215940]

[14]   Chaikof EL, Brewster DC, Dalman RL, *et al.* The care of patients with an abdominal aortic aneurysm: the Society for Vascular Surgery practice guidelines. J Vasc Surg 2009; 50(4) (Suppl.): S2-S49.
[http://dx.doi.org/10.1016/j.jvs.2009.07.002] [PMID: 19786250]

[15]   Chaikof EL, Brewster DC, Dalman RL, *et al.* SVS practice guidelines for the care of patients with an abdominal aortic aneurysm: executive summary. J Vasc Surg 2009; 50(4): 880-96.
[http://dx.doi.org/10.1016/j.jvs.2009.07.001] [PMID: 19786241]

[16]   Lemos DW, Raffetto JD, Moore TC, Menzoian JO. Primary aortoduodenal fistula: a case report and review of the literature. J Vasc Surg 2003; 37(3): 686-9.
[http://dx.doi.org/10.1067/mva.2003.101] [PMID: 12618713]

[17]   Davis PM, Gloviczki P, Cherry KJ Jr, *et al.* Aorto-caval and ilio-iliac arteriovenous fistulae. Am J Surg 1998; 176(2): 115-8.
[http://dx.doi.org/10.1016/S0002-9610(98)00166-4] [PMID: 9737613]

[18]   Lederle FA. Abdominal aortic aneurysm: still no pill. Ann Intern Med 2013; 159(12): 852-3.
[http://dx.doi.org/10.7326/0003-4819-159-12-201312170-00012] [PMID: 24490269]

[19]   Meijer CA, Stijnen T, Wasser MN, Hamming JF, van Bockel JH, Lindeman JH. Doxycycline for stabilization of abdominal aortic aneurysms: a randomized trial. Ann Intern Med 2013; 159(12): 815-23.
[http://dx.doi.org/10.7326/0003-4819-159-12-201312170-00007] [PMID: 24490266]

[20]   Forbes TL, Lawlor DK, DeRose G, Harris KA. Gender differences in relative dilatation of abdominal aortic aneurysms. Ann Vasc Surg 2006; 20(5): 564-8.
[http://dx.doi.org/10.1007/S10016-006-9079-y] [PMID: 16741651]

[21]   Loeys BL, Dietz HC, Braverman AC, *et al.* The revised Ghent nosology for the Marfan syndrome. J Med Genet 2010; 47(7): 476-85.
[http://dx.doi.org/10.1136/jmg.2009.072785] [PMID: 20591885]

[22]   Rayt HS, Bown MJ, Lambert KV, *et al.* Buttock claudication and erectile dysfunction after internal iliac artery embolization in patients prior to endovascular aortic aneurysm repair. Cardiovasc Intervent Radiol 2008; 31(4): 728-34.
[http://dx.doi.org/10.1007/s00270-008-9319-3] [PMID: 18338212]

[23]   Lederle FA, Freischlag JA, Kyriakides TC, *et al.* Long-term comparison of endovascular and open repair of abdominal aortic aneurysm. N Engl J Med 2012; 367(21): 1988-97.
[http://dx.doi.org/10.1056/NEJMoa1207481] [PMID: 23171095]

[24]   Kristensen KE, Torp-Pedersen C, Gislason GH, Egfjord M, Rasmussen HB, Hansen PR. Angiotensin-converting enzyme inhibitors and angiotensin II receptor blockers in patients with abdominal aortic aneurysms: nation-wide cohort study. Arterioscler Thromb Vasc Biol 2015; 35(3): 733-40.
[http://dx.doi.org/10.1161/ATVBAHA.114.304428] [PMID: 25633315]

[25]   Bederson JB, Awad IA, Wiebers DO, *et al.* Recommendations for the management of patients with unruptured intracranial aneurysms: A statement for healthcare professionals from the Stroke Council of the American Heart Association. Circulation 2000; 102(18): 2300-8.
[http://dx.doi.org/10.1161/01.CIR.102.18.2300] [PMID: 11056108]

CHAPTER 10

Stroke

Abstract: Stroke is a clinical condition that is progressed due to the obstruction of blood flow to the brain. The high incidences of stroke can double the burden of disease complications among the affected patients from developed and developing countries. Stroke is a major public health care issue that is associated with multiple risk factors that include physical inactivity, hypertension, smoking, alcohol, diabetes mellitus, stress, and obesity causes occurrence of stroke. Stroke diagnosed through regular physical examination, blood test, CT scan, MRI scan, CSF fluid examination, and cerebral angiogram studies can help to detect and prevent the progression of stroke complications. The management of stroke through prescribing of blood pressure medications, statins, anti platelets, anti coagulants drugs could reduce the future episodes of the occurrence of the stroke.

Keywords: Alcohol, Diabetes Mellitus, Hypertension, MRI Scan, Stroke, Smoking.

INTRODUCTION

Stroke is a medical condition that occurs due to the obstruction of blood flow to the brain. It causes serious clinical symptoms that lead to affects permanent disability for the individual patients. The high incidences of stroke can double the burden of disease complications among the affected patients from developed and developing countries. The presence of a greater incidence of risk factors and poor disease risk screening programmes cause more health care expenditure to the affected population. The poor flow of blood and oxygen supply to the brain cells causes blockage of blood vessels that causes the progression of stroke. The injury of the brain cells causes paralysis of the facial muscles, arms, and impaired cognitive behavior advances the development of stroke clinical complications. Improper treatment of stroke causes serious complications of the disease population which, leads to cause the death of the patient [1, 2].

TYPES OF STROKES

The major types of stroke include ischemic stroke, transient ischemic attack and hemorrhagic stroke. It is shown in Fig. (1).

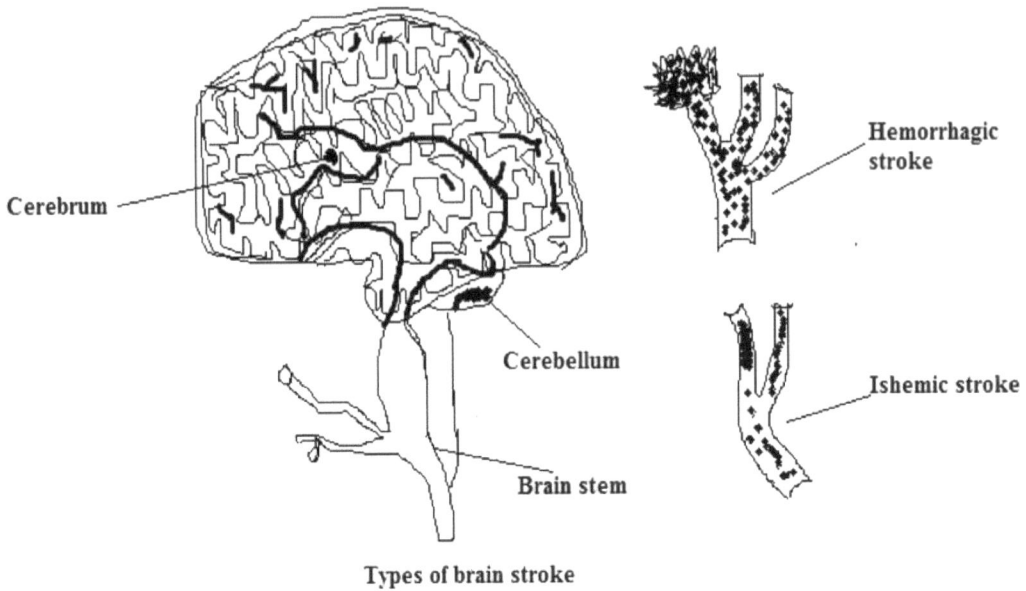

Types of brain stroke

Fig. (1). Types of stroke.

TRANSIENT ISCHEMIC ATTACK

The temporary flow of the blood to the brain cells causes blood clot in brain cells lead to development of transient ischemic attack in the brain.

ISCHEMIC STROKE

The deposition of fatty materials in the inner lining of the blood vessels causes the blood clot which reduces the blood supply to the brain cells cause an ischemic stroke.

HEMORRHAGIC STROKE

The rupture of the blood vessels in the brain causes leaking of the blood in the surrounding tissues leading to the development of hemorrhagic stroke. The development of aneurysm causes weakening of the blood vessels leads to swelling of the arterial walls leads to the rupture of the artery and causes the development of hemorrhagic stroke. The development of high blood pressure in blood vessels results in bleeding into the brain which ultimately results in the progression of stroke complications. The recent statement of the global burden of diseases was predicted that 4.66 million people affected by stroke in 1990 and 5.87 million stroke deaths globally in 2010. These results were showed that 26 per cent of stroke death cases were rising from the past two decades. The detection of stroke diagnosed through physical examination, blood test, CT scan and cerebral angiogram studies can help to identify the detect and prevent the progression of stroke complications. The management of stroke through prescribing of blood pressure medications, statins, anti platelets, anti coagulants drugs can reduce the future episodes of the occurrence of the stroke [3, 4].

RISK FACTORS

• Obesity

• Alcohol

• Use of illicit drugs such as cocaine

• Physical inactivity

• Stress

• Smoking

• High cholesterol

• Diabetes mellitus

• Obstructive sleep apnea

• High blood pressure

• Family history of stroke

• Previous history of cardiovascular disease

• Family history of cardiovascular disease

• Patient having age of 55 years

• Patient receiving hormonal therapy

PREVALENCE OF STROKE

Stroke is a commonly occurring disease in the clinical practice which leads to cause several chronic complications to the individual patients. The incidence of stroke is about 3% of the adult population and increased up to 7 million people among individuals. The stroke is affected about 10% of people are affected with primary hemorrhages, 87% of people are ischemic infarctions and 3% of the people are affected by subarachnoid hemorrhage. Worldwide stroke incidence is estimated that primary hemorrhages represent a higher incidence of stroke ranges from 10% to 25%. African, Asian and Latin American origin has a higher occurrence of developing primary hemorrhage. Western countries origin has 10 to 17% of developing stroke complications. The incidence of stroke is rapidly increased with age and people with age more 55 years may prone to develop a higher rate of stroke incidences [5, 6]. Adult patients with age range from 35 to 44 years; the incidence of stroke is 30 to 120 of 100,000 per year.

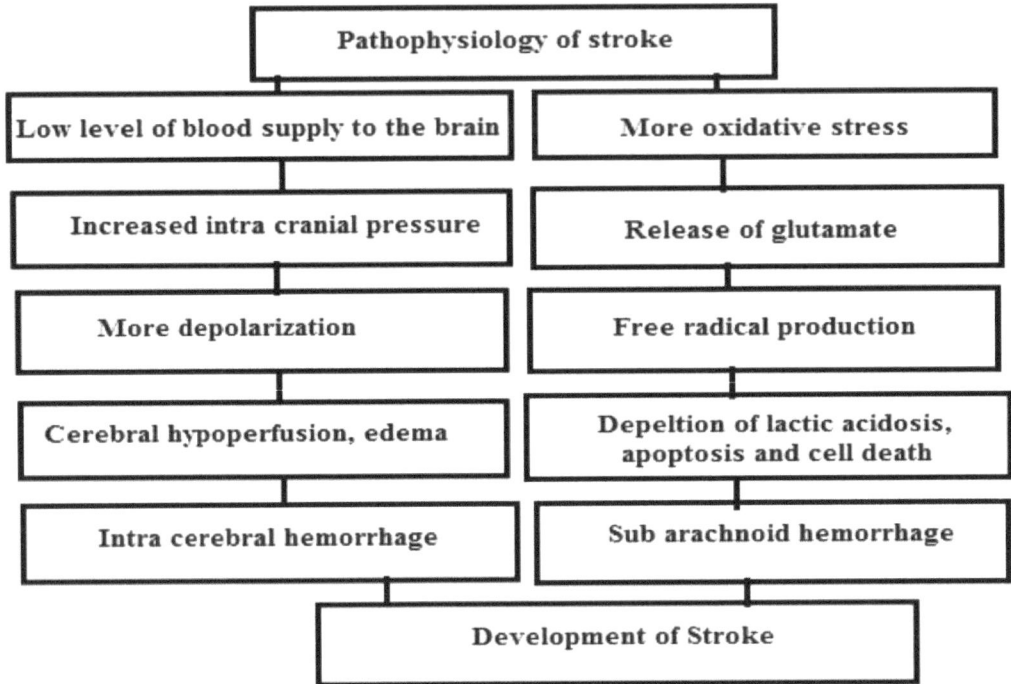

```
                    ┌──────────────────────────────┐
                    │   Pathophysiology of stroke   │
                    └──────────────────────────────┘
```

Low level of blood supply to the brain	More oxidative stress
Increased intra cranial pressure	Release of glutamate
More depolarization	Free radical production
Cerebral hypoperfusion, edema	Depeltion of lactic acidosis, apoptosis and cell death
Intra cerebral hemorrhage	Sub arachnoid hemorrhage
Development of Stroke	

Fig. (2). Pathophysiology of stroke.

PATHOPHYSIOLOGY

The accumulation of toxic substances in the cerebral cells causes damage to the brain which leads to developing the ischemic changes in blood vessel. These results in an imbalance of sodium-potassium pump can increase the free radicals production in the brain cells leads to cause the inflammation. The failure of sodium potassium pump causes the efflux of sodium ions inside cause cytotoxic edema conditions within the cells. The highest concentration of calcium ions can damage the intra cellular cells which results in damage to mitochondrial damage and the occurrence of apoptosis in the cells. The enzymatic conversion reactions of hydrogen peroxide and hydroxyl radicals lead to lipid peroxidation cause damage of the cell membrane results in mutations in the genome. These changes promote cell injury and finally cause cell death. The blood brain barrier protects the brain cell from several inflammatory conditions. The endothelial-astrocyte cell main cells signals and homeostasis in the neuronal region of the brain. Matrix metalloproteinase and plasminogen activator can modulate the brain cells [7, 8]. The low level of blood supply to the brain cells causes hypoxic damage to protection layers of the brain which can damage the brain. The abnormal levels of matrix metalloproteinase cause the inflammation in the brain leads to the development of hemorrhage and ischemia in the brain which results in the progression of stroke. The damage of the blood brain barrier cells causes edema and finally causes hemorrhagic conditions and results in hemorrhagic stroke. The brain cells are sensitive compared with other organs present in the body. The injury of brain cells can affect the brain function which leads to impair the neuronal communication between cells in the brain which leads to inflammation followed a by progression of stroke. The pathophysiology of stroke is shown in Fig. (**2**).

MAJOR STEPS IN PATHOGENESIS OF STROKE

• Poor flow of blood in capillaries in brain cells

• Release of pro inflammatory cells

• Formation of thrombus in brain cells

• Poor response of blood brain barrier function

• Poor endothelial cells function

• Alteration in the physiological changes of the brain

• Injury of brain cells and ischemic events in brain causes the development of stroke

CLINICAL SYMPTOMS OF STROKE

• Poor speech

• Difficulty in walking

• Loss of balance

• Confusion

• Headache

• Numbness in the face and limbs

- Weakness on one side of the body

- Loss of vision

- Face drooping

- Early complications of stroke:

- Bleeding at the infracted area

- Cerebral edema

- Pulmonary embolism

- Pneumonitis

- Myocardial infarction

- Gastrointestinal bleeding

- Gastrointestinal ulcers

- Seizure

- Deep vein thrombosis

- Late complications of stroke

- Aspiration pneumonitis

- Recurrent stroke

- Persistent loss of mobility

- Spasticity of muscles

- Pulmonary embolism

- Ulcers

- Persistent cognitive

- Spasticity of muscles

DIAGNOSIS [9 - 11]

Physical Examination

It includes identification of patient's clinical symptoms and checking blood pressure, respiratory rate, heart rate can help in the detection of individual patient's disease sickness.

Blood Tests

This test is performed to identify the infections, inflammation and clotting conditions in the blood.

CT Scan

This test can produce X-ray images of bleeding, infection, tumors, and other conditions present in the brain.

MRI Scan

The radio waves and electro magnets are used to make an image of the brain to detect the affected parts of the brain.

Carotid Ultrasound

It is an ultrasound scan that is used to check the blood flow pattern in the carotid arteries and to fins the plaque characteristics.

Cerebral Angiogram

This test is used to identify the presence of clotting in the blood vessels.

Echocardiogram

Echocardiogram test is used to produce the images of the heart and blood flow pattern in the arteries and the presence of clotting abnormalities and blood ejection from the ventricles can be detected by this examination.

TREATMENT

Primary Treatment

Previous research studies revealed that hypertension was one of the risk factors for the development of stroke and regular hypertension screening test can helpful for reducing the risk of future progression of stroke. Patients with blood pressure

140/90 mm Hg is considered as normal and above 140/90 mm Hg is a risk for developing hypertensive complications. Dietary modifications and lifestyle modifications and effective drug treatment can lower the burden of hypertension among stroke patients. Patients with diabetes mellitus and hypertension, strict glycemic and blood pressure control can reduce the progression of micro-vascular complications [12 - 17].

Patients diagnosed with dyslipidemia and coronary artery disease were treated with statins and lifestyle modifications can reduce the progression of the future risk of coronary artery disease complications.

Smoking doubles the risk of subarachnoid hemorrhage in the brain. Smoking cessation practices and nicotine replacement therapies can reduce the progression of stroke complications. Diabetes is one of the risk factors for the occurrence of stroke. Strict glycemic control and anti diabetic therapy can reduce the risk of stroke. Regular physical activity at least one hour and 15 minutes walking every week is recommended for stroke patients to improve the health condition and reduce the stroke severity among disease patients. Aspirin therapy is recommended for primary prevention of stroke and also the future risk of developing cardiovascular events.

Secondary Treatment

Risk factors control, lifestyle modifications and antiplatelet therapy is beneficial for secondary prevention of stroke [18 - 22].

Cholesterol Lowering Medications

Statins

These drugs act by inhibiting HMG-CoA reductase enzyme and inhibit the cholesterol biosynthetic pathway and show anti atherosclerotic effect in the blood vessels.

- Atorvastatin

- Fluvastatin

- Lovastatin

- Pitavastatin

- Pravastatin

• Rosuvastatin

• Simvastatin

Adverse effects Headache, dizziness, insomnia, flushing of the skin, drowsiness and myalgia.

THROMBOLYTIC DRUGS

Thrombolytic drugs are prescribed to reduce the formation of blood clot in the blood vessels and also lower the severity of stroke. These drugs will act by conversion of plasminogen which forms plasmin and activates the fibrin bound plasminogen. Fibrin molecules are inhibited by plasmin which leads to breakdown of clot the blood vessels and reduces the stroke complications.

It includes:

• Anistreplase

• Reteplase

• Streptokinase

• T-pa

• Tenecteplase

• Alteplase

• Urokinase

Adverse drug reactions Internal bleeding, damage to the blood vessels, renal damage.

Anti Platelet Drugs

These drugs help to prevent the platelet aggregation and reduce the clot in the blood vessels.

Types of antiplatelet agents:

• Aspirin

• Dipyridamole

• Clopidogrel

• Ticagrelor

Clinical Uses of Antiplatelet Agents

It is used to treat the following disease conditions.

• Coronary artery disease

• Heart attack

• Angina pectoris

• Stroke and transient ischemic attacks

• Peripheral artery disease

Side Effects Nausea, gastric problems, diarrhea, rashes, itching,

Blood Pressure Lowering Medications

Diuretics

<u>*Loop Diuretics*</u>

These drugs will inhibit the sodium potassium co transport mechanism in the ascending loop of henle it leads to an increase in the distal tubular concentration of sodium and reduced levels of hyper tonicity of sodium levels in the intestine cause's diueresis.

Loop diuretics include:

• Bumetanide

• Furosemide

• Ethacrynate

• Torsemide

Adverse effects Hypokalemia, alkalosis, hypomagnesemia, hyperuricemia, dehydration, ototoxicity.

<u>*Thiazides Diuretics*</u>

These drugs inhibit the sodium-chloride transporter in the distal tubule and reabsorption of sodium ions causes the elimination of more water from the body.

• Chlorothiazide

• Chlorthalidone

• Indapamide

• Hydrochlorothiazide

• Methyclothiazide

Adverse effects Hyponatremia, hyperglycemia, dehydration, hypokalemia, hypertriglyceridemia, hyperuricemia, azotemia.

Carbonic Anhydrase Inhibitors

These drugs will inhibit the transport of bicarbonate ions from the proximal convulted tubule which leads to loss of sodium, hydrogen and bicarbonate ions in the urine.

The drugs include

• Acetazolamide

• Methazolamide

Adverse effects Metabolic acidosis and hypokalemia

Potassium Sparing Diuretics

It acts on the distal segment of the distal tubules and causes more water to enter inside the collecting tubule. It will inhibit the aldosterone-sensitive sodium reabsorption thereby loss of potassium and hydrogen from the urine.

• Amiloride

• Spironolactone

• Triamterene

Adverse effects Metabolic acidosis, gynecomastia, hyperkalemia, gastric ulcers.

Calcium Channel Blockers

This drug blocks the entry of calcium ions into the calcium channels and lowers the work load on the heart and dilates the arteries leads to vasodilatation.

These drugs include

- Diltiazem

- Verapamil

- Isradipine

- Nifedipine

- Nicardipine

- Nimopidine

- Amlodipine

- Nisoldipine

- Bepridil

- Felodipine

Adverse effects Rashes, headache, constipation, flushing, edema, drowsiness

BETA BLOCKERS

It reduces the work load on the heart and reduces stress and hormones levels in the body which leads to vasodilatation in the blood vessels.

Commonly prescribed beta blockers include

- Atenolol

- Bisoprolol

- Nadolol

- Nebivolol

- Carvedilol

- Labetalol

- Nebivolol

- Pindolol

• Propranolol

• Timolol

• Metoprolol

Adverse effects Dry mouth, dry skin, feelings of coldness, diarrhea, shortness of breath and insomnia.

Angiotensin Converting Enzyme (ACE) Inhibitors

ACEs block the conversion of angiotensin I to angiotensin II by the action of angiotensinogen in the body and help to lower the vasoconstriction and promote vasodilation [23 - 25].

It includes

• Captopril

• Lisinopril

• Fosinopril

• Ramipril

• Benazepril

• Enalapril

• Perindopril

• Quinapril

• Moexipril

• Trandolapril

Adverse effects Dry cough, hyperkalemia, fatigue, headaches and loss of taste.

Angiotensin II Receptor Blockers

It block the conversion of angiotensin II from its binding to angiotensin II receptors located on the blood vessels and produce vasodialtion in the blood vessels.

These drugs include

• Candesartan

• Telmisartan

• Valsartan

• Eprosartan

• Irbesartan

• Losartan

Adverse effects Hyperkalemia, dizziness, headache, cough, diarrhea, hypotension and angioedema.

CONCLUSION

Abnormal lipid levels in the vascular stream contribute the stroke occurrence. Advance diagnostic investigations such as genomics, genetic profile, and proteomics test helpful for detecting pathophysiological causes associated with stroke patients. Maintaining healthy lifestyle practice, consumption of low fat diet, termination of smoking, alcohol, low level of salt intake, regular physical exercise, and stress management can improve the health outcomes of disease patients. The initiation of conducting awareness programmes on stroke prevention with the health care team in the patient care areas would greatly lower the stroke occurrence. The incidence of risk factors in young stroke patients is differing from geriatric patients. Implementation of clinical pharmacist services with the health care team on detection of stroke risk factors, patient counseling services, and continuous patient follow-up care services and maintaining the controlled lipid, blood pressure, blood sugar levels can lower the disease severity in the health care. Conducting multi centre clinical trials in stroke patients and proper implantation of guidelines, treatment strategies could prevent the progression of stroke risk in clinical settings. The management of stroke through effective prescribing of blood pressure medications such as statins, beta blockers, anti platelets, anti coagulants drugs can reduce the future episodes of the occurrence of the stroke.

REFERENCES

[1]   George MG, Tong X, Kuklina EV, Labarthe DR. Trends in stroke hospitalizations and associated risk factors among children and young adults, 1995-2008. Ann Neurol 2011; 70(5): 713-21.
[http://dx.doi.org/10.1002/ana.22539] [PMID: 21898534]

[2]   Bonita R, Beaglehole R. Stroke prevention in poor countries: time for action. Stroke 2007; 38(11): 2871-2.
[http://dx.doi.org/10.1161/STROKEAHA.107.504589] [PMID: 17954904]

[3]   Seshadri S, Beiser A, Kelly-Hayes M, *et al.* The lifetime risk of stroke: estimates from the Framingham Study. Stroke 2006; 37(2): 345-50.
[http://dx.doi.org/10.1161/01.STR.0000199613.38911.b2] [PMID: 16397184]

[4]   Legos JJ, Barone FC. Update on pharmacological strategies for stroke: prevention, acute intervention and regeneration. Curr Opin Investig Drugs 2003; 4(7): 847-58.
[PMID: 14619407]

[5]   Mattson MP, Culmsee C, Yu ZF. Apoptotic and antiapoptotic mechanisms in stroke. Cell Tissue Res 2000; 301(1): 173-87.
[http://dx.doi.org/10.1007/s004419900154] [PMID: 10928290]

[6]   Allen CL, Bayraktutan U. Oxidative stress and its role in the pathogenesis of ischaemic stroke. Int J Stroke 2009; 4(6): 461-70.
[http://dx.doi.org/10.1111/j.1747-4949.2009.00387.x] [PMID: 19930058]

[7]   McAuley MA. Rodent models of focal ischemia. Cerebrovasc Brain Metab Rev 1995; 7(2): 153-80.
[PMID: 7669493]

[8]   Solenski NJ. Transient ischemic attacks: part I-diagnosis and evaluation. Am Fam Physician 2004; 69(7): 1665-74.

[9]   Fisher M, Ratan R. New perspectives on developing acute stroke therapy. Ann Neurol 2003; 53(1): 10-20.
[http://dx.doi.org/10.1002/ana.10407] [PMID: 12509843]

[10]   Goldstein LB. Neuroprotective therapy for acute ischaemic stroke: down, but not out. Lancet 2004; 363(9407): 414-5.
[http://dx.doi.org/10.1016/S0140-6736(04)15522-0] [PMID: 14962518]

[11]   Grotta J, Pasteur W, Khwaja G, Hamel T, Fisher M, Ramirez A. Elective intubation for neurologic deterioration after stroke. Neurology 1995; 45(4): 640-4.
[http://dx.doi.org/10.1212/WNL.45.4.640] [PMID: 7723948]

[12]   The Interventional Management of Stroke (IMS) II Study. Stroke 2007; 38(7): 2127-35.
[http://dx.doi.org/10.1161/STROKEAHA.107.483131] [PMID: 17525387]

[13]   The stroke prevention in atrial fibrillation III study: rationale, design, and patient features. J Stroke Cerebrovasc Dis 1997; 6(5): 341-53.
[http://dx.doi.org/10.1016/S1052-3057(97)80217-0] [PMID: 17895032]

[14]   Tsai HH, Kim JS, Jouvent E, Gurol ME. Updates on prevention of hemorrhagic and lacunar strokes. J Stroke 2018; 20(2): 167-79.
[http://dx.doi.org/10.5853/jos.2018.00787] [PMID: 29886717]

[15]   Strong K, Mathers C, Bonita R. Preventing stroke: saving lives around the world. Lancet Neurol 2007; 6(2): 182-7.
[http://dx.doi.org/10.1016/S1474-4422(07)70031-5] [PMID: 17239805]

[16]   Durai Pandian J, Padma V, Vijaya P, Sylaja PN, Murthy JM. Stroke and thrombolysis in developing countries. Int J Stroke 2007; 2(1): 17-26.
[http://dx.doi.org/10.1111/j.1747-4949.2007.00089.x] [PMID: 18705983]

[17]   Grise EM, Adeoye O. Blood pressure control for acute ischemic and hemorrhagic stroke. Curr Opin Crit Care 2012; 18(2): 132-8.
[http://dx.doi.org/10.1097/MCC.0b013e3283513279] [PMID: 22322257]

[18]   Topcuoglu MA, Liu L, Kim DE, Gurol ME. Updates on prevention of cardioembolic strokes. J Stroke 2018; 20(2): 180-96.
[http://dx.doi.org/10.5853/jos.2018.00780] [PMID: 29886716]

[19]   Gebremariam SA, Yang HS. Types, risk profiles, and outcomes of stroke patients in a tertiary teaching hospital in northern Ethiopia. eNeurologicalSci 2016; 3: 41-7.

[http://dx.doi.org/10.1016/j.ensci.2016.02.010] [PMID: 29430535]

[20] Greffie ES, Mitiku T, Getahun S. Risk Factors, Clinical Pattern and Outcome of Stroke in a Referral Hospital, Northwest Ethiopia. Clin Med Res 2015; 4(6): 182-8.
[http://dx.doi.org/10.11648/j.cmr.20150406.13]

[21] Kim AS, Johnston SC. Global variation in the relative burden of stroke and ischemic heart disease. Circulation 2011; 124(3): 314-23.
[http://dx.doi.org/10.1161/CIRCULATIONAHA.111.018820] [PMID: 21730306]

[22] Kinlay S, Schwartz GG, Olsson AG, *et al.* Inflammation, statin therapy, and risk of stroke after an acute coronary syndrome in the MIRACL study. Arterioscler Thromb Vasc Biol 2008; 28(1): 142-7.
[http://dx.doi.org/10.1161/ATVBAHA.107.151787] [PMID: 17991875]

[23] Di Tullio MR, Russo C, Jin Z, Sacco RL, Mohr JP, Homma S. Aortic arch plaques and risk of recurrent stroke and death. Circulation 2009; 119(17): 2376-82.
[http://dx.doi.org/10.1161/CIRCULATIONAHA.108.811935] [PMID: 19380621]

[24] Everett BM, Glynn RJ, MacFadyen JG, Ridker PM. Rosuvastatin in the prevention of stroke among men and women with elevated levels of C-reactive protein: justification for the Use of Statins in Prevention: an Intervention Trial Evaluating Rosuvastatin (JUPITER). Circulation 2010; 121(1): 143-50.
[http://dx.doi.org/10.1161/CIRCULATIONAHA.109.874834] [PMID: 20026779]

[25] Fonarow GC, Reeves MJ, Zhao X, *et al.* Age-related differences in characteristics, performance measures, treatment trends, and outcomes in patients with ischemic stroke. Circulation 2010; 121(7): 879-91.
[http://dx.doi.org/10.1161/CIRCULATIONAHA.109.892497] [PMID: 20142445]

CHAPTER 11

Heart Failure

Abstract: Heart failure is a multifaceted disease in which the heart is unable to reach the metabolic demands of the body. The heart failure associated with complex risk factors which include Hypertension, increased salt intake, obesity, diabetes, coronary artery disease alcohol, smoking are the strong risk factors for the development of heart failure. The poor blood circulation lowers the blood pumping to the ventricles and reduces the contraction of the myocardial cells leads to increase the risk of heart failure. The clinical manifestations of heart failure include cough, pedal edema, palpitations, shortness of breath, fatigue, weakness, which can increase the risk of heart failure. The electrocardiogram, chest x-ray, echocardiogram, treadmill test, coronary angiogram test can determine the severity of the cardiovascular disease. The medical management of heart failure includes prescribing diuretics, angiotensin receptor blockers, beta blockers, vasodilators, ACE inhibitors, and digoxin improve the health status of the disease patients and also lowers the future occurrence of heart diseases.

Keywords: Beta Blockers, Coronary Artery Disease, Diabetes Mellitus, Electrocardiogram, Heart Failure, Pedal Edema.

INTRODUCTION

Heart failure is defined as a complex clinical syndrome that is represented with cardiac cell defects which leads to cause poor functioning of the ventricles and lowers the cardiac output. Heart failure is a progressive disorder during this condition heart is unable to send adequate blood to the body demands. The low pumping of the blood leads to lower the blood pumping to the ventricles and contraction of the myocardial cells and causes myocardial infarction. Heart failure is an outcome of cardiac disorders. Heart failure is one of the cardiovascular diseases. A patient diagnosed with myocardial infarction and hypertension causes both systolic and diastolic dysfunction which causes the development of heart failure. The extensive death of the cardiac muscles reduces the blood supply to the mitral valves which cause the damage to the heart leads to develop heart failure conditions. The formation of the atherosclerotic plaques in the blood vessels causes leakage of the blood into the pericardium cells which inhibits the normal function of the heart. The rupture of the intra ventricular septum creates defects in ventricles which lead to cause the poor function of the cardiac muscles.

M.S. Umashankar & A. Bharath Kumar
All rights reserved-© 2020 Bentham Science Publishers

The failure of the body defensive mechanism causes inflammation of the peritoneum cells cause pericarditis. Heart failure may classify into low and high heart failure. The low output heart failure is caused by the low blood supply to the heart. The normal range of the cardiac output can't meet the metabolic demands of the tissues which are known as high cardiac output. The pathophysiology of heart failure is shown in Fig. (**2**). Therefore the cardiac clinical symptoms can manifest with the patients [1 - 4]. The comparison of normal heart and heart failure is shown in Fig. (**1**).

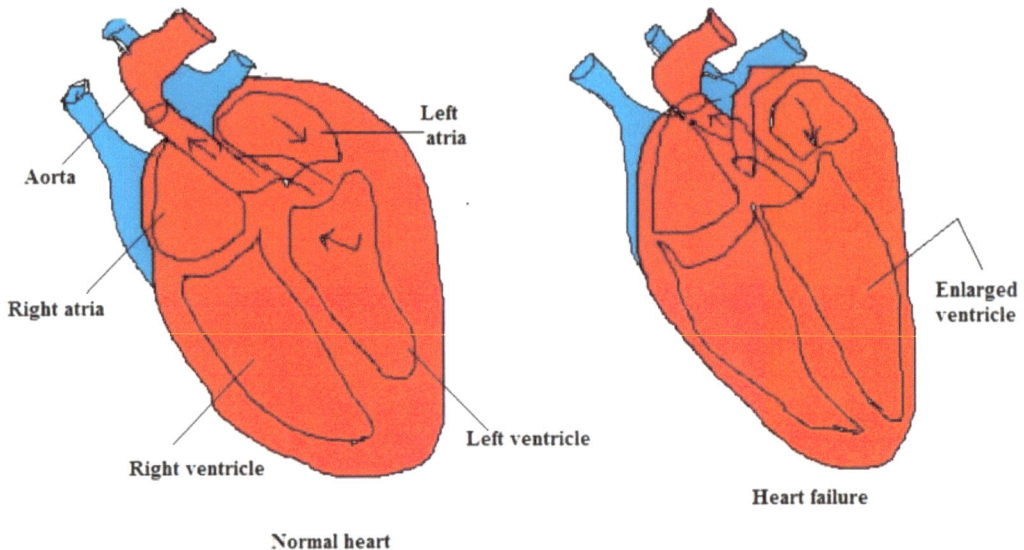

Fig. (1). Comparison of normal heart and heart failure.

Causes of high cardiac output It is caused by severe anemia, hyperthyroidism, vitamins deficiency and paget's disease.

Low cardiac output It is caused by coronary artery disease, cardiomyopathy, myocarditis, HIV infection, Pericarditis, hypertension, cardiomyopathy, asthma, thyrotoxicosis, sepsis and anaemia.

CLASSIFICATION OF HEART FAILURE

The classification of heart failure based on New York Heart Association includes [5, 6]

Class I Heart failure patients having normal physical activity do not cause any symptoms.

Class II Heart failure causes few limitations to physical activity and patients

represent heart failure.

Class III This type of heart classification patient is found to be normal and causes heart failure.

Class IV Heart failure patients are unable to do the physical activity and resting stage the patient may develop the cardiac symptoms.

The classification of heart failure based on American College of Cardiology/American Heart Association [7 - 9]

Stage A Patients are represented with heart failure and the absence of heart failure symptoms.

Stage B Patients are diagnosed with heart failure but the patient has an absence of heart failure symptoms.

Stage C Patients may feel the heart failure symptoms.

Stage D patients who are diagnosed with heart failure need health care interventions.

PREVALENCE

The cardiovascular diseases include hypertension, coronary artery disease, myocardial infarction and congenital heart disease, *etc.* The development of heart failure is associated with various co-morbid and risk factors such as obesity, hypertension, diabetes mellitus, smoking, alcohol and elevated apolipoprotein B/apolipoprotein A ratio can increase the risk of heart failure. At present 5.7 million people affected with heart failure in the world. By the year 2030 more than 8 million people will develop the heart failure condition. Heart failure is identified as one of the commonly occurring disease in elderly patients. The males are more affected as compared with female patients [10, 11]. The heart failure cases are rising very high due to advanced age. Previous research studies stated that in 2013 year 5.1 million people affected globally. By the year 2030, the incidence was expected to increase three folds. Currently, heart failure affecting cases are similar to cancer affecting the population. The heart failure prevalence and mortality were rising exponentially from the year 2000 to 2018.

ETIOLOGY

Systolic dysfunction is usually caused in patients with previous myocardial infarction and the diastolic dysfunction occurs typically in patients with hypertension and diabetes.

In the normal physiological condition when the physiological demand for oxygen increases heart rate increases and in turn the cardiac output is increased as a compensatory mechanism. Where the demand for oxygen and the event of damaged heart or in the physiological condition the heart is unable to pump and as a result the cardiac output decreases. The heart rate as a compensatory mechanism when the heart rate increases for a prolonged period diastolic filling time decreases *i.e.* there is not enough time to fill the heart chamber. The less amount of blood enters the heart. This leads to an increase fill the myocardial oxygen demand further worsening condition. Stroke volume is the amount of blood pump in each contraction. It depends upon there are variables *i.e.* contractility (ability of the heart to contract) preload and after load.

Pathophysiology of Heart failure

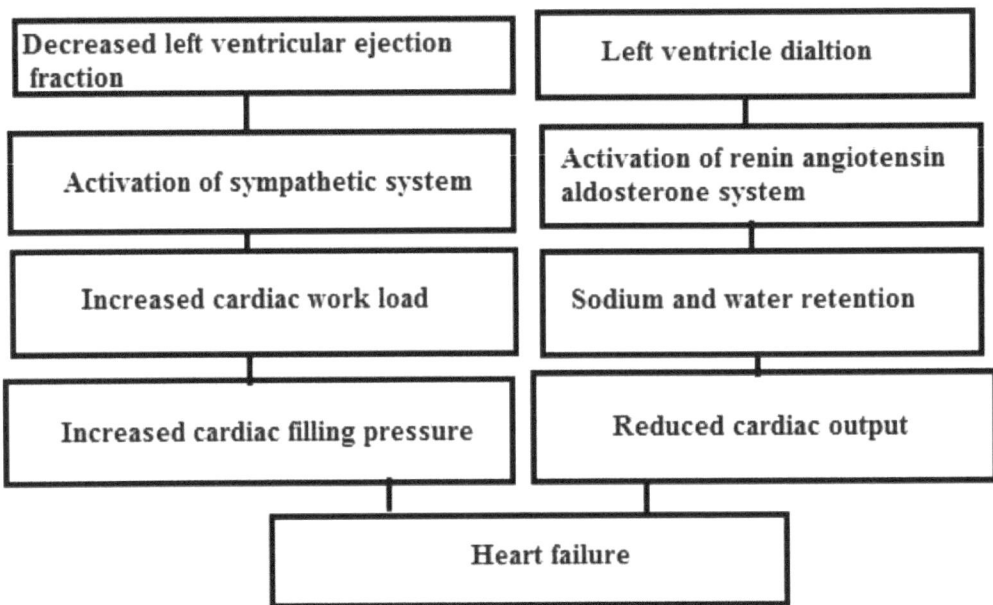

Fig. (2). Pathophysiology of heart failure.

Contractility is the intrinsic ability of the myocardial muscle fiber to contract or shorten. This helps in squeezing the blood or pumping out the blood. The more the fiber is stretched. The more forcefully it will record. In normal conditions, the myocardial fibers stretch to accommodate the incoming blood or pumping out the blood from various parts of the body during diastolic filling. The myocardial fibers shorten during systolic contraction and during the pathological condition part of the ischemic affected muscle fiber loses its elastic nature. This condition forces unaffected healthy muscle fiber to work header as a compensatory mechanism to maintain adequate cardiac output. This compensate mechanism can occur up to some limit. Preload refers to a volume of blood to be accommodated associated with the presence created by the myocardium stretching during diastolic filling.

Preload refers to the volume of blood or venous return or simply filling pressure. Preload is synonymous with frank starlings low of heart *i.e.* when the amount of filling blood increase, the stretching of muscle fiber filling. Thus the stretching and shortening of blood increase. Thus the stretching and shortening of the muscle fibers depending on the stretching of muscle fiber *i.e.* pressures created by myocardial fiber stretches. The increase in the end diastolic volume leads to more forceful, contraction leading to cardiac output. Left ventricular end diastolic volume is the primarily determination of preload. However, the stretching of the muscle fiber to accommodate the pre load can occur only to certain point. In pathological condition, this point is exceeded. *i.e.* volume of the blood filling will over distend the ventricular leading to over stretching of myocardial fiber. This causes a decrease in cardiac output as the full rolling is affected. Thus the damaged impaired heart is unable to handle the increase in preload which automatically results in a decrease in stroke volume. These result in the trapping of blood in the heart causing chamber dilation. After load is a more complex physiological concept. It may be referred to as the sum of forces preventing active forward ejection of blood by the ventricle [12 - 14].

COMPENSATORY MECHANISM

The decrease in the pumping capacity of the heart triggers the compensatory mechanism is an attempt to maintain adequate cardiac output. However, this compensatory mechanism is intended to provide short term responses to maintain cardiac output. But in long term activation of compensatory responses to maintain cardiac output, produces structural biochemical and molecular changes that lead to heart failure.

TACHYCARDIA, CONTRACTILITY AND ADRENERGIC MECHANISM OF HEART

Change in heart rate and contractility is mainly controlled by neither release nor epinephrine. Through the cardiac output must increase with increase heart rate the systolic time intervals change a comparative line with changing heart rate. The systolic time intervals change comparatively little with changing heart rate the systolic time interval changes a comparatively little with changing heart rate. This results in a shortening of diastolic filling. The shortened diastolic filling also results in higher average intra cellular calcium concentration which augments the resistance to fibril stretch generating more response. Increased heart rate myocardial oxygen demand increases. In the presence of ischemia the worsened pathological condition of myocardial ischemia and both diastolic and systolic function may be affected with a result in the drop of the stroke volume. When the heart rate is unable to pump enough blood there occurs a decrease in blood flow and hence the blood pressure low blood pressure activates sympathetic neuro hormones such as nor epinephrine, angiotensin II endothelin and arginin and vasopressin to produce vasoconstriction also impedes forward ejection of blood from the ventricles. This contributes to a reduction in cardiac output which in turn heightens the compensatory responses overtime the failing myocardium becomes less responsive to the stimulatory effect of sympathetic neuro hormones and the compensatory mechanism begins to fail. Then what occurs in the vicious cycle of continued worsening and down of heart's function.

INCREASED PRELOAD /RENAL MECHANISM

The decreased cardiac output leads to a reduction in blood flow to kidneys. as a response to this reduction in blood flow kidney activates the renin angiotensin aldosterone system. Reduce blood flow to the kidneys as well as increased sympathetic tone also stimulates the release of renin. Renin act with angiotensinogen in the plasma to produce angiotensin I. The angiotensin I is converted into angiotensin II by the angiotensin converting enzyme. Angiotensin II acts as a powerful vasoconstrictor which leads to an increase in systemic blood pressure. The released aldosterone act on kidneys and retains salt and water as intra intravascular volume increase secondary to sodium and water retention leading to an increase in systemic blood pressure *i.e.* there is an increase in preload. Further increase in preload will prove detrimental to the heart. Other hormones seems to be active during heart failure are anti diuretic hormone and arterial nartiuretic factor. The anti natriuretic factor which acts as natural diuretic may have a beneficial effect on the failure of the heart [15 - 17].

VENTRICULAR HYPERTROPHY

It refers to an increase in ventricular muscle faced with a chronic increase in workload the ventricular myocardium responds by increasing its muscle mass. Ventricular hypertrophy seems to be the key component in the pathogenesis of progressive wall thickness increases as well as eccentric left ventricular hypertrophy in which there is character enlargement. Venous return increases muscle mass can increase cardiac output in the short term, the efficiency of contraction decreases and thus ventricular hypertrophy play an important role in the progressive nature of heart failure.

Depending on the requirements any or all of the mechanisms can work to compensate for the decrease in cardiac output. However, the compensatory mechanism may sustain the normal cardiac function for only a certain period. But with overtime and increased cardiac workload the compensatory mechanisms may eventually fail and cause greater damage to the heart and the severity of heart failure increases.

MANIFESTATION OF HEART FAILURE

Heart failure mainly manifests as a left sided heart failure and right heart failure there are other divisions also.

Left Heart Failure

The left side of the heart is involved in the pumping of oxygenated blood from the lungs to various tissues in the periphery. In left heart failure there is decreased stroke volume and increased left ventricular diastolic volume producing increased preload. There may be pulmonary edema and cough frothy sputum and crackling sound through stethoscope [18 - 20].

Right Heart Failure

It follows left heart failure, and increased pulmonary vascular pressure occurs in left heart failure offers increased resistance to the pumping of blood by the right ventricle into the lungs and increased work load on the right ventricle leads to dilation and failure of right heart. Right heart failure may also result from chronic obstructive pulmonary disease, systolic fibrosis and adult respiratory syndrome.

Systolic Failure and Diastolic Failure

In systolic failure the ejection of blood from the heart is decreased during diastole, in this condition there is decreased myocardial contractility leading to a decrease in volume of blood, It may occur commonly with ischemic heart disease, myocardial infarction, cardiomyopathy. It has symptoms due to reduced cardiac output. In diastolic failure filing of ventricle is impaired during diastole and reduced ventricular filling coupled with left ventricular systolic function. There may be impaired ventricular relaxation. Diastolic failure is associated with restrictive and hypertrophic cardiomyopathy. Symptoms may include dyspnea and fatigue.

Forward Cardiac Failure

This refers to inability of the right and left ventricles to pump into the pulmonary and systemic circulation respectively. It results from the decreased cardiac output and hypo perfusion of vital organs. It occurs frequently with aortic stenosis and or systemic hypertension.

Backward Cardiac Failure

It results from the inefficiency of the ventricles to empty the blood into arterial circulation. This causes accumulation of fluid in all the chambers of the heart. Backward cardiac failure may result from myocardial infarction and cardiomayopathy.

Acute and chronic cardiac failure

• Rapidly of the onset of heart failure.

• Presence of absence of compensatory mechanisms

• Presence of absence of fluid accumulation in interstitial space.

Acute heart failure has a rapid onset and no structural myocardial changes such as hypertrophy. Chronic heart failure develops gradually. The condition gets worsened or exacerbated by multiple factors. It occurs in hypovolemic with structural myocardial changes such as hypertrophy.

Low Ventricular Output and High Ventricular Output

Low ventricular output cardiac failure refers to insufficient systolic ejection resulting from in adequate blood or cardiac output. It is caused by myocardial infarction, hypotension, cardiomyopathy and hemorrhage.

High Ventricular Output Cardiac Failure

It refers to a condition in which there is increased cardiac output from the ventricles. It is caused by thyrotoxicosis, anemia and pregnancy.

PATHOPHYSIOLOGY

The rhythemic blood pumping of heart which is essentially the constriction and dilation of the rhythemic results from the electrical impulses traveling out the walls of the four chambers of the heart. The impulses originate in SA node which acts as spark plug and travels throughout the atria to AV node. The AV node acts like a relay station sending impulses to more muscles fibres through ventricles.

Cardiac Action Potential

When the stimulated automatically SA node reaches the cardiac cell, specific ions movements of ions across the action potential, such moments ions across the cardiac cells,

Phase 0 is the rapid depolarization of the cell. Phase 1 is the short and rapid depolarization phase. Phase II is prolonged and plateau phase and Phase III is the repolarisation phase and phase IV is a resulting phase.

During phases I and II the cells doses not depolarize in response to another impulse. But in during phases 3, 4, the cells are relatively refractory period and may depolarize in response to another but powerful impulse. The cardiac output is determined by heart rate and stroke volume. The stroke volume in turn depends on preload and after load and contractility. There are main two cellular mechanisms through which certain arrthymia might arise. They are ectopic pacemakers or reentry impulses. The impulses due to the ectopic or re entry impulses may arise in the conduction pathways or muscle cells of atria or ventricles.

Ectopic Pace Makers

The ectopic pace makers refer to the occurrence of other than SA node. These pacemakers may act abnormally in the heart leading to arrhythmias. Under certain conditions, the activity of SA node may fail or be suppressed and the cells of other regions of the myocardium acquiring the property of automaticity take over as the primary pacemaker. Thus they assume control over the rate and rhythm of heart beat. These cardiac cells were unaffected by assuming control over the rate and rhythm of heart beat. They get excited and can act as ectopic pace maker. Hence firing of pacemakers can lead to premature cardiac depolarization's that usually does not follow the normal conduction system of the heart. Premature cardiac depolarization is dissimilarity with impulse origin from SA node leads to develop ectopic arrthymia.

Re Entry Impulses

When the myocardium is under normal functioning, electrical impulses that originate in SA node follow a regular progression through the conduction system of the atria and ventricles. Such polarization impulses cannot re enter cardiac tissue that has been already depolarized but follows the usual conduction path and terminate after ventricles are depolarized. But this may not be followed in a different situation in which the myocardium is affected. Thus in an abnormal myocardium condition may exist in which the myocardium conditions may exist in which there is an area of cardiac tissue with blacked electrical conduction with one way conduction block, it may be possible for depolarization impulses to travel back upward through the one way block to the area already depolarized. Because the polarization process is at a slower rate, the already polarized areas might have some time to repolarise. In this condition, the re entering wave of depolarization may again polarize that area. Thus a single way of depolarization might be involved in causing more than one beat. When the re entry impulses posses again through tissue up after the refractory period has occurred, a self perpetuating a circuitous type of electrical depolarization might occur. End result is arrhythmia. Thus arrhythmias result from abnormal impulses formation or abnormal impulse conduction.

Etiology [21, 22]

An infraction may cause the death of pace maker cells or conducting tissue.

A cardiac tissue disorder such as fibrosis or rheumatic fever or multi system connective tissue disorder.

Sympathetic or parasympathetic control changes

Drugs such as anti arrythmiasis or inotropes or other substances such as caffeine, alcohol affects heart directly.

Hypothyroidism, hyperthyroidism, hypoadrenalism, hyperkalemia, hypokalemia or other electrolytic distribution may one dispose to arrythmiasis.

SYMPTOMS

• Palpitations or rapid heart rate

• Feeling tired or light headache

• Loss of consciousness

• Shortness of breath

• Chest pain, irregular beat

• Bradycardia

• Feeling tired

• Shortness of breath

• Dizziness, weakness and light headache

• Tachycardia symptoms

• Heart beat may be felt like strong impulse

• A fluttering racing beat in the chest

• Shortness of breath

• Fainting

• Dizziness

• Sweating

• Diagnosis

• ECG

• Holter monitoring

• Electrophysiology studies

• Medical and family history

• Physical examination

• Blood test

• X-rays

• Stress test

• Coronary angiogram

• Implantable loop recorder

LIFESTYLE MODIFICATIONS FOR MANAGEMENT OF HEART FAILURE [23]

Many lifestyle and diet factors can improve, or even reverse, congestive heart failure. Cardiac rehabilitation programs can teach people how to make lifestyle changes, as can integrative cardiology clinics.

Some of the lifestyle factors that make a difference include

• Manage stress

• Quit smoking

• Eliminate alcohol

• Eat a healthy Mediterranean, vegetarian, or vegan diet

• Be physically active and become stronger

• Restful sleep

• Manage and treat sleep apnea

• Take dietary supplements including CoQ10, L-carnitine, magnesium, and fish oil

• Avoiding salt and excess fluids

• Meditation Practice

MEDICATIONS FOR MANAGEMENT FOR HEART FAILURE [24, 25]

The Common types of drugs that treat heart failure are:

• Aldosterone inhibitors

• ACE inhibitors

• ARBs (angiotensin II receptor blockers)

• ARNIs (angiotensin receptor-neprilysin inhibitors)

• Beta-blockers

• Blood vessel dilators

• Calcium channel blockers

• Digoxin

• Diuretics

Thrombolytic Drugs

Thrombolytic drugs are prescribed to reduce the formation of blood clot in the blood vessels and also lower the severity of stroke. These drugs will act by conversion of plasminogen which forms plasmin and activates the fibrin bound plasminogen. Fibrin molecules are inhibited by plasmin which leads to breakdown of clot the blood vessels and reduces the stroke complications.

It includes

• Anistreplase

- Reteplase

- Streptokinase

- T-pa

- Tenecteplase

- Alteplase

- Urokinase

Adverse drug reactions Internal bleeding, damage to the blood vessels, renal damage.

Anti Platelet Drugs

These drugs help to prevent the platelet aggregation and reduce the clot in the blood vessels.

Types of antiplatelet agents

- Aspirin

- Dipyridamole

- Clopidogrel

- Ticagrelor

Clinical uses of antiplatelet agents It is used to treat following disease conditions.

- Coronary artery disease

- Heart attack

- Angina (chest pain)

- Stroke and transient ischemic attacks

- Peripheral artery disease

Side Effects Nausea, gastric problems, diarrhea, rashes, itching,

Blood Pressure Lowering Medications

Diuretics

Loop diuretics These drugs will inhibit the sodium potassium co transport mechanism in the ascending loop of henle it leads to an increase the distal tubular concentration of sodium and reduced levels of hyprertonicity of sodium levels in the intestine cause diueresis.

Loop diuretics include

• Bumetanide

• Furosemide

• Ethacrynate

• Torsemide

Adverse effects Hypokalemia, alkalosis, hypomagnesemia, hyperuricemia, dehydration, ototoxicity.

Thiazides Diuretics

These drugs inhibit the sodium-chloride transporter in the distal tubule and reabsorption of sodium ions causes the elimination of more water from the body.

• Chlorothiazide

• Chlorthalidone

• Indapamide

• Hydrochlorothiazide

• Methyclothiazide

Adverse effects Hyponatremia, hyperglycemia, dehydration, hypokalemia, hypertriglyceridemia, hyperuricemia, azotemia.

Carbonic Anhydrase Inhibitors

These drugs will inhibit the transport of bicarbonate ions from the proximal convulted tubule which leads to loss of sodium, hydrogen and bicarbonate ions in the urine.

The drugs include

• Acetazolamide

• Methazolamide

Adverse effects Metabolic acidosis and hypokalemia

Potassium Sparing Diuretics

It acts on the distal segment of the distal tubules and causes more water to enter inside the collecting tubule. It will inhibit the aldosterone-sensitive sodium reabsorption thereby loss of potassium and hydrogen from the urine.

• Amiloride

• spironolactone

• Triamterene

Adverse effects Metabolic acidosis, gynecomastia, hyperkalemia, gastric ulcers.

Calcium Channel Blockers

This drug blocks the entry of calcium ions into the calcium channels and lowers the work load on the heart and dilates the arteries leads to vasodilatation.

These drugs include

• Diltiazem

• Verapamil

• Isradipine

• Nifedipine

• Nicardipine

• Nimopidine

• Amlodipine

• Nisoldipine

• Bepridil

• Felodipine

Adverse effects: Rashes, headache, constipation, flushing, edema, drowsiness

Cholesterol lowering medications include:

Statins

These drugs act by inhibiting HMG-CoA reductase enzyme and inhibit the cholesterol biosynthetic pathway and show anti atherosclerotic effect in the blood vessels.

• Atorvastatin

• Fluvastatin

• Lovastatin

• Pitavastatin

• Pravastatin

• Rosuvastatin

• Simvastatin

Adverse effects Headache, dizziness, insomnia, flushing of the skin, drowsiness and myalgia.

Beta Blockers

It reduces the work load on the heart and reduces stress and hormones levels in the body which leads to vasodilatation in the blood vessels.

Commonly prescribed beta blockers include

• Atenolol

• Bisoprolol

• Nadolol

• Nebivolol

• Carvedilol

• Labetalol

• Nebivolol

• Pindolol

• Propranolol

• Timolol

• Metoprolol

Adverse effects Dry mouth, dry skin, feelings of coldness, diarrhea, shortness of breath and insomnia.

Angiotensin converting enzyme (ACE) inhibitors

ACEs block the conversion of angiotensin I to angiotensin II by the action of angiotensinogen in the body and help to lower the vasoconstriction and promote vasodilation.

It includes

• Captopril

• Lisinopril

• Fosinopril

• Ramipril

• Benazepril

• Enalapril

• Perindopril

• Quinapril

• Moexipril

• Trandolapril

Adverse effects Dry cough, hyperkalemia, fatigue, headaches and loss of taste.

Angiotensin II Receptor Blockers

It blocks the conversion of angiotensin II from its binding to angiotensin II receptors located on the blood vessels and produces vasodialtion in the blood vessels.

These drugs include

• Candesartan

• Telmisartan

• Valsartan

• Eprosartan

• Irbesartan

• Losartan

Adverse effects Hyperkalemia, dizziness, headache, cough, diarrhea, hypotension and angioedema.

Digoxin

It is used to treat the irregular heartbeats which include tachycardia, atrial flutter, and supraventricular tachycardia. Digoxin has an electrophysiological and hemodynamic effect on the cardiovascular system. It will reversibly inhibit the Na-K ATPase enzyme which is responsible for maintaining the intra cellular environment and balance of potassium, sodium and calcium ions into the cells. The inhibition of the sodium pump by Na-K ATPase leads to an increase in the contraction as well as cardiac function of the heart.

Adverse effects Diarrhea, blurred vision, nausea, vomiting, confusion, dizziness and irregular heartbeats.

Nitrates

These drugs are prescribed to treat the angina pectoris. Nitroglycerin is a potent smooth-muscle relaxant and vasodilator. It lowers the systolic blood pressure and dilates the veins and reduces the myocardial wall tension and promotes more blood reaching to the cardiac muscles and decreases the chest pain manifestations.

Classification

Organic nitrates

• Nitroglycerin (glyceryl trinitrate)

• Amyl nitrite

• Isosorbide di-nitrate

• Erythrityl tetra nitrate

• Pentaerythritol tetra nitrate

Arterial Vasodilators

• Hydralazine

• Minoxidil

• Diazoxide

Arterial and venous vasodilators

• Sod. nitroprusside

• Prazosin

• Terazosin

• Doxazosin

Nitrates

Nitrates relax the blood vessels by the release of nitric oxide (NO). It binds with the guanylyl cyclase enzyme which releases cyclic GMP and stimulates the release of cGMP-dependent protein kinase and eventually causes dephosphorylation of myosin light chain to produce the vascular smooth muscle relaxation.

Common side effects of nitrates include

• Headache

• Dizziness

• Tingling under the tongue

• Low blood pressure

• Headache

• Edema

• Pulmonary edema

- Low blood glucose

- Lightheadedness

- Nausea

- Flushing

CONCLUSION

Heart failure is a complex chronic disease that can cause mortality and morbidity in developed and developing countries. Providing effective medical treatment at the early stages of heart failure can lower the risk of heart failure. Severe stage of heart failure requires continuous hospitalized treatment due to complex disease conditions and strict implementation of clinical pharmacist care with the health care team to the heart failure patients on diet, disease, lifestyle modifications, medication adherence, and novel therapeutic and diagnostic tests can lower the hospital readmissions. The non-pharmacological approaches for the management of heart failure include termination of smoking, alcohol, regular physical activity, stress management practices are essential to reduce the heart failure risk.

REFERENCES

[1]   Dassanayaka S, Jones SP. Recent Developments in Heart Failure. Circ Res 2015; 117(7): e58-63.
        [http://dx.doi.org/10.1161/CIRCRESAHA.115.305765] [PMID: 26358111]

[2]   Marti CN, Georgiopoulou VV, Kalogeropoulos AP. Acute heart failure: patient characteristics and pathophysiology. Curr Heart Fail Rep 2013; 10(4): 427-33.
        [http://dx.doi.org/10.1007/s11897-013-0151-y] [PMID: 23918642]

[3]   Ohtani T, Mohammed SF, Yamamoto K, *et al.* Diastolic stiffness as assessed by diastolic wall strain is associated with adverse remodelling and poor outcomes in heart failure with preserved ejection fraction. Eur Heart J 2012; 33(14): 1742-9.
        [http://dx.doi.org/10.1093/eurheartj/ehs135] [PMID: 22645191]

[4]   Ammar KA, Jacobsen SJ, Mahoney DW, *et al.* Prevalence and prognostic significance of heart failure stages: application of the American College of Cardiology/American Heart Association heart failure staging criteria in the community. Circulation 2007; 115(12): 1563-70.
        [http://dx.doi.org/10.1161/CIRCULATIONAHA.106.666818] [PMID: 17353436]

[5]   Zamani P, Rawat D, Shiva-Kumar P, *et al.* Effect of inorganic nitrate on exercise capacity in heart failure with preserved ejection fraction. Circulation 2015; 131(4): 371-80.
        [http://dx.doi.org/10.1161/CIRCULATIONAHA.114.012957] [PMID: 25533966]

[6]   Maeder MT, Thompson BR, Brunner-La Rocca H-P, Kaye DM. Hemodynamic basis of exercise limitation in patients with heart failure and normal ejection fraction. J Am Coll Cardiol 2010; 56(11): 855-63.
        [http://dx.doi.org/10.1016/j.jacc.2010.04.040] [PMID: 20813283]

[7]   Kenchaiah S, Narula J, Vasan RS. Risk factors for heart failure. Med Clin North Am 2004; 88(5): 1145-72.
        [http://dx.doi.org/10.1016/j.mcna.2004.04.016] [PMID: 15331311]

[8]   Yancy CW, Jessup M, Bozkurt B, *et al.* 2013 ACCF/AHA guideline for the management of heart

failure: a report of the American College of Cardiology Foundation/American Heart Association Task Force on Practice Guidelines. J Am Coll Cardiol 2013; 62(16): e147-239.
[http://dx.doi.org/10.1016/j.jacc.2013.05.019] [PMID: 23747642]

[9]   Watson RD, Gibbs CR, Lip GY. ABC of heart failure. Clinical features and complications. BMJ 2000; 320(7229): 236-9.
[http://dx.doi.org/10.1136/bmj.320.7229.236] [PMID: 10642237]

[10]   Triposkiadis F, Karayannis G, Giamouzis G, Skoularigis J, Louridas G, Butler J. The sympathetic nervous system in heart failure physiology, pathophysiology, and clinical implications. J Am Coll Cardiol 2009; 54(19): 1747-62.
[http://dx.doi.org/10.1016/j.jacc.2009.05.015] [PMID: 19874988]

[11]   Anker SD, von Haehling S. Inflammatory mediators in chronic heart failure: an overview. Heart 2004; 90(4): 464-70.
[http://dx.doi.org/10.1136/hrt.2002.007005] [PMID: 15020532]

[12]   Roger VL. Epidemiology of heart failure. Circ Res 2013; 113(6): 646-59.
[http://dx.doi.org/10.1161/CIRCRESAHA.113.300268] [PMID: 23989710]

[13]   Wilhelmsen L, Rosengren A, Eriksson H, Lappas G. Heart failure in the general population of men- -morbidity, risk factors and prognosis. J Intern Med 2001; 249(3): 253-61.
[http://dx.doi.org/10.1046/j.1365-2796.2001.00801.x] [PMID: 11285045]

[14]   Devaux B, Scholz D, Hirche A, Klövekorn WP, Schaper J. Upregulation of cell adhesion molecules and the presence of low grade inflammation in human chronic heart failure. Eur Heart J 1997; 18(3): 470-9.
[http://dx.doi.org/10.1093/oxfordjournals.eurheartj.a015268] [PMID: 9076385]

[15]   Oikonomou E, Tousoulis D, Siasos G, Zaromitidou M, Papavassiliou AG, Stefanadis C. The role of inflammation in heart failure: new therapeutic approaches. Hellenic J Cardiol 2011; 52(1): 30-40.
[PMID: 21292605]

[16]   Paterson I, Mielniczuk LM, O'Meara E, So A, White JA. Imaging heart failure: current and future applications. Can J Cardiol 2013; 29(3): 317-28.
[http://dx.doi.org/10.1016/j.cjca.2013.01.006] [PMID: 23439018]

[17]   Bhatia RS, Tu JV, Lee DS, *et al.* Outcome of heart failure with preserved ejection fraction in a population-based study. N Engl J Med 2006; 355(3): 260-9.
[http://dx.doi.org/10.1056/NEJMoa051530] [PMID: 16855266]

[18]   Owan TE, Hodge DO, Herges RM, Jacobsen SJ, Roger VL, Redfield MM. Trends in prevalence and outcome of heart failure with preserved ejection fraction. N Engl J Med 2006; 355(3): 251-9.
[http://dx.doi.org/10.1056/NEJMoa052256] [PMID: 16855265]

[19]   Mosterd A, Hoes AW. Clinical epidemiology of heart failure. Heart 2007; 93(9): 1137-46.
[http://dx.doi.org/10.1136/hrt.2003.025270] [PMID: 17699180]

[20]   Vasan RS, Levy D. The role of hypertension in the pathogenesis of heart failure. A clinical mechanistic overview. Arch Intern Med 1996; 156(16): 1789-96.
[http://dx.doi.org/10.1001/archinte.1996.00440150033003] [PMID: 8790072]

[21]   Weber KT, Sun Y, Guarda E. Structural remodeling in hypertensive heart disease and the role of hormones. Hypertension 1994; 23(6 Pt 2): 869-77.
[http://dx.doi.org/10.1161/01.HYP.23.6.869] [PMID: 8206620]

[22]   Solomon SD, Dobson J, Pocock S, *et al.* Influence of nonfatal hospitalization for heart failure on subsequent mortality in patients with chronic heart failure. Circulation 2007; 116(13): 1482-7.
[http://dx.doi.org/10.1161/CIRCULATIONAHA.107.696906] [PMID: 17724259]

[23]   Haldeman GA, Croft JB, Giles WH, Rashidee A. Hospitalization of patients with heart failure: National Hospital Discharge Survey, 1985 to 1995. Am Heart J 1999; 137(2): 352-60.
[http://dx.doi.org/10.1053/hj.1999.v137.95495] [PMID: 9924171]

[24]　Brophy JM, Joseph L, Rouleau JL. Beta-blockers in congestive heart failure. A Bayesian meta-analysis. Ann Intern Med 2001; 134(7): 550-60.
[http://dx.doi.org/10.7326/0003-4819-134-7-200104030-00008] [PMID: 11281737]

[25]　Ramani GV, Uber PA, Mehra MR. Chronic heart failure: contemporary diagnosis and management. Mayo Clin Proc 2010; 85(2): 180-95.
[http://dx.doi.org/10.4065/mcp.2009.0494] [PMID: 20118395]

CHAPTER 12

Cardiac Arrhythmia

Abstract: The heart conduction and contraction provide the driving force for the pumping of blood to the heart. The abnormalities in the conduction properties of the heart can lead to arrhythmias. The action potential helps the opening and closing of the ion channels that cause conduction of the cardiac muscles. Atrial fibrillation is most commonly occurs in the cardiac arrhythmia. The arrhythmia prevalence has an incidence of 1%, it is an aging dependent factor and the incidence was raise to ≥ 2.5-fold by the year 2050. Elderly patients the progression of the atrial flutter is related to cardiac disorders. The clinical symptoms of atrial flutter include anxiety, palpitations, dizziness, headache, irregular heartbeat that can impair the quality of life of the patients. The defects in cardiac rhythm are associated with a significant rise in health care cost and also mortality among the affected population. Ventricular arrhythmias are causing about 75% to 80% of the cardiac deaths annually in the world. The ECG devices, echocardiogram, doppler studies, stress test, holter monitoring test are used to identify the risk of developing cardiac arrhythmias among arrhythmias patients. Currently, one third of the patient's exhibit an absence of arrhythmia symptoms and patients were not aware of abnormal heart rhythm. Therefore timely detection of clinical symptoms and prescribing better therapeutic approaches may improve the quality of the patients.

Keywords: Abnormal Heart Rhythm, Arrhythmias Palpitations, Atrial Fibrillation, Irregular Heartbeat.

INTRODUCTION

Arrhythmia is a heterogeneous condition in which disturbance in the rhythm of the heart beat is associated with abnormal electrical action present in the heart. It may vary severity may differ from rate and rhythm affecting the blood supply to the heart. The abnormalities in the heart rhythm can increase the life-threatening conditions to the affected population. SA node and AV node may act as a pacemaker in cardiac muscles which can create electrical impulses and sends to the heart. The abnormalities in the heart rhythms may lead to the development of arrhythmia [1, 2]. The cardiac arrhythmia is shown in Fig. (1).

M.S. Umashankar & A. Bharath Kumar

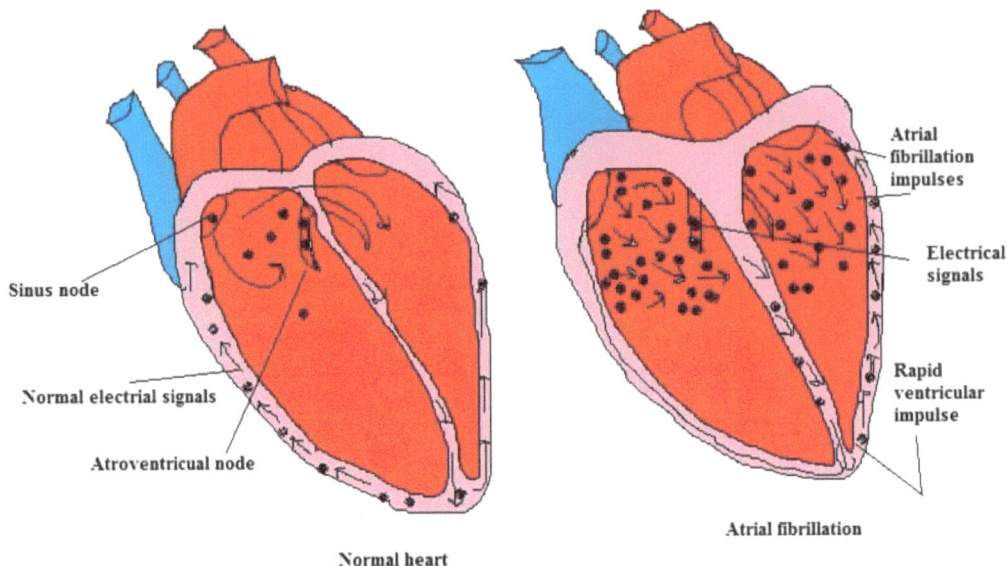

Fig. (1). Cardiac arrhythmia.

CLASSIFICATION OF CARDIAC ARRHYTHMIA

• Normotropic arrhythmia

• Ecotopic arrhythmia

NORMOTROPIC ARRHYTHMIA

It represents an irregular heart beat produced by the SA node. It is classified into following types

Sinus arrhythmia

Sinus tachycardia

Sinus bradycardia

Sinus Arrhythmia

It deals with rhythmical increase or decrease in heart rate is associated with respiratory changes. It is known as respiratory sinus arrhythmia. The normal valve of the heart rate is 72 /minute. Heart rate is changes during inspiration and expiration. Electrocardiogram is used to identify the abnormal rhythms of the heart. The ECG waves vary rhythmically during inspiration and expiration of the heart beats and results change the R-R interval phase which leads to developing arrhythmia. It is caused by abnormal discharge of electrical impulse from SA node, it leads to rise in venous return and inflammation of lungs stimulates the lungs and sends impulse to afferent vagus fibers. It leads to inhibition of vasodilatation in the blood vessels and increase the heart rate [3, 4].

Sinus Tachycardia

The increase in heart rate can cause tachycardia. Heart rate increases more than 100/min can cause tachycardia. The change in physiological and pathological changes may cause tachycardia.

Ectopic Arrhythmia

The development of heart beat from heart except from SA node. The electrical impulse produced from the heart structure is called as ectopic arrhythmia.

Homotropic arrhythmia The impulse for heart beat arise from the cardiac muscles is known as Homotropic arrhythmia.

• Ectopic arrhythmia is classified into varies types which include

• Atrial flutter

• Artial fibrillation

• Ventricular fibrillation

• Heart block

• Extra systole

• Aroxymal tachycardia

Heart Block

The blockage of impulses from the SA node can cause heart block.

Sinoatrial Block

It occurs due to the failure of transmission of impulse from SA node.

Extra Systole

It occurs in various clinical conditions such as excessive smoking, stress and hyperthyroidism *etc.* can increase the risk of premature heart contraction leads to develop the extra systole.

Paroxysmal Tachycardia

The sudden increase in heart rate can cause paroxysmal tachycardia. The presence of ectopic foci which is arising from the AV node can cause supraventricular tachycardia. The clinical symptoms include chest pain, rapid breathing, dizziness and palpitation.

Atrial Flutter

It is a type of arrhythmia characterized by rapid ineffective atrial contraction.

Atrial fibrillation

The rapid irregular atrial contractions at a rate of 300-400 per minute can cause atrial fibrillation. This condition commonly seen in old aged patients affected with cardiac diseases leads to the development of various complications.

Ventricular Fibrillation

The rapid and irregular twitching of the ventricles causes ventricle fibrillation. The ventricle contraction rate more than 400 per minute can cause fibrillation. It is a severe type of cardiac arrhythmia and ventricles cannot pump the blood leads to cause serious arrhythmia.

CARDIAC ACTION POTENTIAL

The resting stage membrane of the cardiac muscles is polarized. This phase sodium, calcium, potassium ion channels are closed. The electrical potential generated by pacemaker cells leads to cardiac cells is depolarized and cause the opening of sodium, potassium, calcium channels in the cells membrane.

Phases of Action Potential in Cardiac Muscle [5 - 8]

Phase 0

The opening of the sodium ion channels facilitates the entry of the sodium ions into the cells causes depolarization of cells.

Phase 1

The sodium ions interacting with the potassium ions cause depolarization in the cell membrane.

Phase 2

The entry of sodium and calcium ions into the calcium ion channels causes prolong plateau peak.

Phase 3

It is the second of rapid repolarization due to the outward movement of potassium ions.

Phase 4

The entry of potassium ions into the cells and sodium and calcium ions exist out of the cells. In this phase slow inward leak of sodium ions from the cells causes depolarization.

INTRODUCTION TO HEART CHAMBERS [9 - 11]

Sino Atrial Node

It is present in the right atrium. The depolarization of the right atrium transfers the impulse to AV node. The depolarization occurs 60 to 100 times per minute.

Atrio Ventricular Node

It is located in the posterior wall of the right atrium and ventricle. It receives an impulse from the SA node and transmits signal to ventricular septum. The defects in SA node can lower the depolarization process.

Left and Right Bundle Branch

The electrical impulse originated from AV node and bundle of hiss and reached to the apex of the ventricles.

Purkinjee Fibers

These fibers are highly branched and carry the electrical impulse to ventricles. The low level of depolarization can decrease the heart rate and cardiac output.

DISEASES OF MYOCARDIUM

It includes the following cardiac diseases.

Cardiomyopathy

It damages the cardiac muscles and causes inflammation in the cardiac chambers.

Types of Cardiomyopathy

Dilated Cardiomyoapthy

It is characterized by the enlargement of cardiac chambers causes inflammation in the cardiac cells is called as dilated cardiomyoapthy.

Hypertrophic Cardiomayopahty

The huge enlargement of ventricles in the septum portion of the heart causes inflammation in the heart.

Constrictive Cardiomyopathy

The excessive strictness of ventricular walls can cause inflammation in the heart.

Rheumatic Heart Disease

The chronic inflammation of the heart may damage the function of myocardium and heart valves leads to develop rheumatic heart disease.

DISORDERS OF HEART FAILURE

The damage of the heart valves may cause infection, inflammation of endothelium leads to poor function of heart valves. The major types of heart valve disorders are stenosis and incompetence.

Stenosis

The narrowing of the heart valves may decrease the blood pumping. Aortic stenosis affects the semi lunar valves and lowers the blood flow to the aorta. Mitral stenosis can decrease the blood flow to the left ventricle into the aorta.

Incompetent Valves

Aortic regurgitation may cause the closing of semi lunar valves and sends the remained blood in the circulation to the left ventricles for contraction. In mitral regurgitation may send the blood to the left atrium for contraction and creates irregular heartbeats which lead to cause arrhythmia.

PREVALENCE

The defects in cardiac rhythm are associated with a significant rise in health care cost and also mortality among the affected population. Atrial fibrillation is causing 2.3 million people in the United States. The ineffective treatment of cardiac arrhythmia leads to an increase in the risk of stroke. Previous research studies revealed that 90,000 cases of supraventricular tachycardia are detected annually in the United States. Ventricular arrhythmias are causing about 75% to 80% of the cardiac deaths annually in the world. The onset of arrhythmia is associated with the development of various chronic diseases such as heart failure, coronary artery disease, stroke *etc.* Atrial fibrillation has a prevalence of 1.5%–3% in the general population [12 - 15]. ECG devices are used to identify the risk of developing cardiac arrhythmias among arrhythmias patients.

PATHOPHYSIOLOGY OF CARDIAC ARRHYTHMIA

The perturbation in the normal activation of the myocardium cells can cause irregular rhythms of heart beat leads to arrhythmia. Sinus node having the properties of automaticity, conduction, contraction, depolarization of atrioventricular node and transmitting through Purkinje fibers causes depolarization of the ventricles. Automaticity is the self production of the cardiac contractions by the myocardial cells. Low level of blood supply to the cardiac cells, electrolyte disturbances, aging, OTC medications can reduce the automaticity property of the cardiac cells. The decreased function of the sinoatrial node can result in dysfunction of the conduction property of the heart which causes irregular heart rhythms production. The suppression of the conduction properties of the SA node can result in dysfunction of the sino atrial node. The delayed ventricular function leads to the cause of ventricular arrhythmias. The blockage of the ventricular function led to the development of myocardial infarction. The abnormalities in the initiation of the electrical impulse from SA node of the heart can cause the development of arrhythmia. The normal production of the heart contraction is associated with sinus node and Purkinje fibers. The abnormal automaticity can occur due to low level membrane potential of cardiac fibers results in irregular heartbeats generation. Abnormal generation of the impulse causes excitation of the muscle fibers. The slow contraction property of the sinus node results in blockage of the blood vessels. The slow conduction and blockage may result in a decrease in the action potential of the cardiac muscles lead to the progression of cardiac arrhythmia [16 - 18]. The pathophysiology of cardiac arrhythmia is shown in Fig. (**2**).

Pathophysiology of cardiac arrythmia

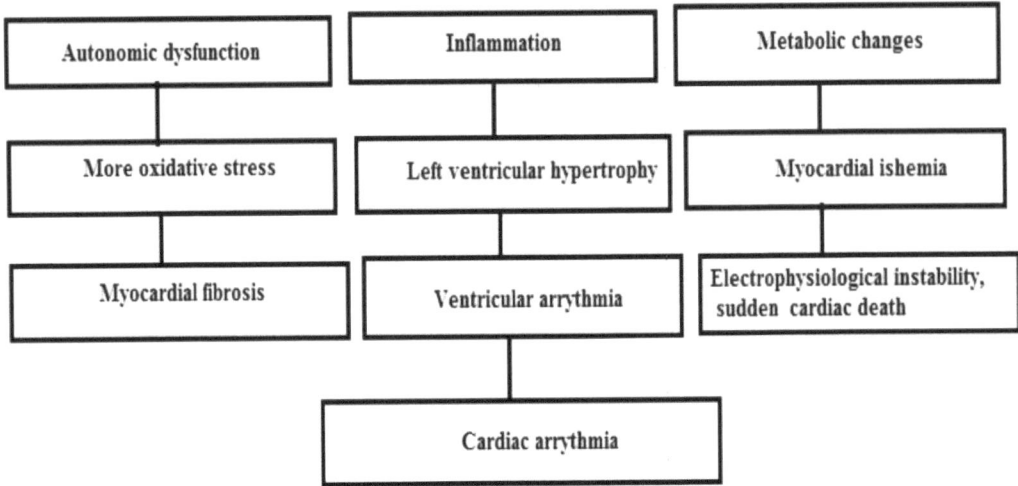

Fig. (2). Pathophysiology of cardiac arrhythmia.

RISK FACTORS FOR ARRHYTHMIA

The following are possible risk factors for arrhythmia

• Hypertension

• Obesity

• Uncontrolled diabetes

• Old age

• Inherited gene defects

• Cardiomyopathy

• Hypothyroidism

• Hyperthyroidism

• Obstructive sleep apnea

• Electrolyte imbalances

• Alcohol

• Caffeine products

DIAGNOSIS OF ARRHYTHMIA

Blood Tests

It is used to identify the infection and inflammatory conditions present in the blood.

Renal Function Test

It is used to detect the defects in renal function.

Liver Function Test

It is used to identify liver complications, and liver infections.

ECG (Electrocardiogram)

This test is performed to record the abnormalities in the rhythm of the heart.

Holter Monitor

It is a device that will record the heart function, rhythms and heart moment and to predict the abnormal heart functions.

Chest X-ray

It is used to detect the inflammatory conditions of the heart.

Electrophysiologic Testing

It is a painless and non surgical test that can help in the determination of the type of arrhythmia.

PREVENTION OF ARRHYTHMIAS [19 - 21]

It includes

• Stress management

• Consumption of the healthy diet

• Smoking cessation

• Alcohol cessation

• Regular physical exercise

• Regular physical examination

• Reduction of salt intake

• Medication adherence

TREATMENT

Implanted Cardioverter Defibrillators

These devices are used to monitor the heart rhythm and heart rate and prevent cardiac arrhythmia.

Cardiac Resynchronization Therapy

It is a device used to coordinate muscle contractions and improve the contraction efficiency of the heart.

CLASSIFICATIONS OF ANTIARRHYTHMIC AGENTS [22 - 25]

It includes

Class 1A Drugs

• Disopryamide

• Quinidine

• Procainamide

Class IB Drugs

• Mexiletine

• Lidocaine

• Tocainide

• Class IC drugs

• Moricizine

• Flecainide

• Propafenone

Class II: Beta Blockers

• Metoprolol

• Atenolol

• Propranolol

• Esmolol

• Timolol

Class III: Potassium Channels Blockers

• Dofetilide

• Sotalol

• Amiodarone

• Ibutilide

Calcium Channel Blockers

This drug blocks the entry of calcium ions into the calcium channels and lowers the work load on the heart and dilates the arteries leads to vasodilatation.

These drugs include

• Diltiazem

• Verapamil

• Isradipine

• Nifedipine

• Nicardipine

• Nimopidine

• Amlodipine

• Nisoldipine

• Bepridil

• Felodipine

Adverse effects Rashes, headache, constipation, flushing, edema, drowsiness

CONCLUSION

The disturbance in the activation of the myocardium may reveal the development of cardiovascular complications. Arrhythmia is one of the potential risk factors among heart failure patients and causes more health care expenditure to the affected population worldwide. The incidence of arrhythmia rises with increasing age. Atrial fibrillation contributes to an increase in the risk of developing stroke and thromboembolism. A better understanding of the electrophysiological base of the electrocardiogram and guides the physician to take the effective decision for the treatment of cardiac arrhythmias. Targeting on recent advances in electrophysiological research studies at the molecular level provides the more effective management of cardiac arrhythmias. Cardiac arrhythmias indicate the structural heart disease and cause an alteration in hemodynamics of the heart. Novel echocardiographic diagnostic tests are useful for a better understanding of arrhythmias and the prediction of cardiac arrhythmias at the early stages. The pharmacological and non-pharmacological interventions may lower the arrhythmia burden in the community. Beta blockers, calcium channel blockers, potassium channel blockers are used to treat the arrhythmia burden. An amalgamation of clinical pharmacist interventions with the health care team on the early stage of arrhythmia detection, identification of clinical symptoms, maintaining healthy weight, mediation adherence, eating low fat diet, smoking and alcohol cessation, regular physical exercises, stress management programmes can lower the development of abnormal heart rhythms.

REFERENCES

[1]   Mirowski M, Reid PR, Mower MM, *et al.* Clinical performance of the implantable cardioverter-defibrillator. Pacing Clin Electrophysiol 1984; 7(6 Pt 2): 1345-50.
      [http://dx.doi.org/10.1111/j.1540-8159.1984.tb05706.x] [PMID: 6209681]

[2]   Hook BG, Marchlinski FE. Value of ventricular electrogram recordings in the diagnosis of arrhythmias precipitating electrical device shock therapy. J Am Coll Cardiol 1991; 17(4): 985-90.
      [http://dx.doi.org/10.1016/0735-1097(91)90884-C] [PMID: 1999638]

[3]   Schwartz PJ, Ackerman MJ. The long QT syndrome: a transatlantic clinical approach to diagnosis and therapy. Eur Heart J 2013; 34(40): 3109-16.
      [http://dx.doi.org/10.1093/eurheartj/eht089] [PMID: 23509228]

[4]   Camm AJ, Al-Khatib SM, Calkins H, *et al.* A proposal for new clinical concepts in the management of atrial fibrillation. Am Heart J 2012; 164(3): 292-302.e1.
      [http://dx.doi.org/10.1016/j.ahj.2012.05.017] [PMID: 22980294]

[5]   Van Gelder I, *et al.* Routine *versus* aggressive upstream rhythm control for prevention of early atrial fibrillation in heart failure, the RACE study. Eur Heart J 2017; 21(7-8): 354-63.

[6]   Heeringa J, van der Kuip DA, Hofman A, *et al.* Prevalence, incidence and lifetime risk of atrial

fibrillation: the Rotterdam study. Eur Heart J 2006; 27(8): 949-53.
[http://dx.doi.org/10.1093/eurheartj/ehi825] [PMID: 16527828]

[7] Kalbfleisch SJ, el-Atassi R, Calkins H, Langberg JJ, Morady F. Association between atrioventricular node reentrant tachycardia and inducible atrial flutter. J Am Coll Cardiol 1993; 22(1): 80-4.
[http://dx.doi.org/10.1016/0735-1097(93)90818-L] [PMID: 8509568]

[8] Haïssaguerre M, Jaïs P, Shah DC, *et al.* Spontaneous initiation of atrial fibrillation by ectopic beats originating in the pulmonary veins. N Engl J Med 1998; 339(10): 659-66.
[http://dx.doi.org/10.1056/NEJM199809033391003] [PMID: 9725923]

[9] Verma A, Jiang CY, Betts TR, *et al.* Approaches to catheter ablation for persistent atrial fibrillation. N Engl J Med 2015; 372(19): 1812-22.
[http://dx.doi.org/10.1056/NEJMoa1408288] [PMID: 25946280]

[10] Ausma J, Wijffels M, Thoné F, Wouters L, Allessie M, Borgers M. Structural changes of atrial myocardium due to sustained atrial fibrillation in the goat. Circulation 1997; 96(9): 3157-63.
[http://dx.doi.org/10.1161/01.CIR.96.9.3157] [PMID: 9386188]

[11] Wellens HJJ, Schwartz PJ, Lindemans FW, *et al.* Risk stratification for sudden cardiac death: current status and challenges for the future. Eur Heart J 2014; 35(25): 1642-51.
[http://dx.doi.org/10.1093/eurheartj/ehu176] [PMID: 24801071]

[12] Lerman BB. Mechanism, diagnosis, and treatment of outflow tract tachycardia. Nat Rev Cardiol 2015; 12(10): 597-608.
[http://dx.doi.org/10.1038/nrcardio.2015.121] [PMID: 26283265]

[13] Wann LS, Curtis AB, January CT, *et al.* 2011 ACCF/AHA/HRS focused update on the management of patients with atrial fibrillation (updating the 2006 guideline): a report of the American College of Cardiology Foundation/American Heart Association Task Force on Practice Guidelines. Circulation 2011; 123(1): 104-23.
[http://dx.doi.org/10.1161/CIR.0b013e3181fa3cf4] [PMID: 21173346]

[14] de Vos CB, Nieuwlaat R, Crijns HJ, *et al.* Autonomic trigger patterns and anti-arrhythmic treatment of paroxysmal atrial fibrillation: data from the Euro Heart Survey. Eur Heart J 2008; 29(5): 632-9.
[http://dx.doi.org/10.1093/eurheartj/ehn025] [PMID: 18270212]

[15] Psaty BM, Manolio TA, Kuller LH, *et al.* Incidence of and risk factors for atrial fibrillation in older adults. Circulation 1997; 96(7): 2455-61.
[http://dx.doi.org/10.1161/01.CIR.96.7.2455] [PMID: 9337224]

[16] Dobrev D, Nattel S. New antiarrhythmic drugs for treatment of atrial fibrillation. Lancet 2010; 375(9721): 1212-23.
[http://dx.doi.org/10.1016/S0140-6736(10)60096-7] [PMID: 20334907]

[17] Ravens U. Novel pharmacological approaches for antiarrhythmic therapy. Naunyn Schmiedebergs Arch Pharmacol 2010; 381(3): 187-93.
[http://dx.doi.org/10.1007/s00210-009-0487-8] [PMID: 20082192]

[18] Cho HC, Marbán E. Biological therapies for cardiac arrhythmias: can genes and cells replace drugs and devices? Circ Res 2010; 106(4): 674-85.
[http://dx.doi.org/10.1161/CIRCRESAHA.109.212936] [PMID: 20203316]

[19] Josephson ME. Electrophysiology at a crossroads: A revisit. Heart Rhythm 2016; 13(12): 2317-22.
[http://dx.doi.org/10.1016/j.hrthm.2016.07.024] [PMID: 27542727]

[20] Coumel P. The management of clinical arrhythmias. An overview on invasive *versus* non-invasive electrophysiology. Eur Heart J 1987; 8(2): 92-9.
[http://dx.doi.org/10.1093/oxfordjournals.eurheartj.a062259] [PMID: 2436917]

[21] Pritchett ELC. Management of atrial fibrillation. N Engl J Med 1992; 326(19): 1264-71.
[http://dx.doi.org/10.1056/NEJM199205073261906] [PMID: 1560803]

[22] Priori SG, Blomström-Lundqvist C, Mazzanti A, *et al.* 2015 ESC Guidelines for the management of patients with ventricular arrhythmias and the prevention of sudden cardiac death. Eur Heart J 2015; 36(41): 2793-867.
[http://dx.doi.org/10.1093/eurheartj/ehv316] [PMID: 26320108]

[23] Zoni-Berisso M, Lercari F, Carazza T, *et al.* Epidemiology 2015 ACC/AHA/HRS Guideline for the Management of Adult Patients With Supraventricular Tachycardia JACC 2016; 67(13) e27e115

[24] Zaza A, Belardinelli L, Shryock JC. Pathophysiology and pharmacology of the cardiac "late sodium current.". Pharmacol Ther 2008; 119(3): 326-39.
[http://dx.doi.org/10.1016/j.pharmthera.2008.06.001] [PMID: 18662720]

[25] Heijman J, Voigt N, Dobrev D. New directions in antiarrhythmic drug therapy for atrial fibrillation. Future Cardiol 2013; 9(1): 71-88.
[http://dx.doi.org/10.2217/fca.12.78] [PMID: 23259476]

CHAPTER 13

Myocardial Infarction

Abstract: Myocardial infarction occurred due to severe myocardial ischemia that leads to myocardial necrosis and cardiac remodeling results in the progression of heart failure. The clinical manifestations of the myocardial infarction include sweating, shortness of breath, abnormal heart beating, vomiting, weakness, nausea, fatigue, stress contribute to the development of myocardial infarction. Cardiovascular diseases are the cause of mortality and morbidity from worldwide countries. Cardiovascular disease incidence is expected to increase by 25 million by the year 2020. The progression of myocardial infarction is associated with various risk factors which include smoking, alcohol, high lipid levels; hypertension can likely increase the risk of myocardial infarction. Every year worldwide more than 3 million people are affected with myocardial infarction. The increasing incidence of myocardial infarction was high in males as compared with females. Previous research studies stated that patients with more than 45 years of age can develop the disease. Atherosclerosis is one of the major risk factors for the development of myocardial infarction. It is a chronic inflammatory condition of the endothelial cells, in which the T lymphocytes, monocytes, macrophages cells can thicken the endothelial cell layers which leads to the progression of atherosclerotic events. Chest x-ray, electrocardiogram, echocardiogram, holter monitoring, coronary angiogram, and stress test is used to detect the severity of disease complications. The pharmacological management of myocardial infarction includes anticoagulants, thrombolytics and percutaneous coronary intervention that can lower the progression of disease complications.

Keywords: Coronary Angiogram, Echocardiogram, Hypertension, Myocardial Infarction, Thrombolytics.

INTRODUCTION

Cardiovascular diseases are the cause of mortality and morbidity from worldwide countries. The improper treatment and screening of cardiovascular risk factors may lead to developing various cardiovascular complications. Cardiovascular disease incidence is expected to increase by 25 million by the year 2020. The progression of myocardial infarction is associated with various risk factors which include smoking, alcohol, high lipid levels; hypertension can likely increase the risk of myocardial infarction. A heart attack occurs when the supply of oxygen is reduced to the cardiac muscles leads to the formation of the block in the blood vessels.

The blood flow is not sufficiently meet the cardiac muscle demands leads to the death of cardiac cells. The myocardial infarction is commonly called a heart attack. The continuous function of the heart requires an adequate amount of oxygen, nutrients in the body. The heart consists of three coronary arteries that supply the oxygenated blood to the cardiac muscles. The blockage of these coronary arteries leads to develop ischemia which triggers the progression of myocardial infarction. The deposition of fatty materials in the blood vessels cause the reduced level of blood flow to the myocardium leads to the formation of blockage in the coronary arteries. A blockage can develop the plaque in the blood vessels can reduce the oxygen supply to the myocardium results in the development of myocardial infarction. The clinical symptoms of myocardial infarction include chest pain which travels to the shoulder, neck, and arm. This condition can be managed through regular medication adherence and lifestyle modification approaches can reduce the myocardial infarction risk complications to the affected patients [1 - 4].

PREVALENCE

Myocardial infarction is a common type of coronary artery disease. The world health organization estimated in 2004 that 12.2% of worldwide deaths were occurred due to ischemic heart disease. Every year worldwide more than 3 million people are affected with myocardial infarction. The increasing incidence of myocardial infarction was high in males as compared with females. Previous research studies stated that patients with more than 45 years of age can develop the disease. The incidence of myocardial infarction in India is 64% in males age ranges from 29-69 years. More than 80% of cardiovascular diseases are occurring from the developing countries. There is a need for new research studies are conducted to identify disease complications among the patients. The rapid urbanization and sedentary life style practices can increase the risk of myocardial infarction. The prevalence of myocardial infarction was found to be high in males as compared with females. The South Asian countries (India, Pakistan, Sri Lanka, Bangladesh, and Nepal) countries have the highest incidence rate was seen in the younger age of 45 years than older people [5 - 7].

RISK FACTORS

• Diabetes

• Family history of coronary artery disease

• Smoking

• Alcohol

• An abnormally high level of blood cholesterol

• An abnormally low level of HDL

• High blood pressure

• Obesity

• Physical inactivity

PATHOGENESIS

Myocardial infarction is associated with the sudden death of myocardial tissue due to lack of blood supply and the formation of the thrombus in the blood vessels leads to the development of myocardial infarction. Ischemia causes metabolic alterations in the body which can alter the blood flow in the blood vessels. Prolong myocardial ischemia causes the death of myocardial cells. The mitochondrial cell dysfunction leads to the development of apoptosis and necrosis of cardiomyocytes in the heart. The clearance of dead cells by the phagocytes, which can stimulate the release of inflammatory cells, inflammatory pathways can alter the blood flow in circulation. Activation of renin□angiotensin□aldosterone system and deposition of extracellular matrix proteins in the blood vessels can impair the function of cardiac cells leads to failure of the protective mechanism of endothelial cells. Plaques are unstable and rupture in nature and formation of blood clot in the blood vessels can block the coronary artery than happens in few minutes. The gradual deposition of cholesterol in the tissues leads to the formation of a plaques in the walls of coronary arteries known as atherosclerosis [8 - 13]. Inflammatory cells such as histamines, bradykines, and cytokines can move into the arterial walls. The cells growth factors are secreted by the smooth muscle, macrophages reach into the plaques acts to stabilize the plaques. A stable plaque may coat with fibrous cap with calcification. The continuous progression of the inflammation causes rupture of the plaques and forms the thrombus in the blood vessels. The lipid particles are associated with plaque formation and inflammation in the blood vessels. The low level of blood flow to the myocardial cells can raise the oxygen demand. Prolong impairment in blood flow to the cardiac cells leads to develop ischemic events. The necrosis and inflammation of the cardiac cells cause the infarction of the coronary arteries. The lack of oxygen supply to the tissues can synthesize the mitochondrial for ATP production. ATP is needed for the maintenance of electrolyte balance. The lack of ATP supplement to the cells can induce necrosis and death of the tissues. Tissue death can alter the conduction pathways of the heart. The rupture of the blood vessels leads to develop the myocardial infarction events. The myocardial infarction is shown in Fig. (**1**).

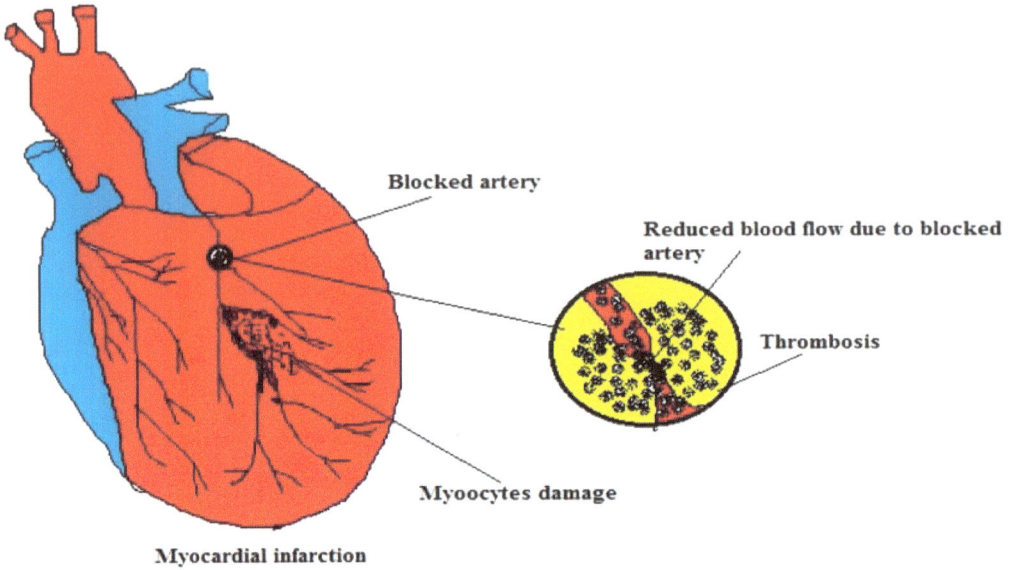

Fig. (1). Myocardial infarction.

CLINICAL SYMPTOMS [14 - 16]

• Tightness in the chest

• Cough

• Dizziness

• Fast heart rate

• Pain in the jaw, and other areas of the upper body that lasts more than a few minutes

• Shortness of breath

• Sweating

• Nausea

• Vomiting

• Anxiety

DIAGNOSIS TEST

• Troponin test

- Complete blood cell count

- Lipid profile

- Chest x-ray

- ECG

- Coronary angiogram

- Electrocardiography

- Doppler studies

- MRI scan

- CT scan

- Creatine Kinase

- Creatine Kinase - MB

- Myoglobin

- B-type natriuretic peptide

- C-reactive protein

- Copeptin

PREVENTION OF MYOCARDIAL INFARCTION [17 - 19]

- Exercising regularly

- Eating healthy foods

- Maintaining a healthy weight

- Smoking cessation

- Alcoholic cessation

- Maintaining controlled blood pressure

- Weight reduction

- Regular medication adherence

• Regular health care visit

PHARMACOTHERAPY [20 - 25]

Cholesterol-lowering agents

Beta-blockers

ACE inhibitors

Angiotensin receptor blockers

Anti-thrombolytic agents

Anti-platelet drugs

Vasodilators

Cholesterol Lowering Medications Include

Statins

These drugs act by inhibiting HMG-CoA reductase enzyme and inhibit the cholesterol biosynthetic pathway and shows anti atherosclerotic effect in the blood vessels.

• Atorvastatin

• Fluvastatin

• Lovastatin

• Pitavastatin

• Pravastatin

• Rosuvastatin

• Simvastatin

Adverse effects Headache, dizziness, insomnia, flushing of the skin, drowsiness and myalgia.

Beta Blockers

It reduces the work load on the heart and reduces stress and hormones levels in the body which leads to vasodilatation in the blood vessels.

• Commonly prescribed beta blockers include

• Atenolol

• Bisoprolol

• Nadolol

• Nebivolol

• Carvedilol

• Labetalol

• Nebivolol

• Pindolol

• Propranolol

• Timolol

• Metoprolol

Adverse effects Dry mouth, dry skin, feelings of coldness, diarrhea, shortness of breath and insomnia.

Angiotensin Converting Enzyme (ACE) Inhibitors

ACEs block the conversion of angiotensin I to angiotensin II by the action of angiotensinogen in the body and help to lower the vasoconstriction and promote vasodilation.

It includes

• Captopril

• Lisinopril

• Fosinopril

• Ramipril

• Benazepril

- Enalapril

- Perindopril

- Quinapril

- Moexipril

- Trandolapril

Adverse effects Dry cough, hyperkalemia, fatigue, headaches and loss of taste.

Angiotensin II Receptor Blockers

It blocks the conversion of angiotensin II from its binding to angiotensin II receptors located on the blood vessels and produces vasodialtion in the blood vessels.

These drugs include

- Candesartan

- Telmisartan

- Valsartan

- Eprosartan

- Irbesartan

- Losartan

Adverse effects Hyperkalemia, dizziness, headache, cough, diarrhea, hypotension and angioedema.

Thrombolytic Drugs

Thrombolytic drugs are prescribed to reduce the formation of a blood clot in the blood vessels and also lower the severity of stroke. These drugs will act by conversion of plasminogen which forms plasmin and activates the fibrin bound plasminogen. Fibrin molecules are inhibited by plasmin which leads to the breakdown of clot the blood vessels and reduces the stroke complications.

It includes

- Anistreplase

• Reteplase

• Streptokinase

• T-pa

• Tenecteplase

• Alteplase

• Urokinase

Adverse drug reactions Internal bleeding, damage to the blood vessels, renal damage.

Anti-platelet Drugs

These drugs help to prevent the platelets aggregation and reduce the clot in the blood vessels.

Types of Antiplatelet Agents

• Aspirin

• Dipyridamole

• Clopidogrel

• Ticagrelor

Adverse effects Headache, dizziness, nausea, vomiting, diarrhea, constipation, dyspepsia, abdominal pain, and nose bleeding.

Vasodilators

These drugs relax the vascular smooth muscles in the blood vessels and leakage of ions cause dilatation of the veins, arteries leads to complete dilation of blood vessels. The dilation of blood vessels can lower the systemic vascular resistance which results in a reduction of blood pressure in the blood vessels.

Classification

Arterial Vasodilators

• Hydralazine

• Minoxidil

• Diazoxide

Arterial and Venous Vasodilators

• Prazosin

• Sod. nitroprusside

• Terazosin

• Organic nitrates

• Isosorbide di-nitrate

• Glyceryl trinitrate

• Amyl nitrite

• Erythrityl tetra nitrate

Side effects Vomiting, flushing, headache, tachycardia, heart palpitations, edema, nausea, joint pain, chest pain

CONCLUSION

Myocardial infarction is associated with the sudden death of myocardial tissue due to lack of blood supply and the formation of thrombus in the blood vessels leads to the development of myocardial infarction. Troponin assays are effective for reduction of the myocardial injury. Identification of patients at the early stage of risk and preventive therapies is beneficial for the reduction of risk burden. Recommendation of the clinical pharmacist services with the health care team on risk factors identification and control, health screening programmes, diet counseling, disease counseling, lifestyle modification counseling, smoking and alcohol cessation, stress management, physical exercises are needed for prevention of ischemic events. Regular monitoring of patients by the health care team which includes physicians, pharmacist, nurse, health care assistant lower the progression of the myocardial ischemic events and proper recommendation of the surgical interventions, cardiac rehabilitation care and new treatment options which targets the reduction of inflammation results in the reduction of progression of the ischemic sequences. The regular prescribing practice of ACE inhibitors, beta-blockers, nitroglycerin, anticoagulants, and thrombolytic drugs can improve the health related outcomes among disease patients in the health care settings.

REFERENCES

[1]   Moran AE, Forouzanfar MH, Roth GA, *et al.* The global burden of ischemic heart disease in 1990 and 2010: the Global Burden of Disease 2010 study. Circulation 2014; 129(14): 1493-501.
[http://dx.doi.org/10.1161/CIRCULATIONAHA.113.004046] [PMID: 24573351]

[2]   Lloyd-Jones DM, Nam BH, D'Agostino RB Sr, *et al.* Parental cardiovascular disease as a risk factor for cardiovascular disease in middle-aged adults: a prospective study of parents and offspring. JAMA 2004; 291(18): 2204-11.
[http://dx.doi.org/10.1001/jama.291.18.2204] [PMID: 15138242]

[3]   Morillas P, Bertomeu V, Pabón P, *et al.* Characteristics and outcome of acute myocardial infarction in young patients. The PRIAMHO II study. Cardiology 2007; 107(4): 217-25.
[http://dx.doi.org/10.1159/000095421] [PMID: 16953107]

[4]   Lu Y, Zhou S, Dreyer RP, *et al.* Sex differences in lipid profiles and treatment utilization among young adults with acute myocardial infarction: Results from the VIRGO study. Am Heart J 2017; 183: 74-84.
[http://dx.doi.org/10.1016/j.ahj.2016.09.012] [PMID: 27979045]

[5]   Iqbal MP, Mehboobali N, Tareen AK, *et al.* Association of body iron status with the risk of premature acute myocardial infarction in a Pakistani population. PLoS One 2013; 8(6): e67981.
[http://dx.doi.org/10.1371/journal.pone.0067981] [PMID: 23840800]

[6]   Javed U, Aftab W, Ambrose JA, *et al.* Frequency of elevated troponin I and diagnosis of acute myocardial infarction. Am J Cardiol 2009; 104(1): 9-13.
[http://dx.doi.org/10.1016/j.amjcard.2009.03.003] [PMID: 19576313]

[7]   Yeh RW, Sidney S, Chandra M, Sorel M, Selby JV, Go AS. Population trends in the incidence and outcomes of acute myocardial infarction. N Engl J Med 2010; 362(23): 2155-65.
[http://dx.doi.org/10.1056/NEJMoa0908610] [PMID: 20558366]

[8]   Avezum A, Makdisse M, Spencer F, *et al.* Impact of age on management and outcome of acute coronary syndrome: observations from the Global Registry of Acute Coronary Events (GRACE). Am Heart J 2005; 149(1): 67-73.
[http://dx.doi.org/10.1016/j.ahj.2004.06.003] [PMID: 15660036]

[9]   Ahmed E, Alhabib KF, El-Menyar A, *et al.* Age and clinical outcomes in patients presenting with acute coronary syndromes. J Cardiovasc Dis Res 2013; 4(2): 134-9.
[http://dx.doi.org/10.1016/j.jcdr.2012.08.005] [PMID: 24027372]

[10]   Al-Khadra AH. Clinical profile of young patients with acute myocardial infarction in Saudi Arabia. Int J Cardiol 2003; 91(1): 9-13.
[http://dx.doi.org/10.1016/S0167-5273(02)00579-X] [PMID: 12957724]

[11]   El-Menyar A, Zubaid M, Shehab A, *et al.* Prevalence and impact of cardiovascular risk factors among patients presenting with acute coronary syndrome in the middle East. Clin Cardiol 2011; 34(1): 51-8.
[http://dx.doi.org/10.1002/clc.20873] [PMID: 21259279]

[12]   Akbari M, Mohammadzadeh M, Rajabpoor M. AzimPoor A. Agents connection with awareness and act of patients that caused acute myocardial infarction encountering with clinical symptoms them to stay in urmia hospitals. Journal of Urmia Nursing and Midwifery Faculty 2009; 7(2): 73-80.

[13]   Anand SS, Islam S, Rosengren A, *et al.* Risk factors for myocardial infarction in women and men: insights from the INTERHEART study. Eur Heart J 2008; 29(7): 932-40.
[http://dx.doi.org/10.1093/eurheartj/ehn018] [PMID: 18334475]

[14]   Banks AD, Dracup K. Factors associated with prolonged prehospital delay of African Americans with acute myocardial infarction. Am J Crit Care 2006; 15(2): 149-57.
[http://dx.doi.org/10.4037/ajcc2006.15.2.149] [PMID: 16501134]

[15]   Ismail J, Jafar TH, Jafary FH, White F, Faruqui AM, Chaturvedi N. Risk factors for non-fatal myocardial infarction in young South Asian adults. Heart 2004; 90(3): 259-63.

[http://dx.doi.org/10.1136/hrt.2003.013631] [PMID: 14966040]

[16]   Janszky I, Ahnve S, Ljung R, *et al.* Daylight saving time shifts and incidence of acute myocardial infarction--Swedish Register of Information and Knowledge About Swedish Heart Intensive Care Admissions (RIKS-HIA). Sleep Med 2012; 13(3): 237-42.
[http://dx.doi.org/10.1016/j.sleep.2011.07.019] [PMID: 22285108]

[17]   Kazemy T, Sharifzadeh GR. Comparisons of acute myocardial infarction (AMI) among women and men. Modern Care Journal 2010; 7(1): 5-11.

[18]   Mirzaei S S, Mohammad A S, Bagherian F. Comparison of signs and symptoms of myocardial infarction and unstable angina in male and female hospitalized patients in coronary care units of kerman medical university hospital 2005 20042005;

[19]   Sari I, Acar Z, Özer O, *et al.* Factors associated with prolonged prehospital delay in patients with acute myocardial infarction. Turk Kardiyol Dern Ars 2008; 36(3): 156-62.
[PMID: 18626207]

[20]   Svensson L, Karlsson T, Nordlander R, Wahlin M, Zedigh C, Herlitz J. Safety and delay time in prehospital thrombolysis of acute myocardial infarction in urban and rural areas in Sweden. Am J Emerg Med 2003; 21(4): 263-70.
[http://dx.doi.org/10.1016/S0735-6757(03)00040-8] [PMID: 12898480]

[21]   Wilson K, Gibson N, Willan A, Cook D. Effect of smoking cessation on mortality after myocardial infarction: meta-analysis of cohort studies. Arch Intern Med 2000; 160(7): 939-44.
[http://dx.doi.org/10.1001/archinte.160.7.939] [PMID: 10761958]

[22]   Jernberg T, Johanson P, Held C, Svennblad B, Lindbäck J, Wallentin L. Association between adoption of evidence-based treatment and survival for patients with ST-elevation myocardial infarction. JAMA 2011; 305(16): 1677-84.
[http://dx.doi.org/10.1001/jama.2011.522] [PMID: 21521849]

[23]   Roe MT, Messenger JC, Weintraub WS, *et al.* Treatments, trends, and outcomes of acute myocardial infarction and percutaneous coronary intervention. J Am Coll Cardiol 2010; 56(4): 254-63.
[http://dx.doi.org/10.1016/j.jacc.2010.05.008] [PMID: 20633817]

[24]   DeWood MA, Spores J, Notske R, *et al.* Prevalence of total coronary occlusion during the early hours of transmural myocardial infarction. N Engl J Med 1980; 303(16): 897-902.
[http://dx.doi.org/10.1056/NEJM198010163031601] [PMID: 7412821]

[25]   Bosch X, Sambola A, Arós F, *et al.* [Use of thrombolytic treatment in patients with acute myocardial infarction in Spain. Observations from the PRIAMHO study]. Rev Esp Cardiol 2000; 53(4): 490-501.
[http://dx.doi.org/10.1016/S0300-8932(00)75118-9] [PMID: 10760231]

CHAPTER 14

Angina Pectoris

Abstract: Angina pectoris is a symptomatic clinical manifestation of myocardial ischemia which is caused by emotional stress. The patients having the age of 65 years and females age 70 years for women are at higher risk of developing angina pectoris. Currently, 4.1 million people are affected by coronary artery disease. The annual death rates of stable angina patients were 1.2% to 2.4. The major risk factors for angina pectoris include hyperlipidemia, hypertension, diabetes mellitus, stress, physical inactivity, smoking; and alcohol contributes to the development of angina pectoris. The clinical manifestations of angina pectoris include chest tightness, chest pain, chest discomfort, burning chest, fatigue, shortness of breath, sweating, dizziness, nausea, vomiting, aching, chest fullness, and more weight on chest. Chest x-ray, electrocardiogram, echocardiogram, holter monitoring, coronary angiogram, and stress test is used to detect the severity of disease complications. The proper understanding of pathophysiological approaches is essential for better management of angina pectoris. The continuous prescribing practice of statins, beta blockers, calcium channel blockers, heparin, anti-platelets, nitrates, ACE inhibitors, thrombolytic medications could improve the heart rate and improve the blood flow in the vascular stream and also lower the cardiovascular complications in primary care settings.

Keywords: Angina Pectoris, Hyperlipidemia, Hypertension, Myocardial Ischemia.

INTRODUCTION

Angina pectoris is the chest pain caused due to low blood and oxygen supply to the heart. Angina pectoris is a clinical syndrome of pericardial discomfort and caused by myocardial infarction. The angina pectoris is occurred due to low oxygen supply and abnormal heart rhythms in the heart. Angina pectoris is the chest discomfort that occurs as a result of reduced blood supply to the cardiac muscles. The stable angina is the one type of angina pectoris. It is a predictable pattern of chest pain. Unstable angina is another form of angina. It occurs due to chest pain for a period of more time. Stable and unstable angina leads to develop a heart attack. Ischemic heart disease is the major cause of death and disability in western countries.

The angina pectoris is the most prevalent manifestation among the high risk of developing angina pectoris patients. The regular lifestyle interventions, anti angina drugs and lifestyle modifications and surgical treatment can lower the progression of angina pectoris complications. The proper understanding of pathophysiological approaches is essential for better management of angina pectoris. The angina pectoris is caused by atherosclerosis [1 - 3]. The progression of angina pectoris is reduced by lifestyle modifications and regular treatment and lifestyle modifications and risk factors control can reduce the progression of angina pectoris. The angina pectoris is shown in Fig. (**1**).

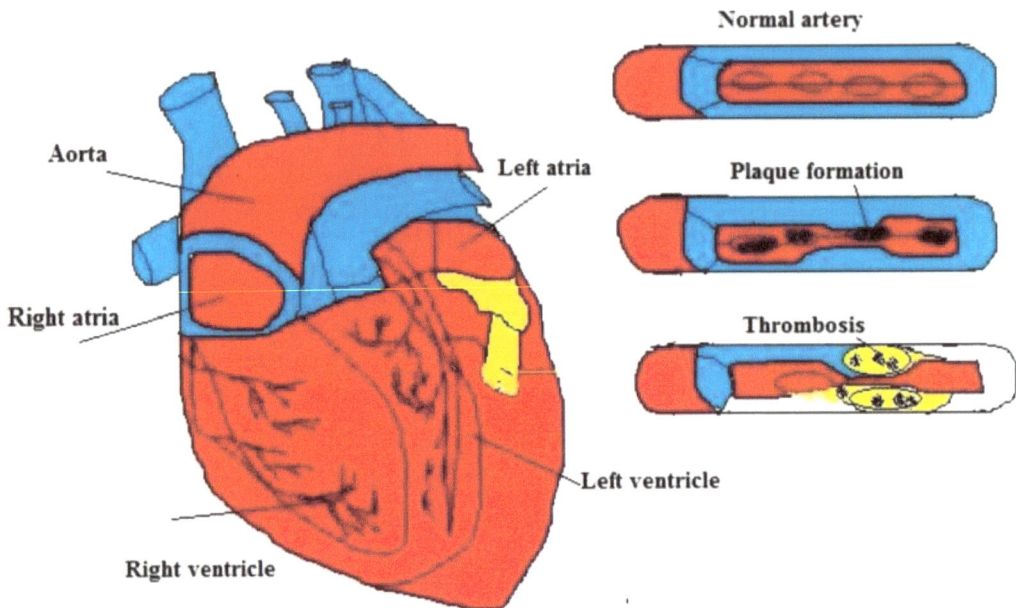

Fig. (1). Angina pectoris.

CHARACTERISTICS OF STABLE ANGINA

• It develops during the exercise

• It is usually predicted

• Chest pain occurs at a short time which ends five minutes

CHARACTERISTICS OF UNSTABLE ANGINA

It occurs even at resting stage

This type of heart attack is unexpected

It is more severe and lasts longer than stable angina

CHARACTERISTICS OF VARIANT ANGINA

It is a severe type of chest pain

It is usually happening in resting stage

HISTORY OF ANGINA PECTORIS

• In the year 1772 William Heberden was identified as the angina pectoris.

• In the year 1452–1519 Leonardo da Vinci was identified as the coronary arteries.

• In the year 1578–1657 William Harvey was described as the blood flow in circulation.

• In the year 1660–1742 Friedrich Hoffman noticed the poor blood flow to the coronary arteries.

• In the year 1776 year Edward Jenner examined the coronary artery disease patients.

• In the year 1776 year Lauder Brunton identified that the coronary artery and its association with the nervous system.

• In the year 1879 W.M. Morrell published a research paper on angina pectoris

• In the year 1879 James black identified the propranolol drug.

• In the year 1964, Albert Fleckenstein and his colleagues identified the calcium channel blockers.

EPIDEMIOLOGY

The incidence of angina pectoris has been gradually rising from the past to current. Previous studies revealed that the angina affecting cases in western countries is 30,000–40,000 per million. The incidence increased with aging in males and females. The patients having the age 65 years and female's age 70 years for women are at higher risk of developing angina pectoris. Currently, 4.1 million people are affected by coronary artery disease. The annual death rates of stable angina patients were 1.2% to 2.4. The presence of high risk factors can increase the risk of angina pectoris. The presence of high risk factors can increase the risk of angina pectoris [4, 5].

RISK FACTORS

It includes

• Age (greater for men over 45 years and women over 55 years)

• Genetics

• Blockage of a coronary artery

• Coronary heart disease

• Diabetes mellitus

• High blood pressure

• Smoking

• Lack of physical activity

• Alcohol

• High cholesterol

• Inflammation

• Injury to one or more coronary arteries

• Obesity

• Family history of heart disease

• Stress

• Anxiety

PATHOPHYSIOLOGY

Angina pectoris shows the clinical symptom of myocardial ischemia. It occurs when the myocytes do not have sufficient oxygen for the oxidation process in the cells and create inequity between myocardial oxygen need and delivery. The angina clinical symptoms can precipitate by ischemia in the coronary arteries. Cardiac hypertrophy, myocardial wall tension, myocardial contractility can affect the myocardial oxygen demand in the cells. Heart is greatly depending on the oxygen delivery to the blood vessels and produces energy in the cells which in turn results in contraction and relaxation of the cardiac muscles. Myocardial ischemia produces anaerobic glycolysis in the liver which increases the release of H^+, K^+, ions into the blood vessels cause acidosis.

The alteration of physical, mechanical and biochemical alterations of cell functions causes vasoconstriction. The vasodilatation of blood vessels can increase blood flow to coronary arteries. The coronary blood flow increases heart rate, contraction of the cardiac muscles. The coronary artery supplies oxygen and nutrients to the heart muscles. The formation of a clot in the blood vessels causes lowers the blood flow to the cardiac muscles leads to ischemia. Oxygen is transported to the heart by epicardial vessels, arteries and arterioles and capillaries. The formation of atherosclerotic plaques in the blood vessels causes impediment in blood flow to the heart which results in demand for oxygen supply in the blood vessels. The release of various inflammatory mediators such as prostaglandins, carbon dioxide, and nitric oxide can initiate the inflammation process in the blood vessels. The poor blood flow to the coronary arteries leads to form the coronary vaso spasm results in atherosclerosis. Endothelial cells also regulate the contraction and relaxation of the cardiac cells. The dysfunction of endothelial cells causes increased oxidative stress with the initiation of inflammation in the blood vessels leads to dysfunction of endothelial cells. The Endothelium dysfunction stimulates the inflammatory response in the circulation. The vasoconstriction of the blood vessels eventually leads to develop the myocardial ischemia. The ischemic condition leads to develop the progression of angina pectoris manifestation in the disease patients [6 - 9].

CLINICAL SYMPTOMS

• Chest pain or discomfort

• Pain in your arms, neck, jaw, shoulder or back accompanying chest pain

• Nausea

• Fatigue

• Shortness of breath

• Sweating

• Dizziness

DIAGNOSIS [10 - 13]

It includes

• Blood test

• Stress test

• Echocardiogram

• Chest X-ray

• Echo cardiogram studies

• Coronary angiography

• Cardiac computerized tomography scan

• Cardiac MRI scan

• Electrocardiogram

PREVENTION [14 - 18]

It includes

• Maintaining a healthy weight

• Eating a healthy diet

• Quitting smoking

• Cessation of alcohol

• Regular blood pressure and lipid monitoring

• Regular medication adherence

• Regular heath care visit

• Maintaining controlled levels of glycemic levels

• Regular physical activity

• Stress management

TREATMENT FOR MANAGEMENT OF ANGINA PECTORIS [19 - 25]

Nitrates

These drugs are prescribed to treat angina pectoris. Nitroglycerin is a potent smooth-muscle relaxant and vasodilator. It lowers the systolic blood pressure and dilates the veins and reduces the myocardial wall tension and promotes more blood reaching to the cardiac muscles and decreases the chest pain manifestations.

Classification

Organic Nitrates

• Nitroglycerin (glyceryl trinitrate)

• Amyl nitrite

• Isosorbide di-nitrate

• Erythrityl tetra nitrate

• Pentaerythritol tetra nitrate

Arterial Vasodilators

• Hydralazine

• Minoxidil

• Diazoxide

Arterial and Venous Vasodilators

Arterial and venous vasodilators

• Sod. nitroprusside

• Prazosin

• Terazosin

• Doxazosin

Nitrates relax the blood vessels by the release of nitric oxide (NO). It binds with the guanylyl cyclase enzyme which releases cyclic GMP and stimulates the release of cGMP-dependent protein kinase and eventually causes dephosphorylation of myosin light chain produce the vascular smooth muscle relaxation.

Common side effects of nitrates include:

- Headache

- Dizziness

- Tingling under the tongue

- Low blood pressure

- Headache

- Edema

- Pulmonary edema

- Low blood glucose

- Lightheadedness

- Nausea

- Flushing

Ranolazine

It blocks the sodium ion channels in the ischemic myocardium and increases intra cellular calcium through sodium calcium exchange in the circulation. Calcium over load increases the ventricular diastole which results in relaxation of the blood vessels. The blockage of the sodium current in the cell membrane leads to improve coronary blood flow and reduces the blockage in the blood vessels.

Side Effects

- Stomach pain

- Dizziness

- Nausea

- Vomiting

- Constipation

- Headache

- Dry mouth

• Revascularization

Percutaneous Coronary Intervention (PCI): It is used to identify the vessel disease and lesions in the blood vessels. It is non surgical procedure that contains a catheter device placed on the coronary arteries to prevent the blood clot and improve the blood flow to the heart.

Coronary artery bypass graft (CABG): It is a surgical procedure which is used to treat atherosclerosis. It will increase the blood flow to the coronary arteries and prevent the fatty plaque formation in the blood vessels. It is effective for angina diagnosed patients. It improves the blood flow to the heart and increases the surveillance rate of the angina patients.

Coronary Artery Bypass Graft (CABG): It is a surgical procedure which is used to treat atherosclerosis. It will increase the blood flow to the coronary arteries and prevent the fatty plaque formation in the blood vessels. It is effective for angina diagnosed patients. It improves the blood flow to the heart and increases the surveillance rate of the angina patients.

ANTI-PLATELET DRUGS

These drugs help to prevent the platelet aggregation and reduce the clot in the blood vessels.

Types of antiplatelet agents

• Aspirin

• Dipyridamole

• Clopidogrel

• Ticagrelor

Clinical uses of antiplatelet agents It is used to treat following disease conditions.

Coronary artery disease

Heart attack

Angina pectoris

Stroke and transient ischemic attacks

Peripheral artery disease

Side Effects Nausea, gastric problems, diarrhea, rashes, itching,

Calcium Channel Blockers This drug blocks the entry of calcium ions into the calcium channels and lowers the work load on the heart and dilates the arteries leads to vasodilatation.

These drugs include

- Diltiazem

- Verapamil

- Isradipine

- Nifedipine

- Nicardipine

- Nimopidine

- Amlodipine

- Nisoldipine

- Bepridil

- Felodipine

Adverse effects Rashes, headache, constipation, flushing, edema, drowsiness

Cholesterol lowering medications include Statins: These drugs act by inhibiting HMG-CoA reductase enzyme and inhibit the cholesterol biosynthetic pathway and show anti atherosclerotic effect in the blood vessels.

- Atorvastatin

- Fluvastatin

- Lovastatin

- Pitavastatin

- Pravastatin

- Rosuvastatin

• Simvastatin

Adverse effects Headache, dizziness, insomnia, flushing of the skin, drowsiness and myalgia.

Beta Blockers

It reduces the work load on the heart and reduces stress and hormones levels in the body which leads to vasodilatation in the blood vessels.

Commonly prescribed beta blockers include

• Atenolol

• Bisoprolol

• Nadolol

• Nebivolol

• Carvedilol

• Labetalol

• Nebivolol

• Pindolol

• Propranolol

• Timolol

Metoprolol

Adverse effects Dry mouth, dry skin, feelings of coldness, diarrhea, shortness of breath and insomnia.

Angiotensin Converting Enzyme (ACE) Inhibitors

ACEs block the conversion of angiotensin I to angiotensin II by the action of angiotensinogen in the body and help to lower the vasoconstriction and promote vasodilation.

It includes

• Captopril

- Lisinopril

- Fosinopril

- Ramipril

- Benazepril

- Enalapril

- Perindopril

- Quinapril

- Moexipril

- Trandolapril

Adverse effects Dry cough, hyperkalemia, fatigue, headaches and loss of taste.

Revascularization

PCI It is used to identify the vessel disease and lesions in the blood vessels.

CABG It is effective for angina diagnosed patients. It improves the blood flow to the heart and increases the surveillance rate of the angina patients.

CONCLUSION

Angina pectoris is a major health care problem and associated with commonly associated with complex risk factors. Among the other medication therapies calcium blockers, beta-blockers, nitrate drugs are considered as first line drugs for effective management of angina pectoris. Clinical pharmacist has to deliver his services with health care team on drug information services, diet counseling, termination of alcohol and smoking, lifestyle modification counseling, weight reduction, risk factors screening and detection, physical exercise, patient referral services, medication adherence and novel therapeutic options can control the angina burden in the clinical practice. Evidence based treatment provided to the chronic stable angina patients and aggressive control of risk factors and strict implementation of guidelines for the early stage of detecting angina pectoris and lowering angina pectoris risk incidences in the health care areas.

REFERENCES

[1]   Arrebola-Moreno A, Dungu J, Kaski JC. Treatment strategies for chronic stable angina. Expert Opin Pharmacother 2011; 12(18): 2833-44.

[http://dx.doi.org/10.1517/14656566.2011.634799] [PMID: 22098227]

[2]   Fox K, Garcia MA, Ardissino D, *et al.* Guidelines on the management of stable angina pectoris: executive summary: The Task Force on the Management of Stable Angina Pectoris of the European Society of Cardiology. Eur Heart J 2006; 27(11): 1341-81.
[http://dx.doi.org/10.1093/eurheartj/ehl001] [PMID: 16735367]

[3]   Campeau L. Letter: Grading of angina pectoris. Circulation 1976; 54(3): 522-3.
[http://dx.doi.org/10.1161/circ.54.3.947585] [PMID: 947585]

[4]   Kones R. Recent advances in the management of chronic stable angina I: approach to the patient, diagnosis, pathophysiology, risk stratification, and gender disparities. Vasc Health Risk Manag 2010; 6: 635-56.
[http://dx.doi.org/10.2147/VHRM.S7564] [PMID: 20730020]

[5]   Maseri A, Chierchia S, Kaski JC. Mixed angina pectoris. Am J Cardiol 1985; 56(9): 30E-3E.
[http://dx.doi.org/10.1016/0002-9149(85)91173-7] [PMID: 3901725]

[6]   Kaski JC. Pathophysiology and management of patients with chest pain and normal coronary arteriograms (cardiac syndrome X). Circulation 2004; 109(5): 568-72.
[http://dx.doi.org/10.1161/01.CIR.0000116601.58103.62] [PMID: 14769677]

[7]   Ong P, Athanasiadis A, Borgulya G, Mahrholdt H, Kaski JC, Sechtem U. High prevalence of a pathological response to acetylcholine testing in patients with stable angina pectoris and unobstructed coronary arteries. The ACOVA Study (Abnormal COronary VAsomotion in patients with stable angina and unobstructed coronary arteries). J Am Coll Cardiol 2012; 59(7): 655-62.
[http://dx.doi.org/10.1016/j.jacc.2011.11.015] [PMID: 22322081]

[8]   Sangareddi V, Chockalingam A, Gnanavelu G, Subramaniam T, Jagannathan V, Elangovan S. Canadian Cardiovascular Society classification of effort angina: an angiographic correlation. Coron Artery Dis 2004; 15(2): 111-4.
[http://dx.doi.org/10.1097/00019501-200403000-00007] [PMID: 15024299]

[9]   Fox KM, Mulcahy D, Findlay I, Ford I, Dargie HJ. The Total Ischaemic Burden European Trial (TIBET). Effects of atenolol, nifedipine SR and their combination on the exercise test and the total ischaemic burden in 608 patients with stable angina. Eur Heart J 1996; 17(1): 96-103.
[http://dx.doi.org/10.1093/oxfordjournals.eurheartj.a014699] [PMID: 8682138]

[10]   Döring G. Antianginal and anti-ischemic efficacy of nicorandil in comparison with isosorbide--mononitrate and isosorbide dinitrate: results from two multicenter, double-blind, randomized studies with stable coronary heart disease patients. J Cardiovasc Pharmacol 1992; 20(3) (Suppl. 3): S74-81.
[http://dx.doi.org/10.1097/00005344-199206203-00013] [PMID: 1282180]

[11]   Di Somma S, Liguori V, Petitto M, *et al.* A double-blind comparison of nicorandil and metoprolol in stable effort angina pectoris. Cardiovasc Drugs Ther 1993; 7(1): 119-23.
[http://dx.doi.org/10.1007/BF00878320] [PMID: 8485067]

[12]   Comparison of the anti-ischemic and anti-anginal effects of nicorandil and amlodipine in patients with stable angina pectoris: the SWAN study. J Clin Basic Cardiol 1999; 2: 213-7.

[13]   Effect of nicorandil on coronary events in patients with stable angina: the Impact Of Nicorandil in Angina (IONA) randomised trial. Lancet 2002; 359(9314): 1269-75.
[http://dx.doi.org/10.1016/S0140-6736(02)08265-X] [PMID: 11965271]

[14]   Chaitman BR, Laddu AA. Stable angina pectoris: antianginal therapies and future directions. Nat Rev Cardiol 2011; 9(1): 40-52.
[http://dx.doi.org/10.1038/nrcardio.2011.129] [PMID: 21878880]

[15]   Tardif J-C. for the INITIATIVE investigators. Efficacy of ivabradine, a new selective I_f inhibitor, compared with atenolol in patients with chronic stable angina. Eur Heart J 2005; 26: 2529-36.
[http://dx.doi.org/10.1093/eurheartj/ehi586] [PMID: 16214830]

[16]   Ruzyllo W, Tendera M, Ford I, Fox KM. Antianginal efficacy and safety of ivabradine compared with

amlodipine in patients with stable effort angina pectoris: a 3-month randomised, double-blind, multicentre, noninferiority trial. Drugs 2007; 67(3): 393-405.
[http://dx.doi.org/10.2165/00003495-200767030-00005] [PMID: 17335297]

[17]   Marzilli M, Klein WW. Efficacy and tolerability of trimetazidine in stable angina: a meta-analysis of randomized, double-blind, controlled trials. Coron Artery Dis 2003; 14(2): 171-9.
[http://dx.doi.org/10.1097/00019501-200304000-00010] [PMID: 12655281]

[18]   Fernandez SF, Tandar A, Boden WE. Emerging medical treatment for angina pectoris. Expert Opin Emerg Drugs 2010; 15(2): 283-98.
[http://dx.doi.org/10.1517/14728210903544482] [PMID: 20384546]

[19]   Montalescot G, Sechtem U, Achenbach S, *et al.* 2013 ESC guidelines on the management of stable coronary artery disease: the Task Force on the management of stable coronary artery disease of the European Society of Cardiology. Eur Heart J 2013; 34(38): 2949-3003.
[http://dx.doi.org/10.1093/eurheartj/eht296] [PMID: 23996286]

[20]   Mancini GB, Gosselin G, Chow B, *et al.* Canadian Cardiovascular Society guidelines for the diagnosis and management of stable ischemic heart disease. Can J Cardiol 2014; 30(8): 837-49.
[http://dx.doi.org/10.1016/j.cjca.2014.05.013] [PMID: 25064578]

[21]   Ambrosio G, Mugelli A, Lopez-Sendón J, Tamargo J, Camm J. Management of stable angina: A commentary on the European Society of Cardiology guidelines. Eur J Prev Cardiol 2016; 23(13): 1401-12.
[http://dx.doi.org/10.1177/2047487316648475] [PMID: 27222385]

[22]   Camm AJ, Manolis A, Ambrosio G, *et al.* Unresolved issues in the management of chronic stable angina. Int J Cardiol 2015; 201: 200-7.
[http://dx.doi.org/10.1016/j.ijcard.2015.08.045] [PMID: 26298381]

[23]   Thadani U. Management of stable angina – current guidelines: a critical appraisal. Cardiovasc Drugs Ther 2016; 30(4): 419-26.
[http://dx.doi.org/10.1007/s10557-016-6681-2] [PMID: 27638354]

[24]   Rousan TA, Mathew ST, Thadani U. Drug therapy for stable angina pectoris. Drugs 2017; 77(3): 265-84.
[http://dx.doi.org/10.1007/s40265-017-0691-7] [PMID: 28120185]

[25]   Tarkin JM, Kaski JC. Pharmacological treatment of chronic stable angina pectoris. Clin Med (Lond) 2013; 13(1): 63-70.
[http://dx.doi.org/10.7861/clinmedicine.13-1-63] [PMID: 23472498]

CHAPTER 15

Congenital Heart Defects

Abstract: Congenital heart disease is congenital anomalies that having heart defects origin form the birth. The structural abnormality of the heart, great vessels is diagnosed at the time of birth. It affects childbirth during pregnancy. Congenital heart defects change the blood flow to the heart. The defect ranges from mild to severe clinical symptoms that can lead to developing life-threatening conditions. The progression of congenital heart disease associated with genetic and non-genetic factors. The risk factors for include diabetes mellitus, viral infections, medications like ACE inhibitors, drinking alcohol and smoking during pregnancy, genetics may increase the more health care burden to diagnosed patients. The improper treatment of congenital heart defects can lead to the development of heart failure, cyanosis, stroke, and arrhythmia. The clinical symptoms of congenital heart defects include shortness of breath, chest pain, cyanosis, rapid heartbeat, cardiac murmur, edema can elevate the risk of heart defects. Physical examination of the patient, echocardiographic investigations are useful for the detection of heart defects. Effective prescribing pattern of ace inhibitors, arrhythmias, beta blockers, antiplatelet, and diuretics is used to enhance health condition of the patients.

Keywords: Alcohol, Congenital Heart Disease, Diabetes Mellitus, Measles Virus, Pregnancy, Smoking.

INTRODUCTION

It is one of the commonly occurring birth defects which are caused by the abnormal working function of the heart during the pregnancy. These defects are occurring from the heart walls cause heart defects. The abnormal blood flow movements from the valves, arteries, and veins to the heart cause congenital heart defects. The blockage of the arteries, veins and valves can modify the direction of blood flow that induces the formation of heart related problem to the affected population. It is usually diagnosed before and after pregnancy. Congenital heart defects occur during the first eight weeks of fetus development that affects 8 out of 1,000 babies. Regular treatment is needed to prevent the risk of developing congenital heart defects. Congenital heart defects were shown in Fig. (1). Congenital heart defects change the blood flow to the heart. The defect ranges from mild to severe clinical symptoms that can lead to developing life-threatening conditions. It is the most commonly occurring birth defect in newborns babies.

M.S. Umashankar & A. Bharath Kumar

Congenital heart defects most commonly seen birth defects in the newborns. Infant heart development occurs at conception and completely developed by eight weeks into the pregnancy [1 - 3].

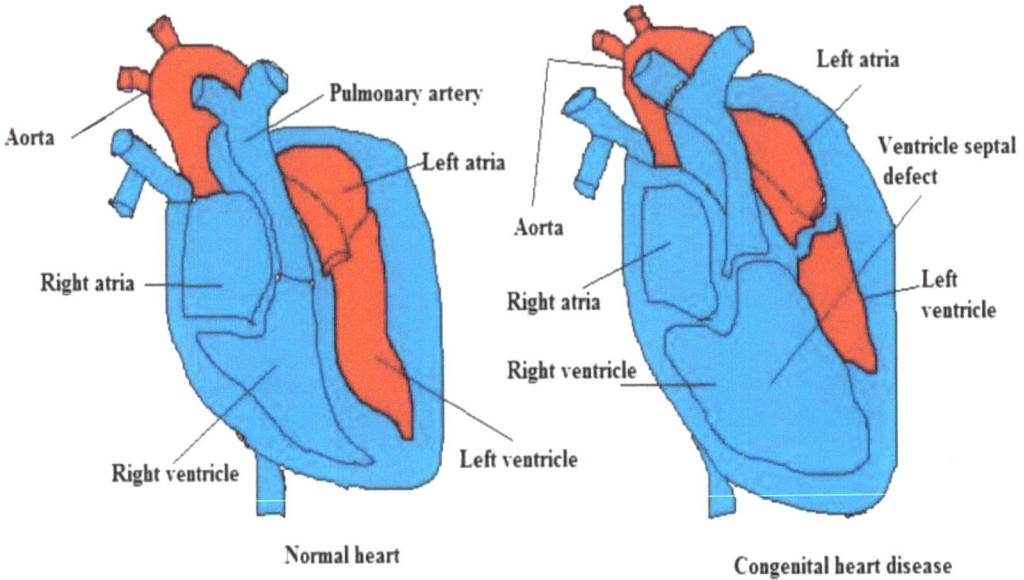

Fig. (1). Congenital heart disease.

TYPES OF CONGENITAL HEART DEFECTS

It Includes the Following Types

• Anomalous pulmonary venous return

• Pulmonary valve stenosis

• Tetralogy of Fallot

• Transposition of the great arteries or vessels

• Tricuspid valve atresia

• Atrial septal defect

• Atrioventricular septal defect

• Aortic valve stenosis

• Coarctation of the aorta

• Ebstein's anomaly

• Patent ductus arteriosus

• Pulmonary valve atresia

• Truncus arteriosus

• Ventricular septal defect

INTRODUCTION TO HEART

The heart is a muscular organ which is situated in the chest. The contraction of the heart muscles causes the pumping of blood to all vital organs in the body. It will distribute the deoxygenated blood to the lungs and collects oxygen thereby sends carbon dioxide to move out of the lungs. The heart and blood vessels are known as the circulatory system. The heat contract about 100,000 times per day and around 5 liters of blood is pumped each minute. Blood vessel sends the blood to reach all parts of the body. **Arteries are stained** with red due to oxygen rich carry ability and **veins are** blue colored due to poor oxygen poor carrying ability and sends the blood to the heart. **Capillaries** are tiny blood vessels and inside of tissues switching of gases can occur. The heart emits about 70 ml of blood during the contraction in an inactive stage which is equivalent to 5.25 liters of fluid per minute and 14,000 liters per day [4 - 6].

Location of Heart

The heart is situated in the medial portion of the lungs is called mediastinum. The heart is separated from the mediastinal structure through a layer is called pericardium. The dorsal surface of the heart located in vertebrae and sternum. The superior and inferior venae cavae, aorta and pulmonary trunk are connected to the heart. The inferior tip of the heart is connected to the left side of the sternum between the fourth and fifth ribs. The right portion of the heart is positioned anteriorly and the left side of the heart was projected towards posterior. The separated part of the apex is attached to the inferior lobe of the left lung is known as notch.

Size and Shape of the Heart

The shape of the heart is similar to a pinecone and heart size ranges from 12 cm in length, 8 cm in wide, and 6 cm in thickness. The human heart weight mostly differs in both sexes. The heart shape is represented with pinecone; the male heart weight ranges from 300–350 grams and female heart weight are approximately 250–300 grams [7, 8].

Chambers and Blood Circulation Process in the Heart

The heart is represented with four chambers which include the left side and the right side one atrium and the ventricle is located. Right and left atrium, acts as collecting chambers and contraction of cardiac muscles to sends the blood to the lower cavity and ventricles distribute blood to all the organs present in the body. Pulmonary value transport blood from the lungs and receives oxygen and delivers carbon dioxide. The right ventricle sends deoxygenated blood to the lungs and finally reaches the pulmonary arteries and oxygenated blood moves to pulmonary veins. It can pump the blood to the left atrium and left ventricle consecutively sends oxygenated blood to the aorta. Oxygen, nutrients present in blood can be utilized by the cells during the metabolic pathways. Carbon dioxide and metabolic fragments can penetrate to the blood. Capillaries are combined to form venules and larger veins connected to superior and inferior vena cava and right atrium. The blood present in the superior and inferior venacava reaches into right atrium and right ventricle.

Heart Chambers

Heart comprises of four chambers which include two atria and ventricles

Receiving chambers: Two atrial cells act as receiving chambers and having an essential role in the pumping of the blood.

Discharging chambers Ventricles are acts as a discharging chamber during its contraction; blood is ejected out of the heart and reaches the blood.

Septum It divides heart longitudinally into inter ventricular septum and interatrial septum.

Blood Vessels

Aorta: Blood move to the left portion of the heart through the arch of the aorta and sends to body tissues.

Pulmonary veins: The oxygenated blood is consumed by the lungs and returns to the left side of the heart.

Pulmonary arteries Pulmonary trunk divides right and left pulmonary arteries, and distributes blood to the lungs.

Superior and inferior vena cava Heart receives oxygen-poor blood from the veins through superior and inferior vena cava and sends to pulmonary circulation.

Heart Valves

It consists of four valves and sends the blood into heart chambers.

Mitral valve It is present between the left atrium and left ventricle.

Pulmonary valve It is situated between the right ventricle and the pulmonary artery.

Tricuspid valve It is positioned between the right atrium and right ventricle.

Aortic valve It is present between the left ventricle and the aorta.

ANATOMY OF HEART

Heart consists of four chambers: It includes atria and ventricle.

Atria It is present in the two upper cavities of the heart.

Ventricles It is situated in two lower chambers of the heart.

The heart wall is covered with three layers: It includes

Epicardium It is a protective layer of the heart and covered with connective tissue.

Myocardium It is covered with muscles of the heart.

Endocardium It is located on the inside of the heart and protects heart valves and chambers.

Pericardium It is enclosed with thin protective membrane known as pericardium.

Left Side of the Heart

Oxygenated blood shifted to the left atrium from pulmonary veins and which results in contraction of the left atrium and leads to the pumping of blood into the left ventricle.

Right Side of the Heart

The right atrium collects deoxygenated blood from superior and inferior vena cava. The contraction of the right atrium pumps the blood into the right ventricle. The complete filling of the right ventricle sends blood to the lungs through the pulmonary artery.

Covering Layers of Heart

The heart is surrounded by three covering layers. It includes pericardium, myocardium, epicardium. The pericardium is connected with strong connective tissue that protects the heart. The pericardium consists of two layers that include parietal pericardium linked to the fibrous pericardium and visceral pericardium is attached to the heart [9 - 11]. The pericardial cavity is located between epicardium and pericardium. A macroscopic layer consisting of the heart is covered with simple squamous epithelial cells known as mesothelium which is linked to the pericardium. Mesothelium cells produce lubricating serous fluid that can lower the rubbing during heart contractions. The heart wall is covered with three layers, which include epicardium, myocardium and endocardium. The middle layer is the myocardium which is made of collagenous fibers and contraction of myocardium membrane causes pumping of blood into the heart. The inner layer of the heart is endocardium connected to the myocardium with a small layer of connective tissue. The endocardium is lined with simple squamous epithelium cells and continues with blood vessels. The endothelium cells may control the growth of the cardiac muscle cells which secretes endothelins can monitor the concentration and relaxation of the heart.

Internal Structural Pattern of Heart

Septa Part of the Heart

Septa divide the heart into chambers. Septa is the other portion of myocardium cells which are covered with endocardium and situated between the two atria. The interatrial septum is represented with oval-shape called fossa ovalis which is connected to fetal heart called foramen ovale. It can permit the blood to the fetal heart through the right and left atrium. The foramen ovale can establish the blood circulation pattern to the heart [12 - 14]. The interventricular septum is positioned between two ventricles. The septum is situated between atria; ventricles are named as atrioventricular septum. It allows blood to pass into atria and ventricles towards the lungs and finally reaches into the pulmonary trunk and aorta.

Right Atrium

It collects blood from systemic circulation and sends to heart. The inferior vena cava receives blood from lower limbs, abdomen and pelvic region of the body. Eventually, superior vena cava drains the blood from coronary artery and move to the systemic circulation. The right atrium is smooth and having prominent ridges. The left atrium does not have ridges. The atria collect the venous blood continuously and to prevent the venous flow during the contraction of ventricles. The ventricular filling occurs during the atria relaxation and contraction blood is pumped into ventricles. The atrium and ventricle valve is controlled by a tricuspid valve.

Left Atrium

The blood can move constantly from pulmonary veins and to the atrium and act as a receiving chamber. The relaxation of the atria and ventricle the blood can move into heart. The completion of the ventricular relaxation phase the contraction of the left atria results in the blood can reach to right ventricle. The left atrium and ventricle valve is guarded by the mitral valve [15, 16].

Right Ventricle

It receives blood from the right atria and both sides of tricuspid valve are connected to connective tissue is known as chordae tendineae. There are many chordae tendineae is attached to each side of the tricuspid valve. The chordae tendineae are composed of collagenous fibers, elastic fibers and endothelium cells. The papillary muscles are enlarging from the ventricular surface and three papillary muscles are located in the right ventricle which is known as anterior, posterior, and septal muscles and connected to the respective valves [17, 18]. Ventricle walls are covered with trabeculae carneae and the edges of the cardiac muscles are enclosed with an endocardium layer known as a moderator band which can help during the cardiac conduction process. During the time of right ventricle contraction, the ventricle delivers blood into the pulmonary trunk. The lower surface of the pulmonary trunk and semi lunar valve can prevent the blood backflow from the pulmonary trunk.

Left Ventricle

The left side of the ventricle delivers blood to the vascular stream and sends blood to aorta through semi lunar valve. The valves provide unidirectional blood flow to the heart. The tricuspid valve situated between the right atrium and right ventricle. The pulmonary valve is situated at the base of the pulmonary trunk. The pulmonary valve lined with endothelial cells and connective tissue. The relaxation of ventricles causes returning blood flow into the ventricle. This blood circulation into the pulmonary valve results in producing heart sounds.

PHYSIOLOGY OF THE HEART

The heart can continuously pump the blood throughout the body. It is covered by muscular layers which help to contract and relax rhythmical manner during the life time of individuals. The cardiovascular system consists of four chambers. The upper part of the heart on both sides atrium is located, which can collect the blood from the heart. Atrium sends blood to the ventricle and it delivers blood to the heart during the cardiac contractions. The right side of the heart allows oxygen-poor blood from several portions of the body and transfer to the lungs. The oxygen is absorption takes place in the lungs and moves into the systemic circulation. The left side of the heart accepts oxygenated blood from the lungs and distribute to the body.

Systole

The contraction of the cardiac muscles in the ventricles is known as systole. During the ventricle contractions, blood reaches arteries. The elevated pressure during astringent of the ventricles is known as systolic pressure.

Diastole

The repose of cardiac muscles located in the ventricles is called diastole. The decrease of pressure during ventricular relaxation is known as diastolic pressure.

BLOOD SUPPLY TO HEART

The deoxygenated blood from superior and inferior vena cava moves to the heart. Blood moves into the right atrium, right ventricle and finally to the pulmonary trunk. Thereby it reaches to systemic circulation takes oxygen and eliminates the carbon dioxide from the in the blood. The blood present in the lungs proceeds to the heart through the pulmonary veins reaches to left atrium and leads to contraction of the left atrium sends the blood into the aorta and finally, it reaches systemic circulation and heart.

EPIDEMIOLOGY

The birth prevalence of congenital heart disease increased significantly from 0.6/1000 live birth between the years 1930 and 1934 to 9.1/1000 births. The incidence of congenital heart disease differed from various geographical locations. The birth prevalence of congenital heart disease was found to be high on Asia, which represents 9.3/1000 live births and a low rate of births found in Africa which includes 1.9/1000 live births. The second-highest rate of birth incidence was seen in Europe which includes 8.2/1000 live births. The high-income countries have high incidence as compared with low income countries. Globally the incidence of congenital heart disease ranges from 3.7 to 17.5/1000 live births which represent 30%–45% of all the birth defects. Previous research studies reported that the adult congenital heart disease diagnosed cases were high than the pediatric diagnosed cases.

It is the most common type of birth defect occurring in infants which can increase the risk of mortality. Previous studies reported that the incidence rate of congenital heart disease was ranging from 4 to 50 per 1000 live births. Congenital heart disease can affect the million of newborns every year. Approximately 20% of the congenital heart disease is caused by genetic syndromes and maternal diabetes and 80% of the congenital heart diseases are caused by the presence of various risk factors. The birth incidence of congenital heart disease was estimated at eight per 1000 live births. The burden of congenital heart disease was high in developing countries. Previous studies stated that the congenital heart disease was steadily increasing from younger adults. Previous studies estimated that every year 180,000 children are affected with congenital heart disease. The 25% of the babies have severe congenital heart disease.

Congenital heart disease is a leading cause of birth defects which is associated with infant illness and increases the death rate. Infant death occurs when the baby's age is less than 28 days. Nearly 48% of the deaths are occurred due to congenital heart disease in one year of age of infants. About 97% of babies born with non critical congenital heart disease are expected to survive one year of age. The 15% of the congenital heart diseases are associated with genetic conditions. About 20% of the people with congenital heart disease patients have a chance of developing cognitive defects [19 - 22]. The burden of congenital heart disease in India is identified to huge due to very high incidence of birth rate. India, it is estimated that every year more than 180,000 children's are born with congenital heart disease. The incidence of congenital heart disease in china was 62.10 per 10,000 patients and 6.5 percentages per 1000 births in Europe. The higher incidence of congenital heart disease may due to socioeconomic factors, environmental, genetic and ethnic factors.

Causes

• Anti-seizure medications.

• Alcohol

• Smoking

• Cocaine

• Diabetes

• Phenylketonuria

• Heredity

• Mutations

• Down syndrome

• Turner syndrome

• Viral infections

COMPLICATIONS [23]

Congenital heart disease may cause various complications which include

Arrhythmias

The abnormal production of the electrical impulses can cause irregular heartbeats which leads to develops cardiac arrhythmias.

Endocarditis

The heart chambers are covered with a thin membrane known as endocardium. The infection of the inner lining of the heart attacked by bacteria and damages the inner membrane of the heart which is called endocarditis.

Stroke

It occurs due to the interruption in the oxygen and blood supply to the brain can cause a stroke.

Heart Failure

The failure of the heart unable to meet the metabolic demands of the body can lead to developing heart failure.

Pulmonary Hypertension

This is a type of uncontrolled blood pressure which can affect the arteries present in the lungs. The congenital heart defects cause poor blood flow to the lungs can cause more pressure on the heart leads to the weakening of the cardiac contractions leads to develop cardiac abnormalities.

Heart Valve Problems

The poor blood flow to the heart valve may cause the progression of valve defects.

DIAGNOSIS

It includes

• Physical examination of the patient

• Echocardiogram studies

• Doppler studies

• Coronary angiogram

• Chest X-ray

• Cardiac catheterization

• Pulse Oximetry

• MRI scan

• CT scan

• Trans esophageal echocardiogram

CLINICAL MANIFESTATIONS

It includes:

• Trouble breathing

• Cyanosis

• Poor eating habits

• Fatigue

• Swelling in the abdomen

• Swelling around the eyes

• Rapid heartbeat

• A heart murmur

• A bluish tint to skin, lips, and fingernails

• Shortness of breath

• Poor weight gain in infants

• Gray or blue skin coloring

• Swollen belly

• Puffiness around the eyes

• Trouble breathing while feeding

• Sweating, especially while feeding

PATHOPHYSIOLOGY

Heart failure occurs due to cardiac output is insufficient to meet the body's metabolic demand which causes pulmonary congestion and edema in the tissues. The ductus arteriosus is a normal connection between the pulmonary artery and aorta which is needed for proper blood flow to the fetus.

Congenital heart disease is associated with shunting lesions. The oxygenated and deoxygenated blood flows in a parallel direction. The deoxygenated blood returns to the right atrium and moved to the lungs. The oxygenated blood returns from the pulmonary veins to the left atrium and pumped to the arch of the aorta. The shunt refers to the abnormality in the flow of the blood from one side to another side. The deoxygenated blood moved to the left heart and reduces the systemic arterial oxygen saturation.

The abnormal hemoglobin levels lead to the cause of the cyanosis. The abnormal levels of cyanosis cause multiple complications to include thromboembolism, bleeding disorders, hyperuricemia occurs in the infants. The reduction in the pulmonary blood flow to the heart can increase the risk of heart murmurs. Depending on the anomaly may reduce the blood flow to the heart and results in cyanosis. The elevated pulmonary blood flow causes high pressure in blood flow which causes the development of pulmonary vascular disease.

The left to right shunts cause abnormal blood pulmonary blood flow which increases the risk of left ventricular volume over load and increases the risk of heart failure. The poor blood flow in the vascular stream obstructs to increase ventricular hypertrophy leads to heart failure. The obstruction of the blood flow in the blood vessel can increase high pressure gradient across the blood vessels cause heart failure.

The blood flow in the circulation in each side of the shunt increases the blood demand on the ventricles. The volume of the shunted blood flow can determine the progression of clinical symptoms. The progression of aortic valve sclerosis occurs from sclerosis to stenosis and the left ventricle difficult to eject the blood from the systole. Higher systolic pressure was produced by the ventricles than the pressure produced by the calcified aortic valve.

The LV becomes physiologically hypertrophied, reflecting its level of work, whereas the RV myocardium remains thin. The abnormal function of the left ventricle can affect the blood flow to the heart and alter the cardiac contractions. Patients with increased right ventricular pressure can increase the risk of congenital obstructions in the pulmonary veins. The higher ventricular resistance in the veins can increase the risk of pulmonary hypertension.

The severe right ventricular pressure can alter the blood circulation to the heart which causes the atrial septal defects. The closing of AV valves can cause blood flow obstruction to atria and alter the systole. The blood volumes in the two atria are equilibrium in systole and result in changes in blood flow to left atria to right atria during the cardiac cycle. Av valve regurgitation can cause atrial septal defects in cardiac cycle events.

Tricuspid regurgitation may slow down the blood flow to the atria. The size of the atria septal defects helps to determine the lesions present in the heart valves. The size of the lesion is high which can resist the blood flow to the heart valves which leads to cause the congenital heart defects.

PREVENTION

• Vaccination against influenza and rubella infections and measles

• Consumption of 400 micrograms of folic acid supplementation during the first trimester of pregnancy

• Avoiding the consumption of OTC medications

• Maintaining controlled levels of hypertension and diabetes mellitus

• Smoking cessation during pregnancy

• Alcoholic cessation during pregnancy

• Genetic screening for congenital heart disease

TREATMENT [24, 25]

Thrombolytic Drugs

Thrombolytic drugs are prescribed to reduce the formation of a blood clot in the blood vessels and also lower the severity of stroke. These drugs will act by conversion of plasminogen which forms plasmin and activates the fibrin bound plasminogen. Fibrin molecules are inhibited by plasmin which leads to the breakdown of clot the blood vessels and reduces the stroke complications.

It includes

•Anistreplase

•Reteplase

•Streptokinase

•T-pa

•Tenecteplase

•Alteplase

•Urokinase

Adverse drug reactions Internal bleeding, damage to the blood vessels, renal damage.

Anti Platelet Drugs

These drugs help to prevent the platelet aggregation and reduce the clot in the blood vessels.

Types of Antiplatelet Agents

• aspirin

• dipyridamole

• clopidogrel

• ticagrelor

Clinical uses of antiplatelet agents It is used to treat following disease conditions.

• Coronary artery disease

• Heart attack

• Angina pectoris

• Stroke and transient ischemic attacks

• Peripheral artery disease

Side Effects Nausea, gastric problems, diarrhea, rashes, itching.

Beta Blockers

It reduces the work load on the heart and reduces stress and hormones levels in the body which leads to vasodilatation in the blood vessels.

Commonly prescribed beta blockers include

• Atenolol

• Bisoprolol

• Nadolol

• Nebivolol

• Carvedilol

• Labetalol

• Nebivolol

• Pindolol

• Propranolol

• Timolol

• Metoprolol

Adverse effects Dry mouth, dry skin, feelings of coldness, diarrhea, shortness of breath and insomnia.

Angiotensin Converting Enzyme (ACE) Inhibitors

ACEs block the conversion of angiotensin I to angiotensin II by the action of angiotensinogen in the body and help to lower the vasoconstriction and promote vasodilation.

It includes

• Captopril

• Lisinopril

- Fosinopril

- Ramipril

- Benazepril

- Enalapril

- Perindopril

- Quinapril

- Moexipril

- Trandolapril

Adverse effects Dry cough, hyperkalemia, fatigue, headaches and loss of taste.

Angiotensin II Receptor Blockers

It blocks the conversion of angiotensin II from its binding to angiotensin II receptors located on the blood vessels and produce vasodialtion in the blood vessels.

These drugs include

- Candesartan

- Telmisartan

- Valsartan

- Eprosartan

- Irbesartan

- Losartan

Adverse effects Hyperkalemia, dizziness, headache, cough, diarrhea, hypotension and angioedema.

Classifications of Antiarrhythmic Agents

It includes

Class IA Drugs

• Disopryamide

• Quinidine

• Procainamide

Class IB Drugs

• Mexiletine

• Lidocaine

• Tocainide

Class IC Drugs

• Moricizine

• Flecainide

• Propafenone

Class II: Beta Blockers

• Metoprolol

• Atenolol

• Propranolol

• Esmolol

• Timolol

Class III: Potassium (K) Channels Blockers

• Dofetilide

• Sotalol

• Amiodarone

• Ibutilide

Calcium Channel Blockers

This drug blocks the entry of calcium ions into the calcium channels and lowers the work load on the heart and dilates the arteries leads to vasodilatation.

These drugs include

• Diltiazem

• Verapamil

• Isradipine

• Nifedipine

• Nicardipine

• Nimopidine

• Amlodipine

• Nisoldipine

• Bepridil

• Felodipine

Adverse effects Rashes, headache, constipation, flushing, edema, drowsiness

Diuretics

Loop diuretics These drugs will inhibit the sodium potassium co transport mechanism in the ascending loop of henle, leads to an increase in the distal tubular concentration of sodium and reduced levels of hyprertonicity of the sodium levels in the intestine cause diueresis.

• Loop diuretics include

• Bumetanide

• Furosemide

• Ethacrynate

• Torsemide

Adverse effects Hypokalemia, alkalosis, hypomagnesemia, hyperuricemia, dehydration, ototoxicity.

Thiazides diuretics These drugs inhibit the sodium-chloride transporter in the distal tubule and reabsorption of sodium ions causes the elimination of more water from the body.

• Chlorothiazide

• Chlorthalidone

• Indapamide

• Hydrochlorothiazide

• Methyclothiazide

Adverse effects Hyponatremia, hyperglycemia, dehydration, hypokalemia, hypertriglyceridemia, hyperuricemia, azotemia.

Carbonic anhydrase inhibitors These drugs will inhibit the transport of bicarbonate ions from the proximal convulted tubule which leads to loss of sodium, hydrogen and bicarbonate ions in the urine.

Drugs include

• Acetazolamide

• Methazolamide

Adverse effects Metabolic acidosis and hypokalemia

Potassium sparing diuretics It acts on the distal segment of the distal tubules and causes more water to enter inside the collecting tubule. It will inhibit the aldosterone-sensitive sodium reabsorption thereby loss of potassium and hydrogen from the urine.

• Amiloride

• Spironolactone

• Triamterene

Adverse effects Metabolic acidosis, gynecomastia, hyperkalemia, gastric ulcers.

Bosentan

It is used to treat pulmonary hypertension in the arteries. It is used to dilate the blood vessels present in the lungs.

Adverse effects Hepatotoxicity, embryo-fetal toxicity and fluid Retention

Digoxin

It is used to treat the irregular heartbeats which include tachycardia, atrial flutter, and supraventricular tachycardia. Digoxin has an electrophysiological and hemodynamic effect on the cardiovascular system. It will reversibly inhibit the Na-K ATPase enzyme which is responsible for maintaining the intra cellular environment and balance of potassium, sodium and calcium ions into the cells. The inhibition of the sodium pump by Na-K ATPase leads to an increase in the contraction as well as cardiac function of the heart.

Adverse effects Diarrhea, blurred vision, nausea, vomiting, confusion, dizziness and irregular heartbeats.

Sildenafil

It is used to treat pulmonary hypertension in the veins. It is a potent inhibitor of phosphodiesterase type 5 (PDE5) in the pulmonary blood vessels. It will increase the cGMP levels in the pulmonary vascular smooth muscle cells results in relaxation of the blood vessels causes vasodilation in the lungs.

Adverse effect Nasal congestion, headache, altered vision, flushing, dizziness and dyspepsia.

Warfarin

Warfarin is a vitamin K antagonist that acts to inhibit the production of vitamin K by epoxide reductase enzyme and also inhibits the carboxylation activity of glutamyl carboxylase that can lower the formation of blood clots in the blood vessels. It will inhibit the carboxylation activity of glutamyl carboxylase which can inhibit the formation of blood clot in the blood vessels.

Adverse effects Ecchymoses, epistaxis, renal bleeding and hepatic bleeding.

CONCLUSION

The heart is a muscular organ which is situated in the chest. The contraction of the heart muscles causes the pumping of blood to all vital organs in the body. It will distribute the deoxygenated blood to the lungs and collects oxygen thereby sends carbon dioxide to move out of the lungs. The higher incidence of congenital heart disease may due to socioeconomic factors, environmental, genetic and ethnic factors. Congenital heart defects are one of the major public health care issuesthat depend on its high prevalence. Congenital heart defects are most commonly affects 1% of the births annually. There is a need for clinical pharmacist care services with the health care team on initiation of awareness programmes on heart defects and educating the patients about disease clinical symptoms, disease screening, risk factors control and lifestyle modification practices that can lower the progression of the heart disease complications. Effective understanding of risk factors, causes, and pathophysiological mechanisms may direct the newer directions for the management of heart defects. Designing public health policies, and novel treatment guidelines and conducting regular screening programmes by the health care team in the patients care areas can reduce the health care expenditure to the patients. Novel ultrasonography examinations are beneficial for early detection and prevention of congenital heart disease in the fetus.

REFERENCES

[1]   Mitchell SC, Korones SB, Berendes HW. Congenital heart disease in 56,109 births. Incidence and natural history. Circulation 1971; 43(3): 323-32.
[http://dx.doi.org/10.1161/01.CIR.43.3.323] [PMID: 5102136]

[2]   Jackson M, *et al.* Epidemiology of congenital heart disease in Merseyside–1979 to 1988. Cardiol Young 1996; 6(4): 272-80.
[http://dx.doi.org/10.1017/S1047951100003899]

[3]   Sullivan ID. Prenatal diagnosis of structural heart disease: does it make a difference to survival? Heart 2002; 87(5): 405-6.
[http://dx.doi.org/10.1136/heart.87.5.405] [PMID: 11997402]

[4]   Tondon A, Sengupta S, Shukla V, Danda S. Risk factors for congenital heart disease in Vellore, India. Curr Res J Biol Sci 2010; 2: 253-8.

[5]   Bolger AP, Coats AJ, Gatzoulis MA. Congenital heart disease: the original heart failure syndrome. Eur Heart J 2003; 24(10): 970-6.
[http://dx.doi.org/10.1016/S0195-668X(03)00005-8] [PMID: 12714029]

[6]   Chadha SL, Singh N, Shukla DK. Epidemiological study of congenital heart disease. Indian J Pediatr 2001; 68(6): 507-10.
[http://dx.doi.org/10.1007/BF02723241] [PMID: 11450379]

[7]   Miller A, Riehle-Colarusso T, Alverson CJ, Frías JL, Correa A. Congenital heart defects and major structural noncardiac anomalies, Atlanta, Georgia, 1968 to 2005. J Pediatr 2011; 159(1): 70-78.e2.
[http://dx.doi.org/10.1016/j.jpeds.2010.12.051] [PMID: 21329942]

[8]   Bruno CJ, Havranek T. Screening for critical congenital heart disease in newborns. Adv Pediatr 2015; 62(1): 211-26.
[http://dx.doi.org/10.1016/j.yapd.2015.04.002] [PMID: 26205115]

[9]   Olney RS, Ailes EC, Sontag MK. Detection of critical congenital heart defects: Review of contributions from prenatal and newborn screening. Semin Perinatol 2015; 39(3): 230-7.
[http://dx.doi.org/10.1053/j.semperi.2015.03.007] [PMID: 25979782]

[10]   Bouma BJ, Mulder BJ. Changing landscape of congenital heart disease. Circ Res 2017; 120(6): 908-22.
[http://dx.doi.org/10.1161/CIRCRESAHA.116.309302] [PMID: 28302739]

[11]   Massaro AN, El-Dib M, Glass P, Aly H. Factors associated with adverse neurodevelopmental outcomes in infants with congenital heart disease. Brain Dev 2008; 30(7): 437-46.
[http://dx.doi.org/10.1016/j.braindev.2007.12.013] [PMID: 18249516]

[12]   McQuillen PS, Miller SP. Congenital heart disease and brain development. Ann N Y Acad Sci 2010; 1184: 68-86.
[http://dx.doi.org/10.1111/j.1749-6632.2009.05116.x] [PMID: 20146691]

[13]   Hoffman JI, Kaplan S. The incidence of congenital heart disease. J Am Coll Cardiol 2002; 39(12): 1890-900.
[http://dx.doi.org/10.1016/S0735-1097(02)01886-7] [PMID: 12084585]

[14]   Moons P, Sluysmans T, De Wolf D, *et al.* Congenital heart disease in 111 225 births in Belgium: birth prevalence, treatment and survival in the 21st century. Acta Paediatr 2009; 98(3): 472-7.
[http://dx.doi.org/10.1111/j.1651-2227.2008.01152.x] [PMID: 19046347]

[15]   Marelli AJ, Mackie AS, Ionescu-Ittu R, Rahme E, Pilote L. Congenital heart disease in the general population: changing prevalence and age distribution. Circulation 2007; 115(2): 163-72.
[http://dx.doi.org/10.1161/CIRCULATIONAHA.106.627224] [PMID: 17210844]

[16]   Brickner ME, Hillis LD, Lange RA. Congenital heart disease in adults. First of two parts. N Engl J Med 2000; 342(4): 256-63.
[http://dx.doi.org/10.1056/NEJM200001273420407] [PMID: 10648769]

[17]   Abqari S, Gupta A, Shahab T, Rabbani MU, Ali SM, Firdaus U. Profile and risk factors for congenital heart defects: A study in a tertiary care hospital. Ann Pediatr Cardiol 2016; 9(3): 216-21.
[http://dx.doi.org/10.4103/0974-2069.189119] [PMID: 27625518]

[18]   Stout KK, Daniels CJ, Aboulhosn JA, *et al.* AHA/ACC Guideline for the Management of Adults With Congenital Heart Disease: Executive Summary: A Report of the American College of Cardiology/American Heart Association Task Force on Clinical Practice Guidelines J Am Coll Cardiol 2018.

[19]   Lui GK, Saidi A, Bhatt AB, *et al.* Diagnosis and Management of Noncardiac Complications in Adults With Congenital Heart Disease: A Scientific Statement From the American Heart Association. Circulation 2017; 136(20): e348-92.
[http://dx.doi.org/10.1161/CIR.0000000000000535] [PMID: 28993401]

[20]   Schmaltz AA, Bauer UM. [Adults with congenital heart disease: treatment and medical problems]. Herz 2013; 38(6): 639-51.
[http://dx.doi.org/10.1007/s00059-013-3927-7] [PMID: 23942735]

[21]   Warnes CA, Williams RG, Bashore TM, *et al.* ACC/AHA 2008 guidelines for the management of adults with congenital heart disease. Circulation 2008; 118: 714-833.

[22]   Van De Bruaene A, Meier L, Droogne W, *et al.* Management of acute heart failure in adult patients with congenital heart disease. Heart Fail Rev 2018; 23(1): 1-14.
[http://dx.doi.org/10.1007/s10741-017-9664-x] [PMID: 29277859]

[23]   Karamlou T, Diggs BS, Person T, Ungerleider RM, Welke KF. National practice patterns for management of adult congenital heart disease: operation by pediatric heart surgeons decreases in-hospital death. Circulation 2008; 118(23): 2345-52.
[http://dx.doi.org/10.1161/CIRCULATIONAHA.108.776963] [PMID: 18997167]

[24]   Chaix MA, Andelfinger G, Khairy P. Genetic testing in congenital heart disease: A clinical approach. World J Cardiol 2016; 8(2): 180-91.
[http://dx.doi.org/10.4330/wjc.v8.i2.180] [PMID: 26981213]

[25]   Vehmeijer JT, Brouwer TF, Limpens J, *et al.* Implantable cardioverter-defibrillators in adults with congenital heart disease: a systematic review and meta-analysis. Eur Heart J 2016; 37(18): 1439-48.
[http://dx.doi.org/10.1093/eurheartj/ehv735] [PMID: 26873095]

CHAPTER 16

Inflammatory Heart Disease

Abstract: The inflammation of the heart muscles is caused by the virus, fungi, bacteria, food, smoke, air, and parasites that increase the inflammatory conditions in the heart muscles known as inflammatory heart disease. Endocarditis is an infection that occurs in the inner lining of the heart valves. Endocarditis commonly occurs by the bacteria, fungi or other microbial species present in the body, reaches the blood stream and leads to damaging the heart. Myocarditis is an inflammation of the myocardium which is present in the middle layer of the heart. It is caused by a viral species infection. The clinical manifestations of the myocarditis include chest pain, fatigue, edema, breathlessness, joint pain, fever, weakness, palpitations and abnormal heart rhythms. Pericarditis is a clinical condition in which the cell membrane around the heart is inflamed. The more amount of fluid deposit around the heart may increase the risk of inflammation and causes pericarditis. The electrocardiogram, chest x-ray, echocardiogram, treadmill test; coronary angiogram test can determine the severity of cardiovascular disease. The management of inflammatory heart disease includes antibiotics, corticosteroids, antiplatelets, diuretics, angiotensin converting enzyme inhibitors, and beta blockers control the progression of inflammatory situations associated with the heart.

Keywords: Antibiotics, Antiplatelets, Electrocardiogram, Endocarditis, Myocarditis, Pericarditis.

ENDOCARDITIS

It is an infection that occurs in the inner lining of the heart valves. Endocarditis was caused by the bacteria, fungi or other microbial species present in the body, reaches the bloodstream and leads to damaging the heart. The ineffective treatment of endocarditis leads to increases in the risk of life threatening conditions. It is also called infective endocarditis, because the inflammation in the heart valves and heart chambers results in the development of risk of inflammatory endocarditis. It is shown in Fig. (**1**).

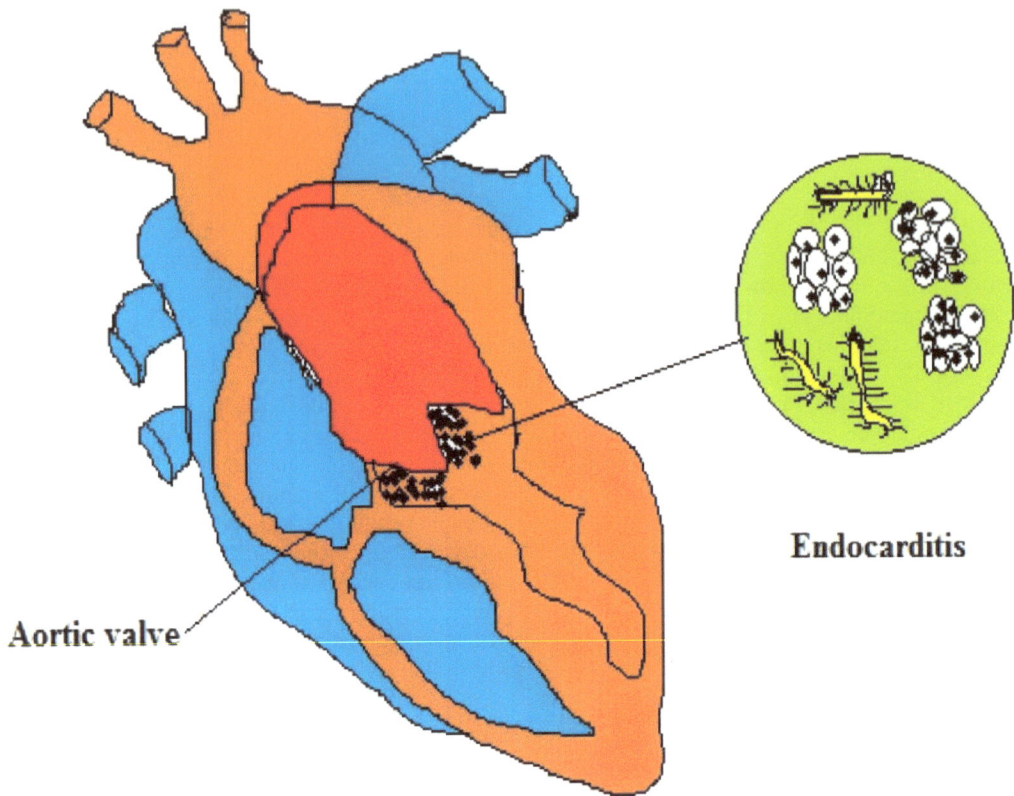

Fig. (1). Endocarditis.

Types of Endocarditis

Depending on the microbial infection is classified into following types

Acute Endocarditis

It is mostly occurred by the aggressive species of staphylococcus bacteria enters into blood stream and damages the heart valve. The entry of the bacteria into the heart valves and multiplies that and forms the septic emboli in the blood stream which leads to damage to the heart valves [1 - 3].

Subacute Endocarditis

It is a type of endocarditis which is caused by the Streptococi group of microbiological species. Streptococus can cause sub-acute endocarditis which also causes gastrointestinal problems. The pathophysiology of inflammatory heart disease is shown in Fig. (**2**).

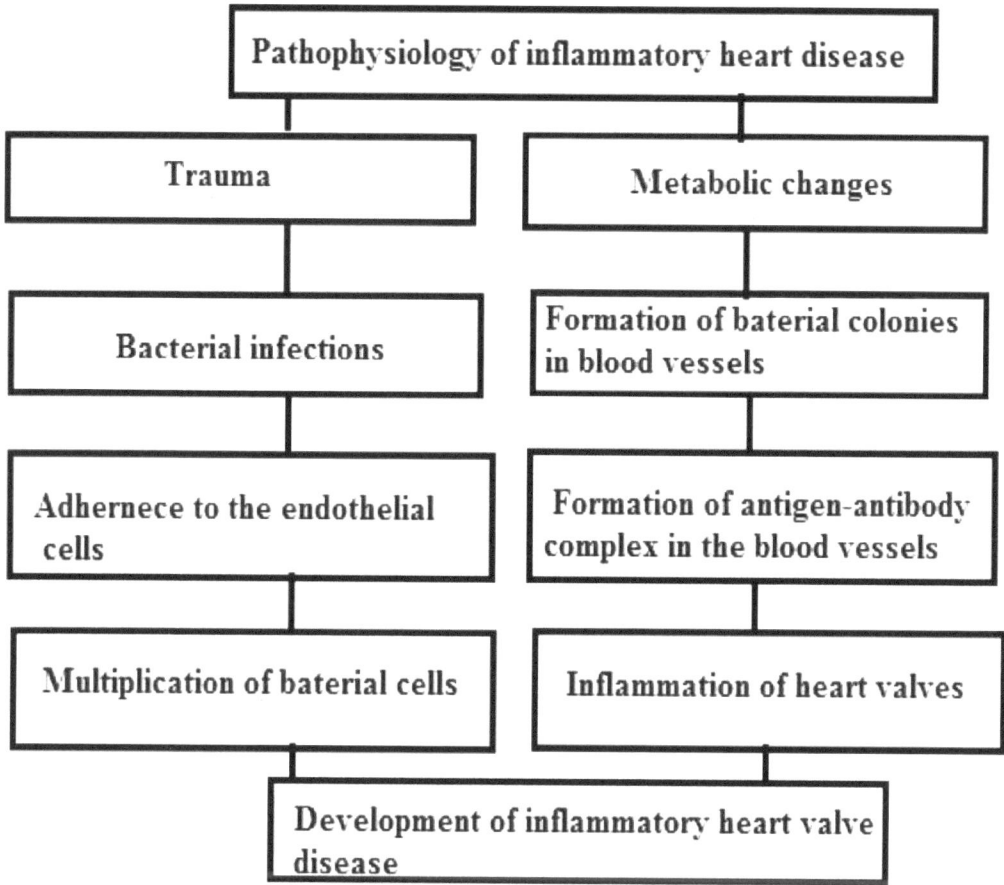

Fig. (2). Pathophysiology of inflammatory heart disease.

Epidemiology

From 1993 to 2003, 3784 patients were affected with infective endocarditis. The incidence of infective endocarditis was <5 per 100,000 patients per year in 50 years of age patients and >15 per 100,000 patients at the age of 65 years. Previous research studies stated that the prevalence of infective endocarditis increased in older aged patients at the age of 50 years. The prevalence of endocarditis is from 0.7 and 6.2 per 10,000 patients per year and it is expected to raise this count in the future.

Clinical Symptoms

It includes

• Fever

- Weakness

- Night sweats

- Shortness of breath

- Fatigue

- Aching joints and muscles

- Paleness

- Swelling in the feet, and legs

- Less common symptoms include

- Weight loss

- Bleeding under the nails

- Blood in urine

- Heart murmur

- Painful, red bumps on the pads of the fingers and toes

COMPLICATIONS [4, 5]

It includes

Cardiovascular disease

Stroke

Enlarged spleen

Seizure

Pulmonary embolism

Kidney damage

Diagnosis

It includes

Physical examination of the patient

Echocardiogram studies

Doppler studies

Coronary angiogram

Chest X-ray

Cardiac catheterization

Pulse Oximetry

MRI scan

CT scan

Trans esophageal echocardiogram

Treatment [6 - 10]

Treatment Regimens for Infectious Endocarditis

• Penicillin G

• Ampicillin

• ceftriaxone

• Gentamicin

• Nafcillin

• Oxacillin

• Vancomycin

• Clindamycin

• Clarithromycin

• Ampicillin

• Vancomycin

• Gentamicin

• Cephalexin

• Cefazolin

• Azithromycin

Myocarditis

It is an inflammation of the myocardium which is present in the middle layer of the heart. It is caused by a viral species infection. The clinical manifestations of the myocarditis include chest pain, breathlessness, palpitations and abnormal heart rhythms. It is a severe clinical condition in which the weakening of the heart muscles not able to supply sufficient blood supply to the body requirements leads to forms the clot in the blood vessels thereby which raise the risk of progression of cardiovascular disease. The global incidence of myocarditis was 22 cases of 100,000 patients annually [11, 12].

Causes

It includes

• Viral species such as adenovirus, parvovirus, and herpes simplex virus, echoviruses, Epstein-Barr virus and german measles virus

• Bacterial species such as staphylococcus, streptococcus

• Parasites as trypanosomacruzi and toxoplasma

• Fungi infections

• Chemicals

• Penicillin allergic reactions

• Radiation

• Wegener's granulomatosis

Pathophysiology

It occurs with the inflammation of the myocardium with necrosis of the cardiac cells. The myocardial injury is caused by the infectious species such as bacteria, virus and fungi may increase the inflammatory reactions in the body lead to an increase in the risk of inflammation.

The entero virus species enter into the gastrointestinal tract cells and attack the heart tissues which increase the risk of inflammation. The early phase of myocarditis is initiated by infection of myocytes through endocytosis. During the inflammation the release of cytokines from macrophages and stimulation of natural killer cells through cell lysis which contributes to altering the myocardial cells function. The stimulation of T-cells, B-cells, and the conscription of leucocytes to the infected areas can elevate the severity of the inflammatory process and finally damage the cardiomyocytes that increase the risk of myocarditis [13, 14].

Clinical Symptoms of Myocarditis

It includes

• Chest pain

• Fever

• Fainting

• Swelling of legs, ankles and feet

• Abnormal heart rhythms

• Shortness of breath

• Fatigue

• Breathing difficulties

• Rapid breathing

• Joint pain

• Diagnosis test

• Electrocardiogram

• Chest X-ray

• Echocardiogram

• Coronary angiogram

• MRI scan

• Blood tests

• Holter monitor

Prevention

It includes

• Consumption of healthy diet

• Proper health hygiene

• Minimize the health risk

• Early immunization

• Avoid illegal sex practice and use of illegal drugs

• Avoid exposure to ticks

TREATMENT

Treatment for myocarditis may include [15, 16]

Anti-platelet Drugs

These drugs help to prevent the platelet aggregation and reduce the clot in the blood vessels.

<u>*Types of Antiplatelet Agents*</u>

• Aspirin

• Dipyridamole

• Clopidogrel

• Ticagrelor

<u>*Clinical Uses of Antiplatelet Agents*</u>

It is used to treat the following disease conditions.

• Angina pectoris

• Heart attack

• Coronary artery disease

• Stroke

• Peripheral artery disease

Side Effects Nausea, gastric problems, diarrhea, rashes, and itching.

Blood Pressure Lowering Medications [17 - 19]

Diuretics

Loop Diuretics

These drugs will inhibit the sodium potassium co transport mechanism in the ascending loop of henle it leads to an increase in the distal tubular concentration of sodium and reduced levels of hyprertonicity of sodium levels in the intestine cause diuresis.

Loop diuretics include

• Bumetanide

• Furosemide

• Ethacrynate

• Torsemide

Adverse effects Hypokalemia, alkalosis, hypomagnesemia, hyperuricemia, dehydration, ototoxicity.

Thiazides Diuretics

These drugs inhibit the sodium-chloride transporter in the distal tubule and reabsorption of sodium ions causes the elimination of more water from the body.

• Chlorothiazide

• Chlorthalidone

• Indapamide

• Hydrochlorothiazide

• Methyclothiazide

Adverse effects Hyponatremia, hyperglycemia, hypokalemia, hyperlipidmeia, hyperuricemia, azotemia.

Carbonic Anhydrase Inhibitors

These drugs will inhibit the transport of bicarbonate ions from the proximal convulted tubule which leads to loss of sodium, hydrogen and bicarbonate ions in the urine.

The drugs include

Acetazolamide

Methazolamide

Adverse effects Metabolic acidosis and hypokalemia

Potassium Sparing Diuretics

It acts on the distal segment of the distal tubules and causes more water to enter inside the collecting tubule. It will inhibit the aldosterone-sensitive sodium reabsorption thereby loss of potassium and hydrogen from the urine.

• Amiloride

• Spironolactone

• Triamterene

• Adverse effects

• Metabolic acidosis

• Gynecomastia

• Hyperkalemia

• Gastric ulcers

Angiotensin Converting Enzyme Inhibitors

ACE inhibitors block the conversion of angiotensin I to angiotensin II by the action of angiotensinogen in the body and help to lower the vasoconstriction and promote vasodilation.

It includes

- Captopril

- Lisinopril

- Fosinopril

- Ramipril

- Benazepril

- Enalapril

- Perindopril

- Quinapril

- Moexipril

- Trandolapril

Adverse effects Dry cough, hyperkalemia, fatigue, headaches and loss of taste.

Angiotensin II Receptor Blockers

It blocks the conversion of angiotensin II from its binding to angiotensin II receptors located on the blood vessels and produces vasodialtion in the blood vessels.

These drugs include

- Candesartan

- Telmisartan

- Valsartan

- Eprosartan

- Irbesartan

- Losartan

Adverse effects Hyperkalemia, dizziness, headache, cough, diarrhea, hypotension and angioedema.

Beta Blockers

It reduces the work load on the heart and reduces stress and hormones levels in the body which leads to vasodilatation in the blood vessels.

Commonly prescribed beta blockers include

• Atenolol

• Bisoprolol

• Nadolol

• Nebivolol

• Carvedilol

• Labetalol

• Nebivolol

• Pindolol

• Propranolol

• Timolol

• Metoprolol

Adverse effects Dry mouth, dry skin, feelings of coldness, diarrhea, shortness of breath and insomnia.

Tetracycilne

It includes chlortetracycline, doxycycline, and minocycline.

Mechanism of action It diffuses into the protein channels present in the bacterial cell membrane and binds to the 30S ribosomal units and prevents the binding of tRNA to mRNA ribosomal units and alters the protein synthesis.

• Adverse effects

• Muscle pain

• Sunburn

• Changes in the amount of urine

• Tooth discoloration

• Numbness of the hands

• Severe stomach abdominal pain

• Dark urine

Corticosteroids

Mechanism of Action of Corticosteroids

These drugs enter into the cells and coupled with steroid receptors in the cytoplasm and regulate the protein synthesis process. Proteins can inhibit the enzyme phospholipaseA2 and control the inflammatory reactions in the body.

Corticosteroids include

• Bethamethasone

• Prednisone

• Prednisolone

• Dexamethasone

• Fludrocortisone

• Prednisolone

• Triamcinolone

• Methylprednisolone

• Dexamethasone

• Hydrocortisone

• Adverse effects

• High blood pressure

• Loss of potassium

• Headache

• swelling of the legs

- Muscle weakness

- weight gain

- Puffiness of the face

- Facial hair growth

- Slow wound healing

- Cataracts

- Glaucoma

- Ulcers in the stomach and duodenum

PERICARDITIS

The pericardium is a covering layer of the heart that holds the heart makes work as normal. Pericarditis is a clinical condition in which the cell membrane around the heart is inflamed. The more amount of fluid deposit around the heart may increase the risk of inflammation and causes pericarditis.It is mainly caused by the infection, trauma, metabolic disorders that can manifest the clinical symptoms of pericarditis [20 - 22].

Types of Pericarditis

It includes

Acute Fibrinous Pericarditis

It occurs when the inflammation of the covering layer of the fibrin causes fibrinous pericarditis.

Acute Purulent Pericarditis

The infection of pericardium covered with pus may cause purulent pericarditis.

Acute Constrictive Pericarditis

The pericardium has a solid mass of calcified fibrosis material that can cause inflammation in the pericardium known as **constrictive pericarditis.**

Chronic Pericarditis

The chronic length of tuberculosis infection causes fluid deposition around the heart muscles causes inflammation of pericarditis.

The incidence of pericarditis was 0.2% to 0.4% in patients with cardiac surgery and idiopathic pericarditis occurs 1 in 100 cases. The idiopathic pericarditis commonly occurs in the developed countries.

Pathophysiology

Acute Pericarditis

It develops a rapid manner and causes inflammation of the pericardial cell membrane causes adverse hemodynamic effects and rhythm disturbances.

Sub-acute Pericarditis

It develops within a week to months. The fibrotic tissue contains calcium leads to lowers the thickness of the pericardium and impairs the ventricular filling and cardiac output causes abnormal heart rhythms and leads to develop the pericarditis.

Causes of Pericarditis

• Infections

• Bronchitis

• Herpes simplex viral infections

• Influenza

• Hepatitis C

• Tuberculosis

• Rheumatoid arthritis

• Radiotherapy

• Kidney Failure

• Symptoms

• Shortness of breath

• Cough

• Fatigue

• Ascites

• Edema

• Heart palpitations

• Difficulty breathing

• Cough

• Leg swelling

• Chest pain

• Anxiety

Diagnostic Test

It includes

• Electrocardiogram

• Chest x ray

• Echocardiography

• MRI scan

• Antinuclear antibody

• Blood culture

• Erythrocyte sedimentation rate

• HIV test

• Tuberculin skin test

Treatment [23 - 25]

NSAIDs

<u>*Mechanism of Action*</u>

It will inhibit the cyclo-oxygenase enzymes and inhibit the production of prostacyclin and lowers the progression of the inflammation.

It includes

• Aspirin

• Celecoxib

• Diclofenac

• Diflunisal

• Etodolac

• Ibuprofen

• Indomethacin

• Ketoprofen

• Ketorolac

• Nabumetone

• Naproxen

• Oxaprozin

• Piroxicam

Adverse effects Nausea, vomiting, diarrhea, constipation, decreased appetite, headache, and drowsiness, kidney failure, and liver failure.

Corticosteroids

Mechanism of Action of Corticosteroids

These drugs enter into the cells and coupled with steroid receptors in the cytoplasm and regulate the protein synthesis process. Proteins can inhibit the enzyme phospholipaseA2 and control the inflammatory reactions in the body.

Corticosteroids include

• Bethamethasone

• Prednisone

- Prednisolone

- Dexamethasone

- Fludrocortisone

- Prednisolone

- Triamcinolone

- Methylprednisolone

- Dexamethasone

- Hydrocortisone

- Adverse effects

- High blood pressure

- Loss of potassium

- Headache

- Swelling of the legs

- Muscle weakness

- Weight gain

- Slow wound healing

- Cataracts

- Glaucoma

- Ulcers in the stomach and duodenum

- Puffiness of the face

- Facial hair growth

CONCLUSION

The cardiovascular disease is associated with complex risk factors which include diabetes, hypertension, obesity, alcohol, smoking, stress increase the risk of cardiovascular complications. Cardiovascular diseases include peripheral arterial disease, coronary artery disease, inflammatory heart disease, myocardial infarction, heart failure, aortic aneurysm, hypertension, cardiac arrhythmias and cause mortality, morbidity among disease population. The cardiovascular disease mostly occurs in males as compared with females due to modified lifestyle practices. Implementation of the clinical pharmacist services with the health care team on risk factors identification and control, health screening programmes, diet counseling, medication usage information, disease counseling, lifestyle modification counseling, smoking and alcohol cessation, stress management, physical exercises and maintaining controlled levels of risk factors can reduce the inflammatory cardiac disease burden in the health care settings.

The early recognition of inflammatory conditions and novel treatment options and diagnostic investigations can help for better control of disease complications. Randomized controlled trials should perform in the health care settings to assess the disease status and also design the newer treatment options for the prevention of inflammatory interactions associated with cardiovascular diseases. The management of inflammatory heart disease includes antibiotics, colchicine, beta blockers, diuretics, anti platelets, corticosteroids, NSAID's; ACE inhibitors could control the progression of cardiovascular inflammatory situations among diagnosed patients.

REFERENCES

[1] Pant S, Patel NJ, Deshmukh A, *et al.* Trends in infective endocarditis incidence, microbiology, and valve replacement in the United States from 2000 to 2011. J Am Coll Cardiol 2015; 65(19): 2070-6.
[http://dx.doi.org/10.1016/j.jacc.2015.03.518] [PMID: 25975469]

[2] Toyoda N, Chikwe J, Itagaki S, Gelijns AC, Adams DH, Egorova NN. Trends in Infective Endocarditis in California and New York State, 1998-2013. JAMA 2017; 317(16): 1652-60.
[http://dx.doi.org/10.1001/jama.2017.4287] [PMID: 28444279]

[3] Hill EE, Herijgers P, Claus P, Vanderschueren S, Herregods MC, Peetermans WE. Infective endocarditis: changing epidemiology and predictors of 6-month mortality: a prospective cohort study. Eur Heart J 2007; 28(2): 196-203.
[http://dx.doi.org/10.1093/eurheartj/ehl427] [PMID: 17158121]

[4] Fernández-Hidalgo N, Almirante B, Tornos P, *et al.* Contemporary epidemiology and prognosis of health care-associated infective endocarditis. Clin Infect Dis 2008; 47(10): 1287-97.
[http://dx.doi.org/10.1086/592576] [PMID: 18834314]

[5] Lefort A, Chartier L, Sendid B, *et al.* Diagnosis, management and outcome of Candida endocarditis. Clin Microbiol Infect 2012; 18(4): E99-E109.
[http://dx.doi.org/10.1111/j.1469-0691.2012.03764.x] [PMID: 22329526]

[6] Murdoch DR, Corey GR, Hoen B, *et al.* Clinical presentation, etiology, and outcome of infective endocarditis in the 21st century: the International Collaboration on Endocarditis-Prospective Cohort Study. Arch Intern Med 2009; 169(5): 463-73.
[http://dx.doi.org/10.1001/archinternmed.2008.603] [PMID: 19273776]

[7] Hoen B, Duval X. Clinical practice. Infective endocarditis. N Engl J Med 2013; 368(15): 1425-33.
[http://dx.doi.org/10.1056/NEJMcp1206782] [PMID: 23574121]

[8] Garg N, Kandpal B, Garg N, *et al.* Characteristics of infective endocarditis in a developing country-

clinical profile and outcome in 192 Indian patients, 1992-2001. Int J Cardiol 2005; 98(2): 253-60.
[http://dx.doi.org/10.1016/j.ijcard.2003.10.043] [PMID: 15686775]

[9]   Bin Abdulhak AA, Baddour LM, Erwin PJ, *et al.* Global and regional burden of infective endocarditis, 1990-2010: a systematic review of the literature. Glob Heart 2014; 9(1): 131-43.
[http://dx.doi.org/10.1016/j.gheart.2014.01.002] [PMID: 25432123]

[10]   García-Cabrera E, Fernández-Hidalgo N, Almirante B, *et al.* Neurological complications of infective endocarditis: risk factors, outcome, and impact of cardiac surgery: a multicenter observational study. Circulation 2013; 127(23): 2272-84.
[http://dx.doi.org/10.1161/CIRCULATIONAHA.112.000813] [PMID: 23648777]

[11]   Spodick DH. Intrapericardial treatment of persistent autoreactive pericarditis/myopericarditis and pericardial effusion. Eur Heart J 2002; 23(19): 1481-2.
[http://dx.doi.org/10.1053/euhj.2002.3228] [PMID: 12242064]

[12]   Caforio AL, Pankuweit S, Arbustini E, *et al.* Current state of knowledge on aetiology, diagnosis, management, and therapy of myocarditis: a position statement of the European Society of Cardiology Working Group on Myocardial and Pericardial Diseases. Eur Heart J 2013; 34(33): 2636-2648, 2648a-2648d.
[http://dx.doi.org/10.1093/eurheartj/eht210] [PMID: 23824828]

[13]   Maisch B, Pankuweit S. Current treatment options in (peri)myocarditis and inflammatory cardiomyopathy. Herz 2012; 37(6): 644-56.
[http://dx.doi.org/10.1007/s00059-012-3679-9] [PMID: 22996288]

[14]   Maisch B, Portig I, Ristic A, Hufnagel G, Pankuweit S. Definition of inflammatory cardiomyopathy (myocarditis): on the way to consensus. A status report. Herz 2000; 25(3): 200-9.
[http://dx.doi.org/10.1007/s000590050007] [PMID: 10904839]

[15]   Maisch B. The sarcolemma as antigen in the secondary immunopathogenesis of myopericarditis. Eur Heart J 1987; 8: 155-65.
[http://dx.doi.org/10.1093/eurheartj/8.suppl_J.155]

[16]   Bock CT, Klingel K, Kandolf R. Human parvovirus B19-associated myocarditis. N Engl J Med 2010; 362(13): 1248-9.
[http://dx.doi.org/10.1056/NEJMc0911362] [PMID: 20357294]

[17]   Shabetai R. Recurrent pericarditis: recent advances and remaining questions. Circulation 2005; 112(13): 1921-3.
[http://dx.doi.org/10.1161/CIRCULATIONAHA.105.569244] [PMID: 16186432]

[18]   Imazio M, Brucato A, Cumetti D, *et al.* Corticosteroids for recurrent pericarditis: high *versus* low doses: a nonrandomized observation. Circulation 2008; 118(6): 667-71.
[http://dx.doi.org/10.1161/CIRCULATIONAHA.107.761064] [PMID: 18645054]

[19]   Murashita T, Schaff HV, Daly RC, *et al.* Experience With Pericardiectomy for Constrictive Pericarditis Over Eight Decades. Ann Thorac Surg 2017; 104(3): 742-50.
[http://dx.doi.org/10.1016/j.athoracsur.2017.05.063] [PMID: 28760468]

[20]   Baughman KL. Diagnosis of myocarditis: death of Dallas criteria. Circulation 2006; 113(4): 593-5.
[http://dx.doi.org/10.1161/CIRCULATIONAHA.105.589663] [PMID: 16449736]

[21]   Maisch B, Portig I, Ristic A, Hufnagel G, Pankuweit S. Definition of inflammatory cardiomyopathy (myocarditis): on the way to consensus. A status report. Herz 2000; 25(3): 200-9.
[http://dx.doi.org/10.1007/s000590050007] [PMID: 10904839]

[22]   Mahrholdt H, Goedecke C, Wagner A, *et al.* Cardiovascular magnetic resonance assessment of human myocarditis: a comparison to histology and molecular pathology. Circulation 2004; 109(10): 1250-8.
[http://dx.doi.org/10.1161/01.CIR.0000118493.13323.81] [PMID: 14993139]

[23]   Maisch B. Effusive-constrictive pericarditis: current perspectives. J Cardiovasc Diagn Interv 2018; 6: 7-14.

[24] Adler Y, Finkelstein Y, Guindo J, *et al.* Colchicine treatment for recurrent pericarditis. A decade of experience. Circulation 1998; 97(21): 2183-5.
[http://dx.doi.org/10.1161/01.CIR.97.21.2183] [PMID: 9626180]

[25] Herzum M, Maisch B, Kochsiek K. Circulating immune complexes in perimyocarditis and infective endocarditis. Eur Heart J 1987; 8: 323-6.
[http://dx.doi.org/10.1093/eurheartj/8.suppl_J.323]

CHAPTER 17

Cardiomyopathy

Abstract: Dilated cardiomyopathy is a heart muscle disease that occurs due to dilation and dysfunction of ventricles. The proper understanding of etiology, pathogenesis can help with determining better therapeutic options for the management of disease complications. The various types of cardiomyopathy include restrictive cardiomyopathy, hypertrophic cardiomyopathy, dilated cardiomyopathy, arrhythmogenic right ventricular cardiomyopathy. Diabetes mellitus, genetic conditions, high blood pressure, heart attack, palpitations, heart valve defects, and pregnancy, smoking, alcohol, and connective tissue disorders are well known risk factors for the development of cardiomyopathy. The clinical manifestations of cardiomyopathy include palpitations, dizziness, headache, chest pain, shortness of breath and edema. The electrocardiogram, chest x-ray, echocardiogram, treadmill test, coronary angiogram test can determine the cardiovascular risk. The clinical management of cardiomyopathy with the prescribing pattern of beta blockers, angiotensin-converting enzyme inhibitors, diuretics, digoxin, angiotensin II receptor blockers, anti-platelet medications can minimize the development of cardiomyopathy complications.

Keywords: Dilated Cardiomyopathy, Heart Attack, High Blood Pressure, Pregnancy, Restrictive Cardiomyopathy.

INTRODUCTION

It is a disease of the cardiac muscles represented with dilation of ventricles and failure of systolic function. The left ventricles walls are weakened and the stoppage of blood flow cannot meet the physiological requirement of the heart which causes the development of dilated cardiomyopathy. Cardiomyopathy is a clinical abnormality of the cardiac muscles. The main types of cardiomyopathy include restrictive cardiomyopathy, hypertrophic and dilated cardiomyopathy. Cardiomyopathy condition the blood can't reach the heart effectively and leads to poor functioning of the heart which causes heart failure. Cardiomyopathy is the disease of the cardiac muscles. The inflammation of the cardiac muscles becomes rigid and weakens the functions of the heart [1 - 3]. The weakening of the cardiac muscles incapability to maintain the electrical rhythm of the heart and shows irregular heartbeats known as arrhythmia.

M.S. Umashankar & A. Bharath Kumar

Types of cardiomyopathy is shown in Fig. (**1**).

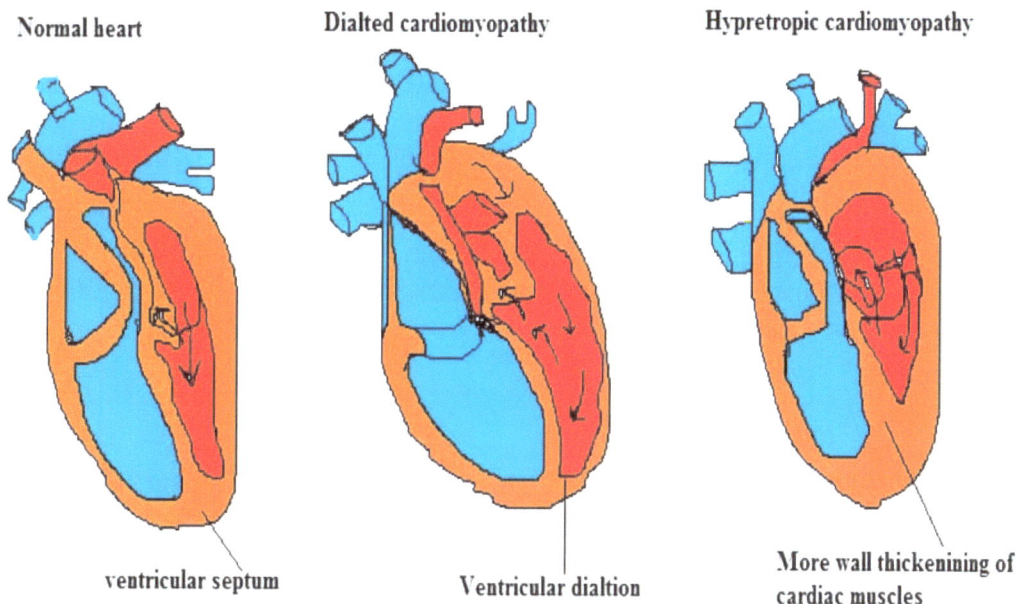

Fig. (1). Types of cardiomyopathy.

There are three main types of inherited cardiomyopathy

• Dilated cardiomyopathy

• Hypertrophic cardiomyopathy

• Restrictive cardiomyopathy

• Arrhythmogenic right ventricular dysplasia

TYPES OF CARDIOMYOPATHY

Dilated cardiomyopathy: It is the most commonly occurring cardiomyopathy in clinical practice. The blood flow from the left ventricle to the heart is less forceful. The dilation of left ventricles causes lowers the blood flow to the heart and increase the risk of developing dilated cardiomyopathy.

Hypertrophic cardiomyopathy: It occurs at any age, the condition is more severe and commonly seen the childhood. The abnormal thickening of the cardiac muscles reduces the blood flow to the heart increase the risk of hypertrophic cardiomyopathy. Previous studies are stated that a family history of cardiomyopathy can increases the risk of hypertrophic cardiomyopathy.

Restrictive cardiomyopathy: The condition is caused by the deposition of iron; proteins in the cardiac muscles cause inflammation can form the abnormal cells to grow in the cardiac muscles. The poor blood supply to the heart during the cardiac contraction and relaxation can develop restrictive cardiomyopathy. The exact cause for restrictive cardiomyopathy is unknown but mostly it occurs in old aged people.

Arrhythmogenic right ventricular dysplasia: This is a rare type of cardiomyopathy, which includes the right ventricle is replaced by the scar tissue that can create abnormal heart rhythms which cause the arrhythmogenic right ventricular dysplasia.

PREVALENCE

The dilated cardiomyopathy progresses at any age in both males and females. Previous research studies stated that DCM has commonly seen in males as compared with females due to unhealthy life style practice. In children, the incidence was found to be 0.57 cases per 100000 and higher in boys as compared with girls. In children, DCM occurrence is idiopathic cause and adults the incidence rate was 1 in 2500 people and annually prevalence was 7 per 100000. In the US the DCM cases were found to be 36 per 100000 of the patients. The familial type of DCM was seen in 20-40% of the affected population. Previous research studies found that the incidence was 1 in 2,700 with men to female [4 - 6]. The HCM has an incidence of 1 in 5,100 patients. Italy the DCM incidence was found 4.5/100,000 cases and total incidence of 7.0/100,000 patients per year. Japan the DCM incidence was found to 3.6/100,000 patients.

PATHOPHYSIOLOGY

The myocyte injury and necrosis of the myocardial cells impair the cardiac contraction functions. The failure of the myocytes and altered cyto skeletal muscles of the heart leads to the dilation of the cardiac chambers can increase the progression of the cardiomyopathy. The myocardial dysfunction cells dysfunction can wane the ventricular remodeling process. The poor functioning of the ventricular filling can increase the risk of heart failure. The primary amyloidal heart disease is induced by the abnormal production of excess production of the immunoglobulin from monoclonal plasma cells can increase the risk of myeloma. Secondary amyloid heart disease is associated with various inflammatory conditions such as tuberculosis, crohn's disease and rheumatoid arthritis *etc*. The dysfunction of myocardial cells can dilate the myocardium can increase the more pressure on the ventricles can increase the risk of heart valve abnormalities. It is represented with the low level of contractile function of myocytes which increases the dilation of cardiomyocytes. Molecular and structural mechanisms are dilating the cardiac muscles. The failure of the cardiac compensatory mechanisms is activated and improves the left ventricular function. Rapid activation of the sympathetic nervous system and the renin-angiotensin-aldosterone system can retain the cardiac output by increasing the heart rate and contractions of the heart. The presence of more pressure in the blood vessels causes hypertrophy and results in vasoconstriction of the blood vessels. The failure of protective mechanisms of heart and changes in the protective mechanism of myocytes causes apoptosis. The excessive activation of adrenergic system shows more toxic effects on the cardiac cells leads to necrosis. The changes in the cardiac myocytes can alter the expression of the genes in protein level which causes the dysfunction of the cardiac muscles. The cardiac functions can influence by various factors such as cytokines, paracrine substances, neurotransmitters and hormones. The changes in the intrinsic function of the myocardial cells can alter the cardiac chamber remodeling. The more stress on the cardiac chambers requires energy for cellular functions and inadequate myocyte energy deficiency leads to dilate the ventricles. The catecholamines can aggravate the apoptosis in heart failure and cause the progression of systolic dysfunction leads to the development of cardiomyopathy [7 - 9].

CAUSES

The possible causes of cardiomyopathy include

• Metabolic disorders, such as obesity, thyroid disease and diabetes mellitus

• Genetic conditions

• Long-term high blood pressure

• Heart tissue damage from a previous heart attack

• Chronic rapid heart rate

• Heart valve problems

• Hemochromatosis

• Nutritional deficiencies

• Pregnancy complications

• Smoking

• Alcohol

• Connective tissue disorders

• Use of anabolic steroids

• Use of some chemotherapy drugs

• Sarcoidosis

• Amyloidosis

DIAGNOSIS

It includes

• Physical examination of the patient

• Chest X-ray

• Electrocardiogram

• Blood test

• Echocardiogram

• Treadmill stress test

• CT scan

• Genetic test

SIGNS AND SYMPTOMS

Cardiomyopathy signs and symptoms may include [10 - 15]

It includes

• Palpitations

• Dizziness

• Lightheadedness

• Chest pain

• Fainting, joint pain

• Shortness of breath

• Swelling of legs, ankles and feet

• Fatigue

• Weight gain

PREVENTION [16 - 19]

It includes

• Avoiding the use of alcohol

• Maintaining controlled levels of high blood pressure, high cholesterol and diabetes

• Eating a healthy diet

• Getting regular exercise

• Getting enough sleep

• Stress management

• Quitting smoking

TREATMENT [20 - 25]

Anti Platelet Drugs

These drugs help to prevent the platelet aggregation and reduce the clot in the blood vessels.

Types of Antiplatelet Agents

• Aspirin

• Dipyridamole

• Clopidogrel

• Ticagrelor

Clinical uses of antiplatelet agents

It is used to treat following disease conditions

It includes

• Coronary artery disease

• Heart attack

• Angina pectoris

• Stroke and transient ischemic attacks

• Peripheral artery disease

Side Effects Nausea, gastric problems, diarrhea, rashes, itching.

Beta Blockers

It reduces the work load on the heart and reduces stress and hormones levels in the body which leads to vasodilatation in the blood vessels.

Commonly prescribed beta blockers include

• Atenolol

• Bisoprolol

• Nadolol

• Nebivolol

• Carvedilol

• Labetalol

• Nebivolol

• Pindolol

• Propranolol

• Timolol

• Metoprolol

Adverse effects Dry mouth, dry skin, feelings of coldness, diarrhea, shortness of breath and insomnia.

Thrombolytic Drugs

Thrombolytic drugs are prescribed to reduce the formation of a blood clot in the blood vessels and also lower the severity of stroke. These drugs will act by conversion of plasminogen which forms plasmin and activates the fibrin bound plasminogen. Fibrin molecules are inhibited by plasmin which leads to the breakdown of clot the blood vessels and reduces the stroke complications.

It includes

• Anistreplase

• Reteplase

• Streptokinase

• T-pa

• Tenecteplase

• Alteplase

• Urokinase

Adverse drug reactions Internal bleeding, damage to the blood vessels, renal damage.

Angiotensin Converting Enzyme (ACE) Inhibitors

ACEs block the conversion of angiotensin I to angiotensin II by the action of angiotensinogen in the body and help to lower the vasoconstriction and promote vasodilation.

It includes

• Captopril

• Lisinopril

• Fosinopril

• Ramipril

• Benazepril

• Enalapril

• Perindopril

• Quinapril

• Moexipril

• Trandolapril

Adverse effects Dry cough, hyperkalemia, fatigue, headaches and loss of taste.

Angiotensin II Receptor Blockers

It blocks the conversion of angiotensin II from its binding to angiotensin II receptors located on the blood vessels and produces vasodialtion in the blood vessels.

These drugs include

• Candesartan

• Telmisartan

• Valsartan

• Eprosartan

• Irbesartan

• Losartan

Adverse effects Hyperkalemia, dizziness, headache, cough, diarrhea, hypotension and angioedema.

Diuretics

Loop Diuretics

These drugs will inhibit the sodium potassium co transport mechanism in the ascending loop of henle it leads to an increase in the distal tubular concentration of sodium and reduced levels of hyprertonicity of the sodium levels in the intestine cause diueresis.

Loop diuretics include

• Bumetanide

- Furosemide

- Ethacrynate

- Torsemide

Adverse effects Hypokalemia, alkalosis, hypomagnesemia, hyperuricemia, dehydration, ototoxicity.

Thiazides Diuretics

These drugs inhibit the sodium-chloride transporter in the distal tubule and reabsorption of sodium ions causes the elimination of more water from the body.

- Chlorothiazide

- Chlorthalidone

- Indapamide

- Hydrochlorothiazide

- Methyclothiazide

Adverse effects Hyponatremia, hyperglycemia, dehydration, hypokalemia, hypertriglyceridemia, hyperuricemia, azotemia.

Carbonic Anhydrase Inhibitors

These drugs will inhibit the transport of bicarbonate ions from the proximal convulted tubule which leads to loss of sodium, hydrogen and bicarbonate ions in the urine.

Drugs include

- Acetazolamide

- Methazolamide

Adverse effects Metabolic acidosis and hypokalemia

Potassium Sparing Diuretics

It acts on the distal segment of the distal tubules and causes more water to enter inside the collecting tubule. It will inhibit the aldosterone-sensitive sodium reabsorption thereby loss of potassium and hydrogen from the urine.

• Amiloride

• spironolactone

• Triamterene

Adverse effects Metabolic acidosis, gynecomastia, hyperkalemia, gastric ulcers.

Digoxin

It is used to treat the irregular heartbeats which include tachycardia, atrial flutter, and supraventricular tachycardia. Digoxin has an electrophysiological and hemodynamic effect on the cardiovascular system. It will reversibly inhibit the Na-K ATPase enzyme which is responsible for the maintaining the intra cellular environment and balance of potassium, sodium and calcium ions into the cells. The inhibition of the sodium pump by Na-K ATPase leads to an increase in the contraction as well as cardiac function of the heart.

Adverse effects Diarrhea, blurred vision, nausea, vomiting, confusion, dizziness and irregular heartbeats.

Warfarin

Warfarin is a vitamin K antagonist that acts to inhibit the production of vitamin K by epoxide reductase enzyme and also inhibits the carboxylation activity of glutamyl carboxylase that can lower the formation of blood clots in the blood vessels. It will inhibit the carboxylation activity of glutamyl carboxylase which can inhibit the formation of blood clot in the blood vessels.

Adverse effects Ecchymoses, epistaxis, renal bleeding and hepatic bleeding.

CONCLUSION

Cardiomyopathy is a heart muscle disorder associated with complex risk factors and pathophysiological mechanisms and symptoms. Dilated cardiomyopathy is an irreversible myocardial disorder that consists of an impaired systole function. The dilated cardiomyopathy progresses at any age in both males and females. The cardiomyopathy incidence was high in males as compared with females due to diverse lifestyle practices. The detection of cardiomyopathy depends on chest x-ray, doppler studies, echocardiogram, electrocardiogram, coronary angiography, MRI scan, holter monitoring studies to assess the cardiovascular disease severity among disease patients. Detailed investigation of family history and genetic profile of individual patients useful for determining personalized therapy can improve the health related quality of life of the affected population. An effective understanding of genetic profile of dilated cardiomyopathy and therapeutic options can minimize the development of cardiac arrhythmias. Evidence based individualized therapies can help for the prevention of disease complications. The implication of newer diagnostic tests like stem cell-derived cardiomyocytes, gene therapy, molecular studies will beneficial for effective treatment of cardiomyopathy and also lowering disease related health care cost to individual patients. Early identification of risk factors, diagnosis and treatment and effective implementation of clinical pharmacist care services with the health care team on risk factors control and patient counseling services can reduce hospital readmission and improves the health status of individual patients.

REFERENCES

[1] Elliott P, Andersson B, Arbustini E, *et al.* Classification of the cardiomyopathies: a position statement from the European Society Of Cardiology Working Group on Myocardial and Pericardial Diseases. Eur Heart J 2008; 29(2): 270-6.
[http://dx.doi.org/10.1093/eurheartj/ehm342] [PMID: 17916581]

[2] Arbustini E, Narula N, Tavazzi L, *et al.* The MOGE(S) classification of cardiomyopathy for clinicians. J Am Coll Cardiol 2014; 64(3): 304-18.
[http://dx.doi.org/10.1016/j.jacc.2014.05.027] [PMID: 25034069]

[3] Elliott P. Cardiomyopathy. Diagnosis and management of dilated cardiomyopathy. Heart 2000; 84(1): 106-12.
[http://dx.doi.org/10.1136/heart.84.1.106] [PMID: 10862601]

[4] Sisakian H. Cardiomyopathies: Evolution of pathogenesis concepts and potential for new therapies. World J Cardiol 2014; 6(6): 478-94.
[http://dx.doi.org/10.4330/wjc.v6.i6.478] [PMID: 24976920]

[5] Pinto YM, Elliott PM, Arbustini E, *et al.* Proposal for a revised definition of dilated cardiomyopathy, hypokinetic non-dilated cardiomyopathy, and its implications for clinical practice: a position statement of the ESC working group on myocardial and pericardial diseases. 2016.
[http://dx.doi.org/10.1093/eurheartj/ehv727]

[6] Abelmann WH. Abelmann WH Classification and natural history of primary myocardial diseaseProg Cardiovasc Dis 1984; 27(2): 73. e94

[7] Christian HA. Clinically the myocardium. AMA Arch Intern Med 1950; 86(4): 491-7.
[http://dx.doi.org/10.1001/archinte.1950.00230160003001] [PMID: 14770575]

[8] Goodwin JF, Oakley CM. The cardiomyopathies. Br Heart J 1972; 34(6): 545-52.
[http://dx.doi.org/10.1136/hrt.34.6.545] [PMID: 4402697]

[9] Richardson P, McKenna W, Bristow M, *et al.* Report of the 1995 World Health Organization/International Society and Federation of Cardiology Task Force on the Definition and Classification of cardiomyopathies. Circulation 1996; 93(5): 841-2.
[http://dx.doi.org/10.1161/01.CIR.93.5.841] [PMID: 8598070]

[10] Dec GW, Fuster V. Idiopathic dilated cardiomyopathy. N Engl J Med 1994; 331(23): 1564-75.
[http://dx.doi.org/10.1056/NEJM199412083312307] [PMID: 7969328]

[11] Elliott PM. Classification of cardiomyopathies: evolution or revolution? J Am Coll Cardiol 2013; 62(22): 2073-4.
[http://dx.doi.org/10.1016/j.jacc.2013.10.008] [PMID: 24263074]

[12] Grünig E, Tasman JA, Kücherer H, Franz W, Kübler W, Katus HA. Frequency and phenotypes of familial dilated cardiomyopathy. J Am Coll Cardiol 1998; 31(1): 186-94.

[http://dx.doi.org/10.1016/S0735-1097(97)00434-8] [PMID: 9426039]

[13] Bozkurt B, Colvin M, Cook J, *et al.* Current Diagnostic and Treatment Strategies for Specific Dilated Cardiomyopathics: A Scientific Statement From the American Heart Association. Circulation 2016; 134(23): e579-646.
[http://dx.doi.org/10.1161/CIR.0000000000000455] [PMID: 27832612]

[14] Japp AG, Gulati A, Cook SA, Cowie MR, Prasad SK. The Diagnosis and Evaluation of Dilated Cardiomyopathy. J Am Coll Cardiol 2016; 67(25): 2996-3010.
[http://dx.doi.org/10.1016/j.jacc.2016.03.590] [PMID: 27339497]

[15] Sinagra G, Di Lenarda A, Brodsky GL, *et al.* Current perspective new insights into the molecular basis of familial dilated cardiomyopathy. Ital Heart J 2001; 2(4): 280-6.
[PMID: 11374497]

[16] McNair WP, Ku L, Taylor MRG, *et al.* SCN5A mutation associated with dilated cardiomyopathy, conduction disorder, and arrhythmia. Circulation 2004; 110(15): 2163-7.
[http://dx.doi.org/10.1161/01.CIR.0000144458.58660.BB] [PMID: 15466643]

[17] Towbin JA, Lowe AM, Colan SD, *et al.* Incidence, causes, and outcomes of dilated cardiomyopathy in children. JAMA 2006; 296(15): 1867-76.
[http://dx.doi.org/10.1001/jama.296.15.1867] [PMID: 17047217]

[18] Moretti M, Merlo M, Barbati G, *et al.* Prognostic impact of familial screening in dilated cardiomyopathy. Eur J Heart Fail 2010; 12(9): 922-7.
[http://dx.doi.org/10.1093/eurjhf/hfq093] [PMID: 20525703]

[19] Mestroni L, Maisch B, McKenna WJ, *et al.* Guidelines for the study of familial dilated cardiomyopathies. Eur Heart J 1999; 20(2): 93-102.
[http://dx.doi.org/10.1053/euhj.1998.1145] [PMID: 10099905]

[20] Iannucci G, Villani M, Alessandri N, Scibilia G, Sciacca A, Baciarello G. Late potentials in idiopathic dilated cardiomyopathy. G Ital Cardiol 1990; 20(6): 549-54.
[PMID: 2227225]

[21] Baig MK, Goldman JH, Caforio ALP, Coonar AS, Keeling PJ, McKenna WJ. Familial dilated cardiomyopathy: cardiac abnormalities are common in asymptomatic relatives and may represent early disease. J Am Coll Cardiol 1998; 31(1): 195-201.
[http://dx.doi.org/10.1016/S0735-1097(97)00433-6] [PMID: 9426040]

[22] Pinto YM, Elliott PM, Arbustini E, *et al.* Proposal for a revised definition of dilated cardiomyopathy, hypokinetic non-dilated cardiomyopathy, and its implications for clinical practice: a position statement of the ESC working group on myocardial and pericardial diseases. Eur Heart J 2016; 37(23): 1850-8.
[http://dx.doi.org/10.1093/eurheartj/ehv727] [PMID: 26792875]

[23] Pitt B, Zannad F, Remme WJ, *et al.* The effect of spironolactone on morbidity and mortality in patients with severe heart failure. N Engl J Med 1999; 341(10): 709-17.
[http://dx.doi.org/10.1056/NEJM199909023411001] [PMID: 10471456]

[24] Yi G, Keeling PJ, Hnatkova K, Goldman JH, Malik M, McKenna WJ. Usefulness of signal-averaged electrocardiography in evaluation of idiopathic-dilated cardiomyopathy in families. Am J Cardiol 1997; 79(9): 1203-7.
[http://dx.doi.org/10.1016/S0002-9149(97)00083-0] [PMID: 9164886]

[25] Rapezzi C, Arbustini E, Caforio AL, *et al.* Diagnostic work-up in cardiomyopathies: bridging the gap between clinical phenotypes and final diagnosis. A position statement from the ESC Working Group on Myocardial and Pericardial Diseases. Eur Heart J 2013; 34(19): 1448-58.
[http://dx.doi.org/10.1093/eurheartj/ehs397] [PMID: 23211230]

CHAPTER 18

Rheumatic Heart Disease

Abstract: The cardiovascular disease affects the heart, blood vessels and blood circulation cause death in adult patients. The cardiovascular diseases include ischemic heart disease, congestive heart failure, hypertension, angina pectoris, stroke, peripheral vascular disease can develop due to a low level of blood flow to the heart can increase the risk of cardiovascular complications. Rheumatic fever is an autoimmune inflammatory disease which can develop with infectious species like bacteria, fungi, virus creates inflammatory conditions and results in the origin of inflammatory mechanisms in the body. It occurs, when the immune system responds abnormally to the inflammation with slow deposition of the calcium crystals in the heart valves increase the risk of developing rheumatic heart disease. Currently, the high prevalence of rheumatic heart disease occurred from low and middle-income countries. Ineffective control of rheumatic fever damages several vital organs such as the heart, brain, kidney, and lungs. The blood test, electrocardiogram, chest x-ray, echocardiogram, cardiac MRI scan, treadmill test, coronary angiogram test can determine the cardiovascular risk. The clinical management of rheumatic heart disease with prescribing antibiotics, anti-inflammatory drugs, and corticosteroids are used to reduce the inflammation and also minimizes the progression of cardiovascular damage.

Keywords: Angina Pectoris, Heart failure, Hypertension, Inflammation, Peripheral Vascular Disease, Rheumatic Fever, Rheumatic Heart Disease.

INTRODUCTION

The cardiovascular disease can affect the heart, blood vessels and blood circulation can cause death in adult patients. The cardiovascular diseases include ischemic heart disease, congestive heart failure, hypertension, angina pectoris, stroke, peripheral vascular disease can develop due to a low level of blood flow to the heart can increase the risk of cardiovascular complications. The heart valves are affected by rheumatic heart disease. Rheumatic heart disease is a severe complication of rheumatic fever. The chronic damage of the heart valves may cause heart failure if untreated properly. Rheumatic fever is an autoimmune inflammatory disease which can develop with ineffective treatment to the diseased patients. It happens, when the immune system responds abnormally to the inflammation with slow deposition of the calcium crystals in the heart valves that can cause rheumatic heart disease.

M.S. Umashankar & A. Bharath Kumar

Rheumatic fever is commonly seen in adolescents and children. Rheumatic heart disease is a chronic valvular disease is caused by cardiac valve damage. Acute rheumatic fever is an auto immune response that is affected by *streptococcus*. The acute illness can be resolved and the presence of lesions may progress overtime leads to develop the chronic condition of rheumatic heart disease. Rheumatic heart disease is a major health care problem and it is highly, the high incidence of Rheumatic heart disease was occurring from the low- and middle-income countries [1 - 4]. Previous studies estimated that affect the 33.4 million individuals currently affected with rheumatic fever. Rheumatic heart disease can be managed through prescribing regular medication to the affected patients can reduce the severity of the progression of the Rheumatic heart disease. The development of rheumatic heart disease is associated with various etiological factors and low and middle income countries have a high incidence rate. Rheumatic heart disease is caused due to streptococcal bacterial infection in the myocytes and the previous history of congenital heart disease can raise the disease severity among the affected population. Rheumatic heart disease progress with infection of bacteria in the musculoskeletal system and atrioventricular valves leads to impair the function of heart. The rheumatic heart disease is shown in Fig. (**1**). Rheumatic heart disease is a chronic condition caused by rheumatic fever. *Streptococcus pyogenes can cause* rheumatic fever and pharyngitis. Rheumatic heart disease can cause chronic heart failure from the impaired function of heart valves. Mostly mitral valves are affected and result in stenosis in the heart valves. In few patients, aortic valves are affected and 50% of the cases rheumatic fever does not have an impression of rheumatic fever in childhood. The rheumatic fever is an inflammatory condition of the body it will originate from throat infections. Rheumatic fever can distress the connective tissues present in the body, especially the brain, heart, skin, joints. Rheumatic fever can hit all the age of people and commonly seen in the children age range between 5 and 15 years old. The rheumatic fever is treated with antibiotics that can reduce the progression of further complications in the infected patients. The recurrent episodes of acute rheumatic fever cause inflammation in the heart valves can reduce the blood flow due to valve dysfunction. The stretching of heart valves impairs the function of blood flow to the heart and surgical options may require improving the function of heart valves. The poor treatment of rheumatic heart disease may enhance the risk of chronic heart failure, arrhythmias, termination of pregnancy, endocarditis and stroke. Rheumatic fever is a clinical condition that develops inflammation in the body [5 - 8]. The clinical manifestation of rheumatic fever includes jerky body movements, bone pain, allergic reactions in the body. The chronic condition of rheumatic fever can cause prolong damage to the heart valves which is called rheumatic heart disease. Rheumatic fever is an inflammatory condition that is triggered by streptococcal bacterial infection.

HEART PROBLEMS LINKED TO RHEUMATIC FEVER [9 - 12]

Valvular Heart Disease

It is the inflammatory condition of the pericardium. The pericardium is a thin layer, protective, bag like membrane surrounded by the heart. It has two layers contains lubricating fluid. During the contraction of the layers, it will move normally without any friction.

Pericarditis

The inflammation of the pericardium causes swelling, pain. Early detection and treatment of pericarditis can prevent the further development of cardiac complications.

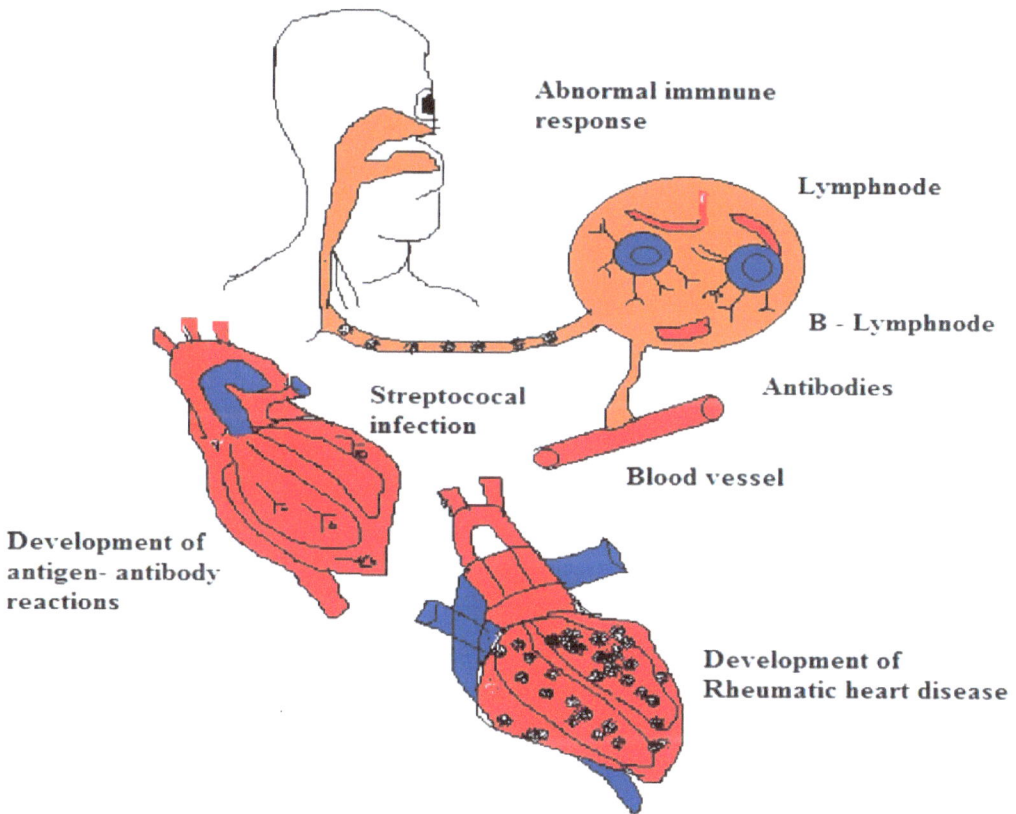

Fig. (1). Rheumatic heart disease.

Endocarditis

Infective endocarditis is the inflammation of the heart which is caused by a

bacterial infection of heart valves. It is one type of cardiac rhythm disorder. It will reduce the electrical signal from atria to ventricles.

Heart Block

The electrical signal causes the contraction of the heart muscles. The slow heart beats which are less than 60 beats per minute is known as bradycardia. Heart block may develop in adults and children. The pregnant women affected with auto immune disease may develop the congenital heart block. Rheumatic heart disease can affect the mitral valve which is located between atria and ventricle in the heart. The damage of the heart valves causes stenosis in the blood vessels. The inflammation of the heart muscles can cause poor pumping of the blood to the heart leads to develop heart failure.

COMPLICATIONS OF RHEUMATIC HEART DISEASE

It includes

• Pregnancy complications

• Bacterial endocarditis

• Heart failure

• Ruptured heart valve

PREVALENCE

Rheumatic heart disease occurs in both endemic and epidemic, endemic cause's high mortality and high incidence in children and non endemic causes low mortality and incidence was high in old age patients. The rheumatic heart disease incidence was 0.15 deaths per 100,000 patients among children age 5 to 9 years in 2015. The high incidence of rheumatic heart disease was seen in South Asia, Africa and Pacific Islands. World heart federation has called for necessary preventive steps to reduce the progression of rheumatic heart disease by the year 2025. In 2015 the rheumatic heart disease was 445 cases per 100,000 populations. In 2015 the prevalence was high in Oceania, South Asia and Saharan Africa [13 - 17]. The comparative prevalence of rheumatic heart disease in various countries includes Pakistan (2.25 million), India (13.17 million cases), Indonesia (1.18 million) and China (7.07 million). Currently, in India 33 million, 13% of the people affected with rheumatic heart disease. In the year 2015, 347000 deaths occurred worldwide. From the year 1990 to 2015, the age related to rheumatic heart disease mortality ranges from 9.2 to 4.8 per 100 000 patients.

RISK FACTORS

• Family history

• Genetics

• Bacterial infections

• Environmental factors

COMMON CLINICAL SYMPTOMS OF RHEUMATIC HEART DISEASE [18, 19]

It may include

• Chest pain

• Fever

• Oedema

• Stroke

• Breathing problems

• Heart palpitations

• Breathlessness

• Fainting (syncope)

COMMON CLINICAL SYMPTOMS OF RHEUMATIC FEVER INCLUDE

It may include

• Chest pain

• Rashes

• Fever

• Palpitations

• Small painless nodules under the skin

• Lethargy

• Fatigue

• Nose bleeding

• Stomach pain

• Joint pain

• Shortness of breath

• Sweating

• Vomiting

• Uncontrollable movements of the face, hands, feet, and face

PATHOPHYSIOLOGY

Acute rheumatic fever is associated with pharyngeal infection. The streptococcal antigens are presented with various cells like dendritic cells; macrophages that produce the antibodies interact with human host cells and initiate the inflammation process in the cells. The initial stage of streptococcal infection in the throat does not cause any episode of rheumatic fever. The chronic progression of the infections may cause immune medicated allergic reactions in the body. Anti bacterial anti bodies are often present in patients infected with streptococcal infections. Mitral valve damage is initiated by the auto antibodies that bind to the heart valves leading to the expression of vascular cell adhesion protein 1 in endothelial cells. The activated endothelium cell promotes the infiltration of T lymphocytes into the valves which increases the more fluid deposition in the heart valves results in edema. The intense valvular tissue stretching leads to an increase the anti bodies in the blood. These antibodies adhere to the heart valves, contribute to the inflammation. The production of auto anti bodies adjacent to the heart valve basement membrane can trigger the initiation of the pathological process that can leads to alter the mitral valve functions. The infiltration of the mono nuclear cells produce cytokines and inflammatory mediators affect the valve functions. The pro inflammatory mediators such as IFN-γ, IL-17, IL-1, and TNF-α cells have been connected with the progression of the rheumatic heart disease. The calcification of heart valves is commonly seen in the mitral valves. Mineralization occurs in the blood vessels which lead to inflammation and expression of the various inflammatory responses in the blood vessels. The macrophages are capable to produce the osteocalcin and osteopontin forms the calcification in the arteries. The calcification of extracellular vesicles originated from smooth muscles, macrophages can create mineralization in the heart valves which induces the development of rheumatic heart disease [20, 21]. The pathophysiology of rheumatic heart disease is shown in Fig. (**2**).

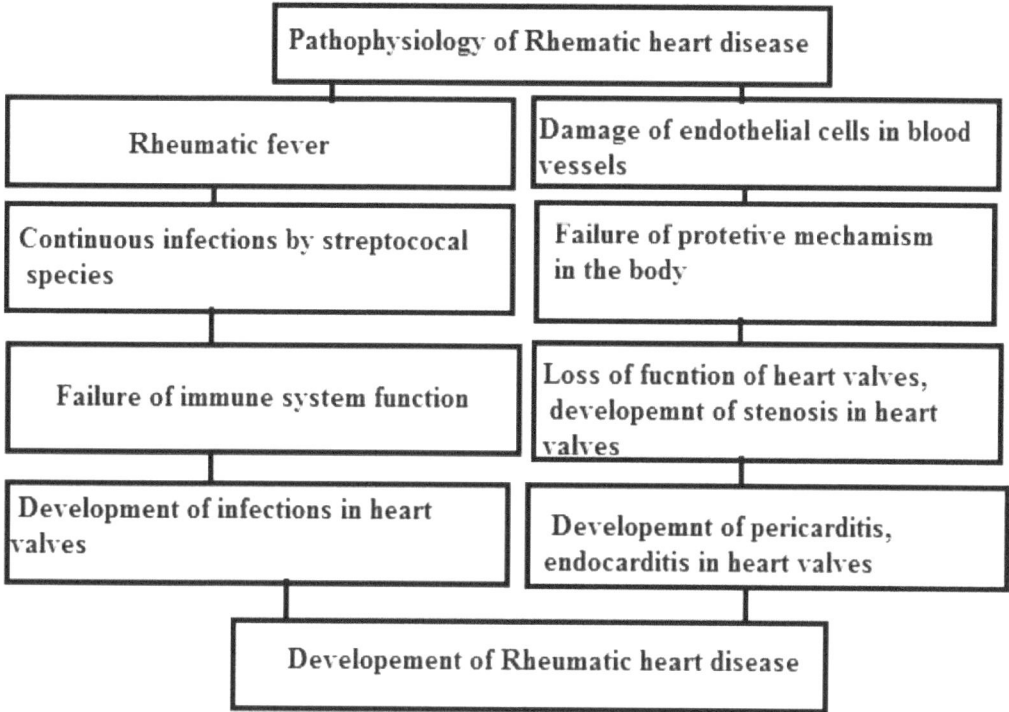

Fig. (2). Pathophysiology of Rheumatic heart disease.

DIAGNOSIS

• Physical examination of the patient

• Blood test

• Coronary angiogram

• Tread mill test

• Echocardiogram

• Electrocardiogram

• Chest X-ray

• Cardiac MRI scan

• CT scan

PREVENTION OF RHEUMATIC HEART DISEASE [22, 23]

• Reduction of risk factors

• Infection control

• Regular health check up

• Good hygiene practice

• Consumption of nutritious diet

• Stress management

• Maintaining good sanitation practice

• Proper washing of hands

• Avoiding consumption of others personal items

TREATMENT

The various types of medications are used to treat rheumatic diseases which include DMARDs, NSAIDs and biological agents [24, 25].

Pain Relievers and Steroids

Narcotic Analgesics

It is used to treat the clinical symptoms of rheumatic diseases includes pain, inflammation. Narcotics drugs include morphine, codeine, hydrocodone, oxycodone are used to lower the deep seated pain.

Side effects Nausea, dry mouth, vomiting, drowsiness and constipation.

Non-steroidal Anti-inflammatory Agents

These drugs are used to treat the acute and chronic management of rheumatic diseases. It will block the activity of the enzyme cycloxygenase (COX) which is mainly involved in the inflammatory pathways.

It includes

• Aspirin

• Tolmetin

- Diclofenac

- Etodolac

- Ibuprofen

- Indomethacin

- Ketorolac

- Celecoxib

- Piroxicam

- Salsalate

- Sulindac

- Ketoprofen

- Nabumetone

- Naproxen

- Oxaprozin

Side effects Nausea, diarrhea, vomiting, constipation, rash, dizziness, headache, and drowsiness, liver damage, kidney damage and ulcers.

Corticosteroids

These drugs are used to reduce the inflammation, pain and swelling of the joints. It can be prescribed orally or injected directly into the affected parts.

- Glucocorticoids

- Hydrocortisone

- Cortisone

- Triamcinolone

- Dexamethasone

- Methylprednisolone

- Beta methasone

- Fludrocortisone

- Ethamethasoneb

- Prednisone

- Prednisolone

Side effects Swelling from fluid retention, weight gain, increased appetite, excessive hair growth, and osteoporosis.

Disease-Modifying Anti-Rheumatic Drugs (DMARDs)

These drugs are used to treat the various types of inflammatory conditions of bones. It will reduce the pain, swelling, inflammation of the joints. It prescribed to take several weeks to months depending on the chronic disease condition of the affected population.

Biologic Response Modifiers

These drugs block the inflammatory pathways by regulating the actions of the immune system. It will block the inflammation associated molecules which is known as cytokines and prevents progressive bone damage. Tumor necrosis factor alpha (TNF-alpha) inhibitors include etanercept, adalimumab, and infliximab.

- Side effects

- Headache

- Cough

- Nausea

- Vomiting

- Heartburn

- Stomach pain

- Weakness

- Antibiotics

- Penicillin V

- Amoxicillin

• Benzathine

Cephalosporins

First-generation Cephalosporins

First-generation cephalosporins include

• Cephalexin

• Cephradine

• Cefadroxil

Second-generation Cephalosporins

• Cefprozil

• Cefaclor

• Cefuroxime

Third-generation Cephalosporins

• Ceftibuten

• Cefpodoxime

• Ceftazidime

• Cefixime

Fourth-generation Cephalosporins

• Cefepime

• Cefozopran

• Cefpirome

Clinical Uses of Cephalosporins

• Abdominal Infections

• Skin and soft tissue infections

• UTI

- Meningitis

- Pneumonia

- Sepsis

- Macrolides

- Erythromycin

- Azithromycin

- Telithromycin

- Clarithromycin

- Spiramycin

- Side effects

- Abdominal pain

- Vomiting

- Diarrhea

- Nausea

- Dizziness

- Dyspepsia

- Skin Rash

CONCLUSION

Rheumatic heart disease is a type of cardiovascular disease that mostly occurs in adults in developed and developing countries. Streptococcal infections induce the development of rheumatic fever which leads to causes of cardiovascular abnormalities. Rheumatic heart disease is a chronic inflammatory condition associated with complex etiological factors and causes more health care expenditure to individual patients. Rheumatic heart disease can cause chronic heart failure from the impaired function of heart valves. The rheumatic heart disease is prevented with the position of clinical pharmacist in the health care areas to counsel the patients on diet, disease, life style modification practices, stress management, conducting awareness porgrammes on disease prevention, risk factors detection and physical exercise for daily 40 minutes, medication adherence and patient follow-up care services could lower the cardiovascular risk incidences in hospitals. There is a lack of awareness about rheumatic fever complications that can worsen the health condition of infected patients and finally increase the premature death of patients. There is a need for the design of a population based monitoring system in every hospital in the country for identification of chronic disease burden, development of newer guidelines for better control of the progression of rheumatic heart disease cases in health care settings. Clinical research studies are implicated for better understanding of rheumatic heart disease chronic disease complications and newer therapeutic and diagnostic tools can prevent the acceleration of rheumatic heart disease risk in clinical settings.

REFERENCES

[1]   Lyons JG, Stewart S. Prevention: Convergent communicable and noncommunicable heart disease. Nat Rev Cardiol 2011; 9(1): 12-4.
        [http://dx.doi.org/10.1038/nrcardio.2011.180] [PMID: 22105675]

[2]   Carapetis JR. Rheumatic heart disease in Asia. Circulation 2008; 118(25): 2748-53.
        [http://dx.doi.org/10.1161/CIRCULATIONAHA.108.774307] [PMID: 19106399]

[3]   Remenyi B, Carapetis J, Wyber R, Taubert K, Mayosi BM. Position statement of the World Heart Federation on the prevention and control of rheumatic heart disease. Nat Rev Cardiol 2013; 10(5): 284-92.
        [http://dx.doi.org/10.1038/nrcardio.2013.34] [PMID: 23546444]

[4]   Watkins DA, Johnson CO, Colquhoun SM, *et al.* Global, regional and national burden of rheumatic heart disease, 1990-2015. N Engl J Med 2017; 377(8): 713-22.
        [http://dx.doi.org/10.1056/NEJMoa1603693] [PMID: 28834488]

[5]   Kaplan E. Global assessment of rheumtatic fever and rheumatic heart disease at the close of the century. Circulation 1993; 88(4): 1.
        [http://dx.doi.org/10.1161/01.CIR.88.4.1964]

[6]   Zühlke LJ, Steer AC. Estimates of the global burden of rheumatic heart disease. Glob Heart 2013; 8(3): 189-95.
        [http://dx.doi.org/10.1016/j.gheart.2013.08.008] [PMID: 25690495]

[7]   Reményi B, Wilson N, Steer A, *et al.* World Heart Federation criteria for echocardiographic diagnosis of rheumatic heart disease--an evidence-based guideline. Nat Rev Cardiol 2012; 9(5): 297-309.
        [http://dx.doi.org/10.1038/nrcardio.2012.7] [PMID: 22371105]

[8]   Zühlke L, Mayosi BM. Echocardiographic screening for subclinical rheumatic heart disease remains a research tool pending studies of impact on prognosis. Curr Cardiol Rep 2013; 15(3): 343.
        [http://dx.doi.org/10.1007/s11886-012-0343-1] [PMID: 23338725]

[9]   Roberts K, Colquhoun S, Steer A, Reményi B, Carapetis J. Screening for rheumatic heart disease: current approaches and controversies. Nat Rev Cardiol 2013; 10(1): 49-58.
        [http://dx.doi.org/10.1038/nrcardio.2012.157] [PMID: 23149830]

[10]   Parks T, Smeesters PR, Steer AC. Streptococcal skin infection and rheumatic heart disease. Curr Opin Infect Dis 2012; 25(2): 145-53.
        [http://dx.doi.org/10.1097/QCO.0b013e3283511d27] [PMID: 22327467]

[11]   Reményi B, Wilson N, Steer A, *et al.* World Heart Federation criteria for echocardiographic diagnosis of rheumatic heart disease--an evidence-based guideline. Nat Rev Cardiol 2012; 9(5): 297-309.

[http://dx.doi.org/10.1038/nrcardio.2012.7] [PMID: 22371105]

[12]   Arguedas A, Mohs E. Prevention of rheumatic fever in Costa Rica. J Pediatr 1992; 121(4): 569-72.
[http://dx.doi.org/10.1016/S0022-3476(05)81146-1] [PMID: 1403390]

[13]   Rammelkamp CH, Wannamaker LW, Denny FW. The epidemiology and prevention of rheumatic fever. Bull N Y Acad Med 1952; 28(5): 321-34.
[PMID: 19312604]

[14]   Watkins DA, Johnson CO, Colquhoun SM, *et al.* Global, regional, and national burden of rheumatic heart disease, 1990-2015. N Engl J Med 2017; 377(8): 713-22.
[http://dx.doi.org/10.1056/NEJMoa1603693] [PMID: 28834488]

[15]   Dougherty S, Khorsandi M, Herbst P. Rheumatic heart disease screening: Current concepts and challenges. Ann Pediatr Cardiol 2017; 10(1): 39-49.
[http://dx.doi.org/10.4103/0974-2069.197051] [PMID: 28163427]

[16]   Beniwal R, Bhaya M, Panwar RB, Panwar S, Singh A. Diagnostic criteria in rheumatic heart disease. Glob Heart 2015; 10(1): 81-2.
[http://dx.doi.org/10.1016/j.gheart.2014.07.001] [PMID: 25754572]

[17]   Marijon E, Ou P, Celermajer DS, *et al.* Prevalence of rheumatic heart disease detected by echocardiographic screening. N Engl J Med 2007; 357(5): 470-6.
[http://dx.doi.org/10.1056/NEJMoa065085] [PMID: 17671255]

[18]   Sliwa K, Carrington M, Mayosi BM, Zigiriadis E, Mvungi R, Stewart S. Incidence and characteristics of newly diagnosed rheumatic heart disease in urban African adults: insights from the heart of Soweto study. Eur Heart J 2010; 31(6): 719-27.
[http://dx.doi.org/10.1093/eurheartj/ehp530] [PMID: 19995873]

[19]   Nkgudi B, Robertson KA, Volmink J, Mayosi BM. Notification of rheumatic fever in South Africa -- evidence for underreporting by health care professionals and administrators. S Afr Med J 2006; 96(3): 206-8.
[PMID: 16607429]

[20]   Robertson KA, Volmink JA, Mayosi BM. Lack of adherence to the national guidelines on the prevention of rheumatic fever. S Afr Med J 2005; 95(1): 52-6.
[PMID: 15762250]

[21]   Karthikeyan G, Mayosi BM. Is primary prevention of rheumatic fever the missing link in the control of rheumatic heart disease in Africa? Circulation 2009; 120(8): 709-13.
[http://dx.doi.org/10.1161/CIRCULATIONAHA.108.836510] [PMID: 19667233]

[22]   Manyemba J, Mayosi BM. Intramuscular penicillin is more effective than oral penicillin in secondary prevention of rheumatic fever--a systematic review. S Afr Med J 2003; 93(3): 212-8.
[PMID: 12768947]

[23]   Nordet P, Lopez R, Dueñas A, Sarmiento L. Prevention and control of rheumatic fever and rheumatic heart disease: the Cuban experience (1986-1996-2002). Cardiovasc J Afr 2008; 19(3): 135-40.
[PMID: 18568172]

[24]   Bach JF, Chalons S, Forier E, *et al.* 10-year educational programme aimed at rheumatic fever in two French Caribbean islands. Lancet 1996; 347(9002): 644-8.
[http://dx.doi.org/10.1016/S0140-6736(96)91202-7] [PMID: 8596378]

[25]   McDonald M, Brown A, Noonan S, Carapetis JR. Preventing recurrent rheumatic fever: the role of register based programmes. Heart 2005; 91(9): 1131-3.
[http://dx.doi.org/10.1136/hrt.2004.057570] [PMID: 16103536]

CHAPTER 19

Management of Cardiovascular Disease in Diabetic Complications

Abstract: Diabetes mellitus is a complex metabolic disorder affecting more than 330 million people around the globe. Diabetes mellitus is identified as the fifth leading cause of death worldwide and causes various complications. The prevalence of diabetes mellitus is rising substantially from worldwide. Over the past few years, the global burden of diabetes mellitus has enlarged 382 million and this count may increase in the future. Cardiovascular disease is a group of numerous diseases such as heart failure, cardiomyopathy, congenital heart disease, coronary heart disease *etc.* causes severe health complications to the affected patients. The deposition of lipid particles inside the arteries can cause clot and favor for the progression of cardiovascular diseases which led to damage to the function of vital organs. Several risk factors are shared with the development of cardiovascular diseases include smoking, alcohol, stress, insufficient physical activity, poor diet, high blood pressure, high lipid profile, diabetes mellitus can greatly advance the risk of cardiovascular disease. Chest x ray, electrocardiogram, stress test, echocardiogram, holter monitoring, coronary angiogram, blood sugar test, lipid profile, investigations are used to detect the progression of cardiovascular disease in diabetic patients. Cardiovascular disease in diabetes mellitus can be prevented through lifestyle modification counseling and regular medication adherence and advance diagnostic and therapeutic management could reduce the progression of cardiovascular disease among diabetic patients.

Keywords: Cardiomyopathy, Coronary heart disease, Diabetes mellitus, Heart failure, High blood pressure, High lipid profile.

INTRODUCTION

Diabetes mellitus is a distressing disease that affects more than 330 million people around the globe. The centers for disease control predicted that 26% of the population is having obesity and 8% of the population having diabetes in the United States. Diabetes mellitus is identified to be the fifth leading cause of death worldwide and causes various complications. Diabetes mellitus can be prevented through lifestyle modification counseling and regular medication adherence could reduce the progression of the complications.

Poor glycemic control can lead to an increase in the risk of developing cardiovascular disease which includes hypertension, congestive cardiac failure,

M.S. Umashankar & A. Bharath Kumar

and coronary artery disease, stroke *etc*. The high mortality rate was seen in the 2000 year it was 2.9 million worldwide [1 - 3]. Several research studies stated that the control of glycemic levels, cholesterol, hypertension and medication therapy can beneficial for improving the health outcomes among diabetes associated cardiovascular disease.

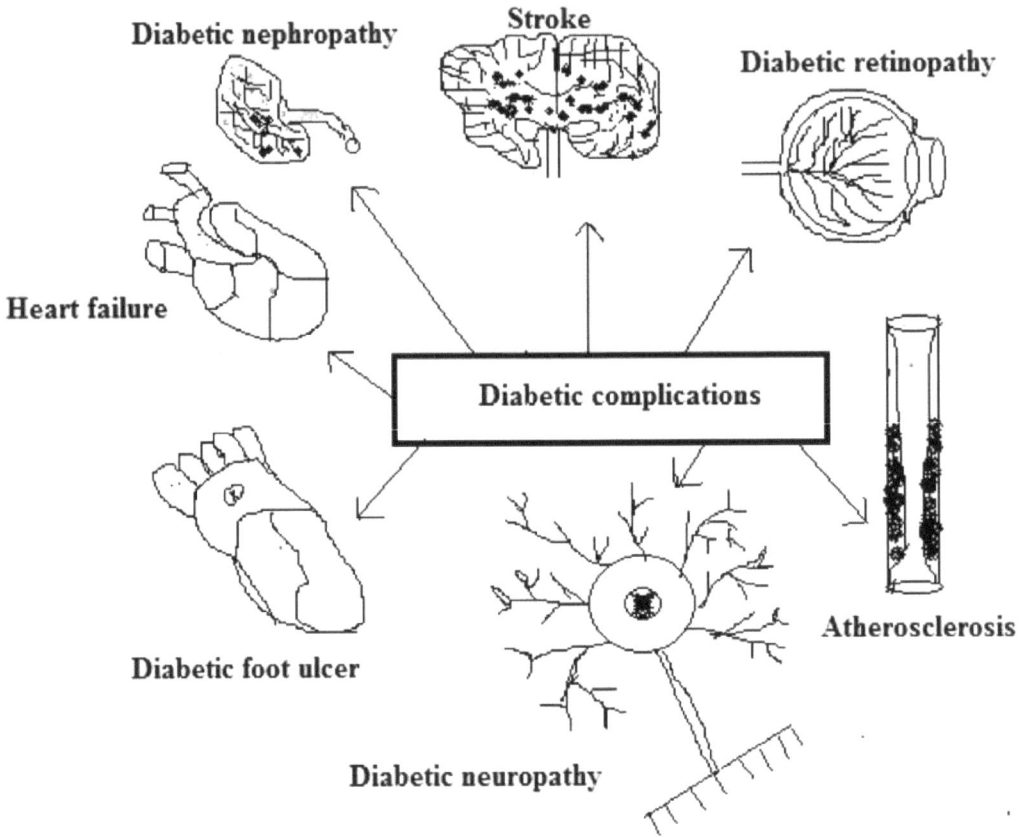

Fig. (1). Diabetic complications.

The prevalence of diabetes mellitus is rising substantially from worldwide. Over the past few years, the global burden of diabetes mellitus has enlarged 382 million and this count may increase in the future. The international diabetes federation estimated that 592 million people worldwide will have DM by 2035. Type 2 diabetes mellitus affected patients were more as compared with type 1 diabetes mellitus. The uncontrolled levels of glycemic levels can contribute to developing macrovascular and microvascular complications such as, hypertension, coronary artery disease, peripheral vascular disease, myocardial infarction, renal failure, neuropathy, retinopathy *etc*. which can cause more economic burden to the individual patients. Diabetic complications were shown in Fig. (**1**). The increased risk of the cardiovascular disease mortality rate was very high in males as compared with females. Effective therapeutic options can lower the progression of incidences of diabetic complications. Previous studies stated that high oxidative stress, abnormal glycemic levels, insulin resistance, coagulation abnormalities, autonomic neuropathy, and endothelial cell dysfunction can contribute to the progression of cardiovascular disease among diabetic patients [4 - 6].

INCIDENCE

The incidence of diabetes mellitus has been raised from developed and developing countries. Diabetes mellitus is a major risk factor for coronary artery disease. Diabetic patients may have 2- to 4-folds greater risk of developing coronary artery disease. The diabetes mellitus incidence was raised from all countries in the world. The global incidence of diabetes mellitus has bulged from 1985 to 2014. The 30 million patients are affected by diabetes mellitus in 1985 and 382 million people are affected in 2014. International diabetes federation predicted that 592 million patients are affected with diabetes mellitus by 2030. The international diabetes federation estimated that 415 million people affected with diabetes mellitus. Currently, diabetes mellitus patients were 8.8% worldwide. The international diabetes federation predicted that diabetic incidence may rise to 642 million by 2040. Cardiovascular disease is a major cause of death among the diabetic population. Diabetic patients may have a high incidence of cardiovascular disease as compared with non diabetic patients. Coronary artery disease is causing more deaths in the western population. The increase in the prevalence may due to the presence of various risk factors such as diabetes mellitus, hypertension, stress; physical inactivity can increase the risk of disease complications [7 - 9].

MODIFIABLE RISK FACTORS FOR CORONARY ARTERY DISEASE

• High blood cholesterol level

• Cigarette smoking

• Alcohol

• Hypertension

• Diabetes mellitus

• Physical activity

• Obesity

• Stress

NON MODIFIABLE RISK FACTORS

Family history of coronary artery disease and diabetes mellitus

Increasing age

Gender(male)

PATHOGENESIS

The pathophysiology of the association between diabetes mellitus and cardiovascular disease is multi factorial. Diabetes is a primary risk factor for developing cardiovascular disease. The abnormal level of LDL particles can penetrate the arterial wall causes oxidation. The oxidized LDL is atherogenic and attracts the various inflammatory cells to the blood vessels. The proliferation of various inflammatory cells forms the atherosclerotic plaques. The glycation process of LDL increases the high lipid levels in the blood. Hypertriglyceridemia can elevate the cholesterol levels can elevate the LDL and reduce the HDL levels. The healthy endothelial cells regulate the platelet cell functions, blood vessel tone, and leukocyte cell adhesion. The dysfunction of the endothelial cells leads to cause the inflammation and thrombogenesis in the blood vessels. The increased oxidation and trigycerides abnormality can cause insulin deficiency and insulin resistance increases the risk of atherogenicity in diabetic patients. Pro-inflammatory causes the injury mechanisms to increase vascular permeability and promote the more reactive oxygen species and ultimately lead to causes apoptosis. The increased levels of adipokines including interleukin 1β, tumor necrosis factor-α, plasminogen activator inhibitor 1 (PAI-1) are involved in the origin of the inflammation process. The high levels of platelet aggregation and clotting factor abnormalities make the hypercoagulation in the blood vessels. Hyperglycemia is the most common clinical feature of diabetes mellitus and uncontrolled diabetes mellitus can increase the risk of ischemic events. Hyperglycemia reduces the nicotinamide adenine dinucleotide (NAD+) to NADH and increases the synthesis of uridine diphosphate (UDP) N-acetyl glucosamine can modify the cellular functions. The gycosylation of the proteins in the coronary artery walls can contribute the atherosclerosis. The abnormal blood sugar level, proteins result in the formation of the advanced glycation end products which can increase the hyperglycemia. The hyperglycemia increases the formation of reactive oxygen species which inhibits the endothelial production of the nitric oxide and blocks the migration of the reactive oxygen species ions into the plaque area and increases the rupture of the coronary arteries. The presence of thrombogenesis and platelet dysfunction in coronary artery disease can worsen the clinical consequences of plaque formation. The abnormal glucose concentration in the blood vessels can activate the protein kinase C, which increases the expression of the glycoprotein Ib enhances the thrombosis in the blood vessels [10 - 14].

DIAGNOSIS

• Glycated hemoglobin (A1C) test

• Fasting blood sugar test

• Postprandial glucose test

• Random blood sugar test

• Electrocardiogram

• Exercise stress test

• Chest X-ray

• Echocardiogram

• Doppler studies

• Blood test

• Coronary angiography

• Magnetic resonance imaging (MRI) scan

• Computerized tomography (CT) scan

SYMPTOMS

Clinical symptoms of coronary heart disease

It includes

• Chest pain

• Chest tightness

• Chest discomfort

• Shortness of breath

• Pain, numbness, weakness

• Coldness in legs or arms

• Pain in the neck, jaw, throat, upper abdomen

CLINICAL SYMPTOMS OF HEART ARRHYTHMIAS

It includes

• Flutters in chest

• Tachycardia

• Bradycardia

• Chest pain or discomfort

• Shortness of breath

• Lightheadedness

• Dizziness

• Fainting

CLINICAL SYMPTOMS OF HEART DEFECTS

It includes

• Pale gray or blue skin color

• Swelling in the legs, abdomen

• Shortness of breath

• Life-threatening symptoms of heart defects include

• Easily getting short of breath during exercise or activity

• Easily tiring during exercise or activity

• Swelling in the hands, ankles or feet

CLINICAL SYMPTOMS OF DILATED CARDIOMYOPATHY

It includes

• Breathlessness with exertion or at rest

• Swelling of the legs, ankles and feet

• Fatigue

• Irregular heartbeats that feel rapid, pounding or fluttering

• Dizziness, light headedness

• Fainting

CLINICAL SYMPTOMS OF HEART INFECTIONS

It includes

• Fever

• Shortness of breath

• Weakness or fatigue

• Swelling in legs

• Dry or persistent cough

• Skin rashes

CLINICAL SYMPTOMS OF VALVULAR HEART DISEASE

It includes

• Fatigue

• Shortness of breath

• Irregular heartbeat

• Swollen feet or ankles

• Chest pain

• Fainting

TREATMENT

Cardiovascular disease incidence is more prevalent and causes mortality and morbidity in patients with diabetes mellitus and effective treatment strategies can lower the risk of cardiovascular events. The disease causative risk factors such as diabetes mellitus, hypertension, obesity, stress, physical inactivity can raise the progression of disease complications. The risk factors should kept control to initiate a better therapeutic regimen that can reduce the burden of cardiovascular disease amongst diabetic patients [15 - 20].

DPP-4 Inhibitors

These drugs can increase the incretin levels and lowers the glucagon release leads to increases the insulin secretion and decrease the blood glucose levels.

It includes

• Sitagliptin

• Vildagliptin

• Saxagliptin

• Linagliptin

Side effects Nausea, diarrhea, stomach pain, headache, runny nose, sore throat, skin reactions and purple rashes.

SGLT2 Inhibitors

Mechanism of action SGLT inhibitor blocks the SGLT2 protein absorption from proximal renal tubule, increases the renal glucose excretion and lowers the blood glucose levels. These agents increase insulin sensitivity and enhance the insulin sensitivity release from the pancreatic beta islets.

It includes

• Canagliflozin

• Dapagliflozin

• Empagliflozin

• Ertugliflozin

Side effects

Urinary tract infections

• Increased urination

• Skin infections

• Kidney problems

• Flu like symptoms

• Constipation

• Nasal congestion

• Urinary discomfort

Metformin

Metformin decreases blood glucose levels by inhibiting hepatic blood glucose production. It will decrease the intestinal absorption of glucose and raises peripheral glucose utilization. Metformin inhibits the mitochondrial complex I activity and prevent the production of mitochondrial ATP and activate the AMP-activated protein kinase can decreases the gluconeogenesis formation. In the liver metformin increases, the anaerobic glucose metabolism in erythrocytes reduces the glucose uptake in the liver and increases insulin sensitivity [21 - 23].

Adverse effects Lactic acidosis, malaise, myalgias, abdominal pain and respiratory distress.

Thiazolidinediones

Mechanism of Action

It increases the insulin sensitivity in the cell tissues and acts on the peroxisome proliferator-activated receptor-γ (PPARγ). PPAR-γ stimulates the transcription for many of the genes responsive to insulin. It decreases the hepatic gluconeogenesis and increases the insulin dependent glucose uptake in the muscles. These drugs are commonly called as insulin sensitizers which can increase the insulin in muscles. It is used in the treatment of insulin resistance which can improve the insulin secretion activity.

Drugs include

• Pioglitazone

• Rosiglitazone

• Ciglitazone

- Lobeglitazone

- Rivoglitazone

- Netoglitazone

- Balaglitazone

- Troglitazone

Side effects

Side effects of glitazones may include

- Water retention

- Weight gain

- Eye sight problems

- Reduced sense of touch

- Chest pain and infections

- Allergic skin reactions

GLP1 Analogues

These are the class of injectable h hypoglycemic medications which can stimulate the Glucagon-like peptide 1 receptor.

Mechanism of Action

GLP-1 is originated from the L cells of the small intestine. GLP-1 binds to a specific GLP-1 receptor which was located in the pancreatic beta cells, gastric mucosa, kidney and heart. GLP-1 stimulates the glucose-dependent insulin release from the pancreatic islets. GLP-1 activates the GLP-1 receptor by activating the adenylyl cyclase in the pancreatic beta cells. It will decrease the glucagon secretion and lowers the blood glucose levels in the blood.

Glucagon-like peptide-1 analogues include

Exenatide

Liraglutide

Adverse effects Nausea, vomiting, diarrhea, headache, weakness, or dizziness, pancreatitis.

Beta Blockers

It reduces the work load on the heart and reduces stress and hormones levels in the body which leads to vasodilatation in the blood vessels.

Commonly prescribed beta blockers include

• Atenolol

• Bisoprolol

• Nadolol

• Nebivolol

• Carvedilol

• Labetalol

• Nebivolol

• Pindolol

• Propranolol

• Timolol

• Metoprolol

Adverse effects Dry mouth, dry skin, feelings of coldness, diarrhea, shortness of breath and insomnia.

Cholesterol Lowering Medications

Statins

These drugs act by inhibiting HMG-CoA reductase enzyme and inhibit the cholesterol biosynthetic pathway and show anti atherosclerotic effect in the blood vessels.

• Atorvastatin

• Fluvastatin

- Lovastatin

- Pitavastatin

- Pravastatin

- Rosuvastatin

- Simvastatin

Adverse effects Headache, dizziness, insomnia, flushing of the skin, drowsiness and myalgia.

Thrombolytic Drugs

Thrombolytic drugs are prescribed to reduce the formation of a blood clot in the blood vessels and also lower the severity of stroke. These drugs will act by conversion of plasminogen which forms plasmin and activates the fibrin bound plasminogen. Fibrin molecules are inhibited by plasmin which leads to the breakdown of clot the blood vessels and reduces the stroke complications [24].

It includes

- Anistreplase

- Reteplase

- Streptokinase

- T-pa

- Tenecteplase

- Alteplase

- Urokinase

Adverse drug reactions Internal bleeding, damage to the blood vessels, renal damage.

ANGIOTENSIN CONVERTING ENZYME (ACE) INHIBITORS

ACEs block the conversion of angiotensin I to angiotensin II by the action of angiotensinogen in the body and help to lower the vasoconstriction and promote vasodilation.

It includes

• Captopril

• Lisinopril

• Fosinopril

• Ramipril

• Benazepril

• Enalapril

• Perindopril

• Quinapril

• Moexipril

• Trandolapril

Adverse effects Dry cough, hyperkalemia, fatigue, headaches and loss of taste.

LIFESTYLE MODIFICATIONS FOR PREVENTION OF CARDIOVASCULAR DISEASE IN DIABETES MELLITUS [25]

• Regular physical exercise for about 30 minutes every day

• Avoid consumption of sugar products

• Limit the intake of sodium not more than 2-4gms per day

• Regular consumption of DASH (Dietary Approaches to Stop Hypertension) diet

• Stress management

• Smoking cessation

• Alcohol cessation

• Maintaining scheduled sleep

• Avoiding consumption of fatty foods

• Eating high fiber food

- Maintaining healthy weight

- Regular meditation practice

- Restriction of salt intake

- Avoiding consumption of sea and sweet foods

- Regular medication adherence

- Regular foot and eye care

CONCLUSION

Diabetes mellitus is a leading risk factor for developing cardiovascular disease. The incidence of diabetes mellitus has risen from developed and developing countries. Diabetic patients may have 2- to 4-folds greater risk of developing coronary artery disease. The development of cardiovascular disease is connected with various risk factors that can be considered to establish prevention programmes in hospitals to reduce the occurrence of cardiovascular disease in diabetic patients. The pathophysiological liaison between cardiovascular disease and diabetes mellitus includes high oxidative stress, abnormal glycemic levels, insulin resistance, coagulation abnormalities, autonomic neuropathy, and endothelial cell dysfunction can contribute to the progression of cardiovascular disease among diabetic patients.

Maintain the controlled levels of blood glucose levels can prevent the acceleration of diabetic complications. The prevention of cardiovascular disease in diabetes mellitus with prescribing of aspirin and satins, blood pressure medications, glucose reduction therapies and maintaining the controlled levels of risk factors could reduce the cardiovascular disease risk among diabetic patients. Incorporation of clinical pharmacist interventions with the health care team on providing diet counseling, disease counseling, lifestyle modification counseling, drug information services, medication adherence, stress management, regular physical exercises, eating low fat diet, smoking and alcohol cessation, patient follow-up care services, can reduce the progression of disease burden in the health care settings. A better understanding of pathophysiological approaches is essential to design the new therapeutic targets and novel blood sugar lowering drugs to control the origin of cardiovascular risk among diabetic patients.

REFERENCES

[1]   Hiatt WR, Kaul S, Smith RJ. The cardiovascular safety of diabetes drugs--insights from the rosiglitazone experience. N Engl J Med 2013; 369(14): 1285-7.
[http://dx.doi.org/10.1056/NEJMp1309610] [PMID: 23992603]

[2]   Zhong J, Maiseyeu A, Davis SN, Rajagopalan S. DPP4 in cardiometabolic disease: recent insights from the laboratory and clinical trials of DPP4 inhibition. Circ Res 2015; 116(8): 1491-504.
[http://dx.doi.org/10.1161/CIRCRESAHA.116.305665] [PMID: 25858071]

[3]   Scirica BM, Bhatt DL, Braunwald E, *et al.* Saxagliptin and cardiovascular outcomes in patients with type 2 diabetes mellitus. N Engl J Med 2013; 369(14): 1317-26.
[http://dx.doi.org/10.1056/NEJMoa1307684] [PMID: 23992601]

[4]   Gupta A, Jelinek HF, Al-Aubaidy H. Glucagon like peptide-1 and its receptor agonists: Their roles in management of Type 2 diabetes mellitus. Diabetes Metab Syndr 2017; 11(3): 225-30.
[http://dx.doi.org/10.1016/j.dsx.2016.09.003] [PMID: 27884496]

[5]   Pfeffer MA, Claggett B, Diaz R, *et al.* Lixisenatide in patients with type 2 diabetes and acute coronary syndrome. N Engl J Med 2015; 373(23): 2247-57.
[http://dx.doi.org/10.1056/NEJMoa1509225] [PMID: 26630143]

[6]   Marso SP, Daniels GH, Brown-Frandsen K, *et al.* Liraglutide and cardiovascular outcomes in type 2 diabetes. N Engl J Med 2016; 375(4): 311-22.
[http://dx.doi.org/10.1056/NEJMoa1603827] [PMID: 27295427]

[7]   Cariou B, Charbonnel B, Staels B. Thiazolidinediones and PPARγ agonists: time for a reassessment. Trends Endocrinol Metab 2012; 23(5): 205-15.
[http://dx.doi.org/10.1016/j.tem.2012.03.001] [PMID: 22513163]

[8]   Kern DM, Devore S, Kim J, *et al.* Mortality, outcomes, and healthcare costs in T2DM patients at risk for cardiovascular disease. Am J Accountable Care 2015; 44(9): 1118-20.

[9]   Rehman MB, Tudrej BV, Soustre J, *et al.* Efficacy and safety of DPP-4 inhibitors in patients with type 2 diabetes: Meta-analysis of placebo-controlled randomized clinical trials. Diabetes Metab 2017; 43(1): 48-58.
[http://dx.doi.org/10.1016/j.diabet.2016.09.005] [PMID: 27745828]

[10]   Solano MP, Goldberg RB. Management of dyslipidemia in diabetes. Cardiol Rev 2006; 14(3): 125-35.
[http://dx.doi.org/10.1097/01.crd.0000188034.76283.5e] [PMID: 16628021]

[11]   Franco OH, Steyerberg EW, Hu FB, Mackenbach J, Nusselder W. Associations of diabetes mellitus with total life expectancy and life expectancy with and without cardiovascular disease. Arch Intern Med 2007; 167(11): 1145-51.
[http://dx.doi.org/10.1001/archinte.167.11.1145] [PMID: 17563022]

[12]   Gaede P, Lund-Andersen H, Parving HH, Pedersen O. Effect of a multifactorial intervention on mortality in type 2 diabetes. N Engl J Med 2008; 358(6): 580-91.
[http://dx.doi.org/10.1056/NEJMoa0706245] [PMID: 18256393]

[13]   Redmon JB, Bertoni AG, Connelly S, *et al.* Effect of the look AHEAD study intervention on medication use and related cost to treat cardiovascular disease risk factors in individuals with type 2 diabetes. Diabetes Care 2010; 33(6): 1153-8.
[http://dx.doi.org/10.2337/dc09-2090] [PMID: 20332353]

[14]   Hu FB, Stampfer MJ, Haffner SM, Solomon CG, Willett WC, Manson JE. Elevated risk of cardiovascular disease prior to clinical diagnosis of type 2 diabetes. Diabetes Care 2002; 25(7): 1129-34.
[http://dx.doi.org/10.2337/diacare.25.7.1129] [PMID: 12087009]

[15]   Kengne AP, Patel A, Marre M, *et al.* Contemporary model for cardiovascular risk prediction in people with type 2 diabetes. Eur J Cardiovasc Prev Rehabil 2011; 18(3): 393-8.
[http://dx.doi.org/10.1177/1741826710394270] [PMID: 21450612]

[16]   Tight blood pressure control and risk of macrovascular and microvascular complications in type 2 diabetes: UKPDS 38. BMJ 1998; 317(7160): 703-13.
[http://dx.doi.org/10.1136/bmj.317.7160.703] [PMID: 9732337]

[17]   Kuusisto J, Mykkänen L, Pyörälä K, Laakso M. NIDDM and its metabolic control predict coronary heart disease in elderly subjects. Diabetes 1994; 43(8): 960-7.
[http://dx.doi.org/10.2337/diab.43.8.960] [PMID: 8039603]

[18]   Nadeau KJ, Regensteiner JG, Bauer TA, *et al.* Insulin resistance in adolescents with type 1 diabetes and its relationship to cardiovascular function. J Clin Endocrinol Metab 2010; 95(2): 513-21.
[http://dx.doi.org/10.1210/jc.2009-1756] [PMID: 19915016]

[19]   Nathan DM, Genuth S, Lachin J, *et al.* The effect of intensive treatment of diabetes on the development and progression of long-term complications in insulin-dependent diabetes mellitus. N Engl J Med 1993; 329(14): 977-86.
[http://dx.doi.org/10.1056/NEJM199309303291401] [PMID: 8366922]

[20]   Duckworth W, Abraira C, Moritz T, *et al.* Glucose control and vascular complications in veterans with type 2 diabetes. N Engl J Med 2009; 360(2): 129-39.
[http://dx.doi.org/10.1056/NEJMoa0808431] [PMID: 19092145]

[21]   Hamilton SJ, Watts GF. Endothelial dysfunction in diabetes: pathogenesis, significance, and treatment. Rev Diabet Stud 2013; 10(2-3): 133-56.
[http://dx.doi.org/10.1900/RDS.2013.10.133] [PMID: 24380089]

[22]   Eguchi K, Boden-Albala B, Jin Z, *et al.* Association between diabetes mellitus and left ventricular hypertrophy in a multiethnic population. Am J Cardiol 2008; 101(12): 1787-91.
[http://dx.doi.org/10.1016/j.amjcard.2008.02.082] [PMID: 18549860]

[23]   Brooks BA, Franjic B, Ban CR, *et al.* Diastolic dysfunction and abnormalities of the microcirculation in type 2 diabetes. Diabetes Obes Metab 2008; 10(9): 739-46.
[http://dx.doi.org/10.1111/j.1463-1326.2007.00803.x] [PMID: 17941867]

[24]   Patil VC, Patil HV, Shah KB, Vasani JD, Shetty P. Diastolic dysfunction in asymptomatic type 2 diabetes mellitus with normal systolic function. J Cardiovasc Dis Res 2011; 2(4): 213-22.
[http://dx.doi.org/10.4103/0975-3583.89805] [PMID: 22135479]

[25]   Kannel WB. Lipids, diabetes, and coronary heart disease: insights from the Framingham Study. Am Heart J 1985; 110(5): 1100-7.
[http://dx.doi.org/10.1016/0002-8703(85)90224-8] [PMID: 4061265]

CHAPTER 20

Management of Cardiovascular Disease in Diabetic Nephropathy

Abstract: Diabetes mellitus is a complex metabolic disorder that is represented with a defect in insulin secretion and insulin action. Diabetic nephropathy is a well-known complication of diabetes that occurs in 20% to 40% of the diabetic population. Kidney failure is categorized into acute and chronic renal disease. Acute renal disease may origin rapidly which is reversible. Chronic kidney disease develops in a slow manner at least three months of duration which leads to cause kidney failure. The permanent damage to the kidney cells by the multiple risk factors that result in loss of renal function which leads to cause renal failure. Chronic renal failure is a well-established risk factor for developing cardiovascular disease complications. Renal failure patients may develop ten to twenty folds risk of developing cardiovascular disease. Dialysis is performed to normalize the health condition of chronic renal failure patients. The progression of kidney failure with cardiovascular disease has been associated with various risk factors such as obesity, hypertension, diabetes, smoking, and alcohol enhances the risk of cardiovascular disease with renal failure. The chest x-ray, electrocardiogram, echocardiogram, coronary angiogram, urine culture test, MRI scan, CT scan, blood test, renal biopsy, fasting blood sugar, random blood sugar, serum creatinine, creatine clearance, uric acid, total proteins, glomerular filtration rate was used to detect the severity of cardiovascular disease in diabetic nephropathy. Early identification of causative factors detection and effective prescribing practice of blood lowering medications, statins, hyperlipidemic drugs, diuretics, and erythropoietin drugs can improve the health outcomes of cardiovascular disease in diabetic nephropathy patients.

Keywords: Acute Renal Disease, Chronic Renal Failure, Diabetes Mellitus, Dialysis, Hypertension.

INTRODUCTION

Cardiovascular disease patients who are diagnosed with diabetic nephropathy can cause more health care expenditure. The increase in the incidence of diabetes mellitus, hypertension clinical conditions are more common among renal failure patients. Diabetic nephropathy has a high risk of developing cardiac death in young patients as compared with old aged patients.

M.S. Umashankar & A. Bharath Kumar

The recent statement from the center for disease control explained that heart disease is the leading cause of death among renal failure patients. Cardiovascular disease is the most common in renal failure patients. The presence of more stress, diabetes mellitus, alcohol, smoking and blood pressure doubles the progression of cardiac risk incidences. The stoppage of the blood flow to the heart leads to the death of the myocardial tissues. Chronic kidney disease is a major health care issue in the community. Chronic renal failure is defined as a glomerular filtration rate of less than 60 mL/min/1.73 m² at least the last three months. The permanent damage to the kidney cells by the multiple risk factors that result in loss of renal function which leads to cause renal failure. Kidney failure is classified into acute and chronic renal disease. Acute renal disease may origin rapidly which is reversible. Chronic kidney disease develops in a slow manner at least three months of duration which leads to cause kidney failure. Chronic renal failure is a well established risk factor for developing cardiovascular disease complications. Patients who diagnosed with renal failure may have ten to twenty folds increases the risk of cardiovascular disease [1 - 3]. Dialysis is performed to improve the health status of chronic renal failure patients. Patients diagnosed with various stages of renal dysfunction and not under dialysis treatment have a greater risk of mortality and morbidity from cardiovascular disease. The risk incidences of cardiovascular disease differ from renal failure patients. The improper blood supply to the heart develops the high pressure in the veins that are connected to the kidneys which result in the poor blood supply to the kidney causes the blockage and results in kidney failure.

COMPLICATIONS OF RENAL FAILURE [4 - 7]

Anemia

Red blood cells consist of a protein called hemoglobin that transports the oxygen to the overall body. Anemia causes the heart to pump more blood to all parts of the body. The more pressure on the chambers of the heart causes the failure of the heart function. The body is insufficient to produce red blood cells, which lowers the oxygen supply to the body tissues and organs and increases the risk of heart failure. Imbalance of the calcium and phosphorus levels: the abnormal deposition of the calcium and phosphorous in the blood increases the risk of progressing kidney failure with cardiovascular disease.

Hypertension

The more pressure that is deposited in the arteries of the blood vessels that raise the more heart contractions and pumps more blood to the cardiac muscles. The contraction of the heart rate is high called systolic blood pressure and lowest contractions of the heart called diastolic blood pressure. The elevated blood pressure which is above the normal range is known as hypertension. Hypertension increases the risk of developing various complications such as coronary artery disease, stroke, and congestive heart failure,*etc.* The rennin enzyme controls the blood pressure. The low level of the blood pressure, rennin stimulates the hormones to increase the blood pressure. The failure of the kidneys releases an excess of rennin leads to more rise in the blood pressure. The uncontrolled blood pressure increases the risk of developing chronic heart failure, stroke and coronary artery disease.

Abnormal Homocysteine Levels

Homocysteine is an amino acid that is commonly present in the blood. Healthy condition kidney controls the homocysteine in the blood and excess will be removed from the circulation. The failure of kidney function cannot remove the homocysteine from the blood. The high level of homocysteine connected to plaques in the blood vessels leads to the origin of coronary artery disease. The presence of abnormal levels of proteins in the blood called homocysteine. The normal function of the kidneys can remove the proteins from the blood circulation. The abnormal deposition of the proteins in the blood can cause the risk of developing various complications such as heart attack, stroke, and coronary artery disease [8 - 10].

Coronary Artery Disease

A low level of blood flow to the arteries increases the risk of heart attack. Coronary artery disease is manifested with various clinical symptoms. The over accumulation of the fatty substances in the arteries restrict the blood flow to the coronary artery results on the progression of coronary artery disease. The arteries distribute the oxygen and blood to the heart muscles. The lack of oxygen supply to the heart muscles leads to develop chest pain.

Atherosclerosis

The accumulation of fatty materials and calcium in the coronary arteries that lead to forms the plaque in arteries causes atherosclerosis. The progression of kidney failure with cardiovascular disease has been associated with various risk factors such as obesity, hypertension, diabetes, smoking, and alcohol enhances the risk of cardiovascular disease with renal failure.

The identification of early stages of renal failure and treatment strategies can prevent the risk of developing cardiovascular disease among diabetic patients. Most of the patients with renal failure die from cardiovascular disease. Renal replacement therapy can reduce the risk of progression of renal failure among cardiovascular disease patients. The low level of glomerular filtration rate which is less than 15 ml/min/1.73m^2, can increase the risk of cardiovascular events, and hospital readmission. The microalbuminuria decreases kidney function, which raises the risk of developing cardiovascular disease. Patients with a previous medical history of chronic renal failure can increase premature cardiac death and increases the need of renal transplantation. Acute kidney injury is the rapid damage to the kidneys. The kidney damage is a short term that leads to cause the long term damage to the long term complications among affected patients. Acute renal injury is characterized by the deterioration in renal function more than two months of kidney failure. Acute kidney injury is caused by hypovolemia, dehydration, and inflammation. The failure of the kidney to eliminate the waste materials such as urea, creatinine from the blood through the urine leads to develop kidney failure. Kidney failure is treated with hemodialysis, peritoneal dialysis, and kidney transplantation. The chronic failure condition the glomerular filtration rate differs from stage 1 to stage 5 and causes permanent renal damage [11 - 15]. The stages of kidney disease are shown in Table **1**.

Table 1. The stages of kidney disease are based on the eGFR number.

Stage	Condition	GFR Rate
Stage 1	Normal	GFR > 90 mL/min
Stage 2	Mild	GFR = 60-89 mL/min
Stage 3A	Moderate CKD	GFR = 45-59 mL/min
Stage 3B	Moderate CKD	GFR = 30-44 mL/min
Stage 4	Severe CKD	GFR = 15-29 mL/min
Stage 5	End Stage CKD	GFR <15 mL/min

PREVALENCE

The cardiovascular diseases include ischemic heart disease, heart failure, cardiac arrhythmias, coronary artery disease and hypertension. Chronic kidney disease affects patients who are diagnosed with cardiovascular disease. Previous research studies stated that end stage renal disease patients 20 to 30 times likely to die from cardiovascular disease. The low level of glomerular filtration rate and albuminuria was greatly associated with the death of renal disease patients with cardiac disease. Globally, the incidence of diabetes mellitus has been raised. Diabetes mellitus is predicted to grow 550 million people by the year 2035. Diabetic nephropathy is a well known complication of diabetes that occurs in 20% to 40% of the diabetic population. Cardiovascular disease is the major cause of death among patients is receiving dialysis. Cardiac failure is the most common among renal failure patients in the general population. Among dialysis patients, the incidence was 40%. In 2015, 1.2 million people died from kidney failure and increased up to 25% in 2005. Currently, 26 million people are affected by chronic kidney disease. Diabetes mellitus is a complex metabolic disorder that is represented with a defect in insulin secretion and insulin action. Worldwide 422 million people are affected with diabetes mellitus. Diabetic nephropathy is a major public health problem that can lower the life expectancy of diabetes mellitus patients. The risk of diabetic nephropathy developed with micro albuminuria, and macro albuminuria. United States, 2016 the incidence of heart failure was at the age of 66 years, 28.8% in chronic kidney disease patients. In 2010, 2.62 million patients were treated with dialysis worldwide and this count may rise to 9.24 million by 2030. Worldwide the health care expenditure for chronic kidney disease was predicted to much greater as compared with treatment for end-stage kidney disease. Low socio-economical status and poverty are identified as risk factors for developing chronic kidney disease. In 2015, worldwide 415 million people affected with diabetes mellitus. By the year 2040, the incidence rate was raised to 642 million with a significant increase from low to middle income countries. Oman the prevalence of diabetic nephropathy was found to be 42.5%, Yemen 21.2%, Iraq 16.1%, Sudan 44%, Egypt 34.2%, United Kingdom 30.8%, mexican Americans was 31%,11.2% in Thailand, and 12.7% in Taiwan, 9% in Germany, and 16% in Italy and Sweden. The incidence of diabetic nephropathy in United States was 9.8% in 1988–1994 periods to 12.3% in 2011–2012. National Kidney Foundation predicted that the 8 million people having glomerular filtration rate less than 60 mL/min which raises the incidence of renal failure among cardiac disease patients worldwide. The incidence of cardiovascular disease in renal failure was 47.2% in UK, and 39.1% Spain, 26.8% in Japan and 33.4% in US respectively. Worldwide the mortality rate of end-stage renal disease was more than 20% per year. Previous research studies stated that diabetes mellitus, hypertension, albuminuria, dyslipidemia, and anemia contribute to increasing the risk of diabetic nephropathy among cardiovascular disease patients [16, 17].

CAUSES OF RENAL FAILURE

It includes

• Diabetes mellitus

• High blood pressure

• Urinary tract problems

• Autoimmune diseases

- Genetic diseases

- Glomerulonephritis

- Interstitial nephritis

- Kidney infection

- Heart attack

- Illegal drug use and drug abuse

- Tobacco and alcohol use

OTHER CAUSES OF RENAL FAILURE

It includes

- Infections

- Heavy metal toxins

- Vasculitis

- Multiple myeloma

- Scleroderma

- Blood clot in kidneys

- Chemotherapy drugs

- Hemolytic uremic syndrome

- Risk factors for cardiovascular disease

- Modifiable Risk factors include

- High blood cholesterol level

- Cigarette smoking

- Alcohol

- Physical activity

- Hypertension

• Obesity

• Diabetes mellitus

• Stress

• Non Modifiable Risk factors

• Family history of coronary artery disease or diabetes mellitus

• Increasing age

• Gender(male)

PATHOGENESIS

Cardiac disease complications are identified to cause high mortality among renal disease patients. The progression of high cardiovascular disease risk in renal patients is associated with complex causative factors which include metabolic, endocrine and hemodynamic factors that can increase the hyper urecemia. The low levels of blood supply to the ventricles and more pressure on the ventricles causes hypertrophy of the ventricles. The left ventricular hypertrophy lowers the hemodynamic function leads to impair the heart function. The altered left ventricular function alters the myocyte function which results in the development of cardiovascular disease. The left ventricular hypertrophy induces the myocytes death and reduces the capillary density leads to diastolic dysfunction. The cardiac myocytes death causes left ventricular hypertrophy which results in cardiovascular conduction abnormalities. Patients with prolong uremia increase the risk of coronary artery disease. The left ventricular hypertrophy increases the risk of end stage renal disease. The left ventricular hypertrophy reduces the capillary density which creates an inequality between oxygen demands and supply that causes ischemia. The ischemic changes impair the systolic and diastolic dysfunction. The poor function of the heart increases the risk of ventricular arrhythmia and cardiac death among renal failure patients. The increased preload cause's hypovolemia leads to develop the left ventricular dilation. After load and pre load causes left ventricular hypertrophy that is commonly seen in the renal failure patients. Higher aldosterone activates the renin-angiotensin system which induces myocardial fibrosis. The excess of sympathetic over activity may cause left ventricular dysfunction [18, 19].

The pathogenesis of cardiovascular disease in renal disease patients is a complex process that is linked with multiple risk factors such as diabetes mellitus, dyslipidemia, and hypertension are contributes to the origin of kidney failure. The abnormal hemoglobin levels, mineral metabolism and more oxidative stress and systemic inflammation increase the risk of developing renal failure among cardiac disease patients. The more oxidative stress reduces the antioxidant capacity which can elevate the metabolic function. The activation of rennin angiotensin aldosterone system results in higher levels of angiotensin II causes vasoconstriction and increases the risk of albuminuria among renal failure patients. The higher levels of endothelin-1 cause vasoconstriction in the blood vessels which lowers the blood flow to the renal tubules. The higher levels of endothelin-1 cause hypertrophy and proliferation of the extra cellular matrix and alter the function of glomerular cells leads to an increase in albuminuria and finally cause the development of kidney disease among cardiovascular disease patients. The imbalance of polyol pathway increases the glycemic levels in the blood. The conversion of glucose to sorbitol occurs in the presence of NADPH-dependent enzyme. The reduction of glucose to sorbitol decreases the intracellular NADPH levels can raise more oxidative stress and causes cell apoptosis. The higher level of NADH forms the methylglyoxal and finally forms the fructose which damages the renal tubules. Advanced glycation end products cause glycation of proteins which increase the glycemic levels in the blood. The cytokines modify the vascular endothelial cells permeability which alters the permeability of the glomerular cells and causes the death of endothelial cells which is highly toxic and damages the renal cells. Advanced glycation end products attached to pro inflammatory receptors and activate the release of cytokines such as IL-6, IL-1, and TNF-α and increase the more production of reactive oxygen species which damages the nephrons leads to the development of diabetic nephropathy. Pathogenesis of diabetic nephropathy is shown in Fig. (**1**).

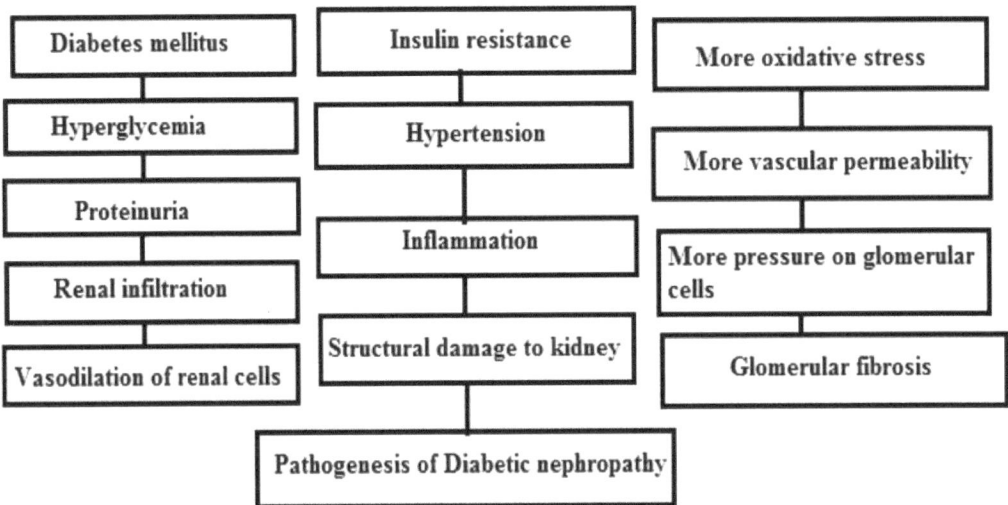

Fig. (1). Pathogenesis of diabetic nephropathy.

SYMPTOMS

Clinical Symptoms of Coronary Heart Disease

It includes

- Chest pain

- Shortness of breath

- Chest discomfort

- Pain, numbness, weakness

- Coldness in legs or arms

- Abdominal pain

Clinical Symptoms of Heart Arrhythmias

It includes

- Tachycardia

- Bradycardia

- Chest pain or discomfort

- Lightheadedness

- Dizziness

- Syncope

- Fluttering in chest

- Shortness of breath

Clinical Symptoms of Heart Defects

It includes

- Swelling in the legs, and abdomen

- shortness of breath during feedings

- Life-threatening symptoms of heart defects include

- Short of breath

- Swelling in the hands, ankles

Clinical Symptoms of Dilated Cardiomyopathy

- Fatigue

- Breathlessness

- Padal edema

- Irregular heartbeats

- Dizziness

- Light headedness

- Fainting

Clinical Symptoms of Heart Infections

- Swelling in legs

- Fever

- Dry cough

- Shortness of breath

- Weakness

- Skin rashes

Clinical Symptoms of Valvular Heart Disease

- Chest pain

- Fatigue

- Shortness of breath

- Padal edema

- Irregular heartbeat

- Fainting

Clinical Symptoms of Renal Failure

- Nausea and vomiting
- Loss of appetite
- Fluid retention
- High blood pressure
- Decreased mental sharpness
- Fatigue
- Confusion
- Weakness
- Fatigue and weakness
- Sleep problems
- Muscle cramps
- Chest pain
- Shortness of breath
- Decreased urine output
- Irregular heartbeat
- Chest pain
- Seizure
- Diagnosis
- Fasting blood sugar test
- Postprandial glucose test
- Random blood sugar test
- Glycated hemoglobin test
- Electrocardiogram

- Exercise Stress tests

- Chest X-rays

- Echocardiogram

- Doppler studies

- Coronary Angiography

- Magnetic Resonance Imaging scan

- Computerized Tomography scan

- Blood test

- Urine tests

- Ultrasound scan of kidney

- Renal biopsy

- Blood urea nitrogen test

- Electrolyte test

- Blood urea test

- Serum creatinine test

- Glomerular filtration test

- Phosphorus and calcium test

- Albumin test

- Creatinine clearance test

- Parathyroid hormone test

- Hemoglobin test

- Uric acid test

- Urine albumin and albumin/creatinine ratio

- Urine total protein or urine protein to creatinine ratio

LIFESTYLE MODIFICATIONS FOR PREVENTION OF CARDIOVASCULAR DISEASE IN DIABETES MELLITUS [20, 21]

- Regular physical exercise for about 30 minutes every day

- Avoid consumption of sugar products

- Limit the intake of sodium not more than 2-4gms per day

- Regular consumption of DASH (Dietary Approaches to Stop Hypertension) diet

- Stress management

- Smoking cessation

- Alcohol cessation

- Maintaining scheduled sleep

- Avoiding consumption of fatty foods

- Eating high fiber food

- Maintaining healthy weight

- Regular meditation practice

- Restriction of salt intake

- Avoiding consumption of sea and sweet foods

- Regular medication adherence

- Regular foot and eye care

- Eating low fat especially saturated fat

- Consumption of low in dietary cholesterol

- Minimize the consumption of trans fat

- Regular intake of high dietary fibre foods

MANAGEMENT OF CARDIOVASCULAR DISEASE RISK [22 - 25]

Anti Platelet Drugs

These drugs help to prevent the platelet aggregation and reduce the clot in the blood vessels.

Types of Antiplatelet Agents

• aspirin

• dipyridamole

• clopidogrel

• ticagrelor

Clinical Uses of Antiplatelet Agents

It is used to treat following disease conditions.

• Angina pectoris

• Heart attack

• Coronary artery disease

• Stroke

• Peripheral artery disease

Side Effects Nausea, gastric problems, diarrhea, rashes, and itching.

Blood Pressure Lowering Medications

Diuretics

Loop diuretics These drugs will inhibit the sodium potassium co transport mechanism in the ascending loop of henle it leads to an increase in the distal tubular concentration of sodium and reduced levels of hyprertonicity of sodium levels in the intestine cause diueresis.

Loop diuretics include

• Bumetanide

- Furosemide

- Ethacrynate

- Torsemide

Adverse Effects Hypokalemia, alkalosis, hypomagnesemia, hyperuricemia, dehydration, ototoxicity.

Thiazides Diuretics

These drugs inhibit the sodium-chloride transporter in the distal tubule and reabsorption of sodium ions causes the elimination of more water from the body.

- Chlorothiazide

- Chlorthalidone

- Indapamide

- Hydrochlorothiazide

- Methyclothiazide

Adverse Effects Hyponatremia, hyperglycemia, dehydration, hypokalemia, hypertriglyceridemia, hyperuricemia, azotemia.

Carbonic Anhydrase Inhibitors

These drugs will inhibit the transport of bicarbonate ions from the proximal convulted tubule which leads to loss of sodium, hydrogen and bicarbonate ions in the urine.

The drugs include

Acetazolamide

Methazolamide

Adverse Effects Metabolic acidosis and hypokalemia

Potassium Sparing Diuretics

It acts on the distal segment of the distal tubules and causes more water to enter inside the collecting tubule. It will inhibit the aldosterone-sensitive sodium reabsorption thereby loss of potassium and hydrogen from the urine.

Amiloride

spironolactone

Triamterene

Adverse effects Metabolic acidosis, gynecomastia, hyperkalemia, gastric ulcers.

Cholesterol Lowering Medications Include

Statins

These drugs act by inhibiting HMG-CoA reductase enzyme and inhibit the cholesterol biosynthetic pathway and show anti atherosclerotic effect in the blood vessels.

• Atorvastatin

• Fluvastatin

• Lovastatin

• Pitavastatin

• Pravastatin

• Rosuvastatin

• Simvastatin

Adverse effects Headache, dizziness, insomnia, flushing of the skin, drowsiness, and myalgia.

Angiotensin Converting Enzyme Inhibitors

ACEs block the conversion of angiotensin I to angiotensin II by the action of angiotensinogen in the body and help to lower the vasoconstriction and promote vasodilation.

It includes

• Captopril

• Lisinopril

• Fosinopril

- Ramipril

- Benazepril

- Enalapril

- Perindopril

- Quinapril

- Moexipril

- Trandolapril

Adverse effects Dry cough, hyperkalemia, fatigue, headaches and loss of taste.

Angiotensin II Receptor Blockers

It blocks the conversion of angiotensin II from its binding to angiotensin II receptors located on the blood vessels and produces vasodialtion in the blood vessels.

These drugs include

- Candesartan

- Telmisartan

- Valsartan

- Eprosartan

- Irbesartan

- Losartan

Adverse effects Hyperkalemia, dizziness, headache, cough, diarrhea, hypotension and angioedema.

Beta Blockers

It reduces the work load on the heart and reduces stress and hormones levels in the body which leads to vasodilatation in the blood vessels.

Commonly prescribed beta blockers include

- Atenolol

- Bisoprolol

- Nadolol

- Nebivolol

- Carvedilol

- Labetalol

- Nebivolol

- Pindolol

- Propranolol

- Timolol

- Metoprolol

Adverse effects Dry mouth, dry skin, feelings of coldness, diarrhea, shortness of breath and insomnia.

Calcium Channel Blockers

This drug blocks the entry of calcium ions into the calcium channels and lowers the work load on the heart and dilates the arteries leads to vasodilatation.

These drugs include

- Diltiazem

- Verapamil

- Isradipine

- Nifedipine

- Nicardipine

- Nimopidine

- Amlodipine

- Nisoldipine

- Bepridil

• Felodipine

Adverse effects Rashes, headache, constipation, flushing, edema, drowsiness

MANAGEMENT OF KIDNEY FAILURE

Erythropoietin

Red blood cells are formed in the bone marrow. Erythropoietin can synthesize red blood cells in the kidneys. This agent is used to treat the anemia in renal failure patients. Hemoglobin is the protein in red blood cells that helps blood carry oxygen throughout the body. Erythropoietin contains more red blood cells which increase the hemoglobin levels in the body. Hemoglobin is the protein that is present in the red blood cells helps to supply the oxygen throughout the body. The low level of hemoglobin increases the risk of developing anemia. The iron supplements and Erythropoietin is used to prevent the anemia complications.

Side Effects of Erythropoietin

It includes

• High blood pressure

• Nausea

• Injection site reactions

• Swelling

• Fever

• Dizziness

Phosphate Binders

These medications are used to control the blood phosphate levels. It will remove the excess amount of phosphate in the body through stools and lowers the phosphate quantity in the blood.

Adverse effects

It includes

• Nausea

• Vomiting

- Constipation

- Diarrhea

- Indigestion

- Abdominal pain

Sodium Bicarbonate

It is a blood alkalizer, that raises the plasma bircarbonate levels and blood pH leads to lowers the acidosis. It is also used as a urinary alkalizer, which removes the free bicarbonate ions present in the urine. Sodium bicarbonate is an antacid that chemically neutralizes the excess quantity of acid levels present in the stomach.

Adverse Effects

- Breathlessness

- Headache

- Nausea

- Vomiting

- Nervousness

- Loss of appetite

- Frequent urination

- Muscle pain

- Twitching

- Restlessness

- Mental changes

Vitamin D Supplements

The chemically active form of vitamin D binds to intracellular receptors which contain DNA that can modulate the gene expression.

Adverse Effects

It includes

• Bone pain

• Extreme thirst

• Confusion

• Weight loss

• Frequent urination

• Muscle weakness

• Kidney stones

• Nausea

• vomiting

• constipation

DIALYSIS

Hemodialysis

Hemodialysis is the most commonly performed with renal failure patients. This process depends on hemodialyzer to eliminate the excess of waste fluids present in the blood. The blood is eliminated from the body through the artificial mechanical device and returns to the body. The process is performed with dialysis solution and AV graft and fistula which is inserted into the veins to continue the dialysis process.

Peritoneal Dialysis

This process involves a catheter is inserted into the abdomen that can help to filter the blood through the peritoneum. The dialysis fluid passes into the peritoneum and absorbs the waste materials and filleted blood reached the abdomen.

Continuous Renal Replacement Therapy (CRRT)

This therapy is continued for 24hours per day in specialized conditions in the renal care units. The removal of waste materials from the blood is achieved by hemo filtration, and hemo dialysis process.

Dialysis Complications

Hemodialysis Complications

- Sepsis

- Pericarditis

- Insomnia

- Hyperkalemia

- Bacterial infections

- Irregular heartbeats

- Hypotension

- Anemia

- Muscle cramps

- Sudden cardiac death

Peritoneal Dialysis Complications

- Stomach pain

- Hernia

- Fever

- Abdominal muscles weakness

- High blood sugar

- Weight gain

CONCLUSION

The high incidence of diabetes mellitus and renal failure has been an increase in developed and developing countries. The improper control of diabetic nephropathy escalates the risk of developing end stage renal disease in renal failure patients. The chronic duration of diabetes mellitus increases the risk of renal failure. The pathophysiological association between diabetes and diabetic nephropathy is metabolic and hemodynamic pathways, more oxidative stress, and release of various inflammatory cells leads to cause the renal damage. Microalbuminuria is the earliest clinical symptom of renal failure. Maintaining the controlled levels of blood glucose and blood pressure can lower the risk of microalbuminuria mediated risk among renal failure patients. The development of diabetic complications is associated with several risk factors which include environmental factors, genetics, hypertension, alcohol, smoking, diabetes mellitus; stress, and obesity can accelerate renal failure complications.

The management of cardiovascular disease in renal failure includes lipid control, blood pressure control, low protein intake, low level of salt intake, weight management, smoking and alcoholic cessation can minimize the occurrence of cardiovascular events among renal failure patients. Clinical pharmacist should be positioned in the clinical areas to address risk factors control, providing patient counseling services on diet, disease, lifestyle modification, dietary restriction, weight control, stress management, physical exercise, initiation of awareness programmes on renal failure prevention and novel therapeutic drugs can prevent the occurrence of renal failure among cardiac patients.

Early detection of renal failure stage and aggressive therapeutic interventions are lowering the adverse outcomes of the disease. The clinical management of renal failure in cardiovascular disease involves prescribing of ACE inhibitors, statins, diuretics, erythropoietin, angiotensin receptor blockers, anti-diabetic medications that can lower the progression of cardiovascular events among renal failure patients.

REFERENCES

[1]   Pradel FG, Jain R, Mullins CD, Vassalotti JA, Bartlett ST. A survey of nephrologists' views on preemptive transplantation. Clin J Am Soc Nephrol 2008; 3(6): 1837-45.
       [http://dx.doi.org/10.2215/CJN.00150108] [PMID: 18832107]

[2]   Herzog CA, Asinger RW, Berger AK, *et al*. Cardiovascular disease in chronic kidney disease. A clinical update from Kidney Disease: Improving Global Outcomes (KDIGO). Kidney Int 2011; 80(6): 572-86.
       [http://dx.doi.org/10.1038/ki.2011.223] [PMID: 21750584]

[3]   Konstantinidis I, Nadkarni GN, Yacoub R, *et al*. Representation of patients with kidney disease in trials of cardiovascular interventions: an updated systematic review. JAMA Intern Med 2016; 176(1): 121-4.
       [http://dx.doi.org/10.1001/jamainternmed.2015.6102] [PMID: 26619332]

[4]   Gansevoort RT, Correa-Rotter R, Hemmelgarn BR, *et al*. Chronic kidney disease and cardiovascular risk: epidemiology, mechanisms, and prevention. Lancet 2013; 382(9889): 339-52.
       [http://dx.doi.org/10.1016/S0140-6736(13)60595-4] [PMID: 23727170]

[5]   Wang LW, Fahim MA, Hayen A, *et al*. Cardiac testing for coronary artery disease in potential kidney transplant recipients: a systematic review of test accuracy studies. Am J Kidney Dis 2011; 57(3): 476-87.
       [http://dx.doi.org/10.1053/j.ajkd.2010.11.018] [PMID: 21257239]

[6]   Go AS, Chertow GM, Fan D, McCulloch CE, Hsu C-Y. Chronic kidney disease and the risks of death, cardiovascular events, and hospitalization. N Engl J Med 2004; 351(13): 1296-305.
[http://dx.doi.org/10.1056/NEJMoa041031] [PMID: 15385656]

[7]   Baumeister SE, Böger CA, Krämer BK, *et al.* Effect of chronic kidney disease and comorbid conditions on health care costs: A 10-year observational study in a general population. Am J Nephrol 2010; 31(3): 222-9.
[http://dx.doi.org/10.1159/000272937] [PMID: 20068286]

[8]   Weir MR. Recognizing the link between chronic kidney disease and cardiovascular disease. Am J Manag Care 2011; 17 (Suppl. 15): S396-402.
[PMID: 22214474]

[9]   Leoncini G, Viazzi F, Pontremoli R. Chronic kidney disease and albuminuria in arterial hypertension. Curr Hypertens Rep 2010; 12(5): 335-41.
[http://dx.doi.org/10.1007/s11906-010-0141-3] [PMID: 20694530]

[10]   Acquarone N, Castello C, Antonucci G, Lione S, Bellotti P. Pharmacologic therapy in patients with chronic heart failure and chronic kidney disease: a complex issue. J Cardiovasc Med (Hagerstown) 2009; 10(1): 13-21.
[http://dx.doi.org/10.2459/JCM.0b013e3283189533] [PMID: 19708224]

[11]   Frankenfield DL, Howell BL, Wei II, Anderson KK. Cost-related nonadherence to prescribed medication therapy among Medicare Part D beneficiaries with end-stage renal disease. Am J Health Syst Pharm 2011; 68(14): 1339-48.
[http://dx.doi.org/10.2146/ajhp100400] [PMID: 21719594]

[12]   Davis JW, Fujimoto RY, Chan H, Juarez DT. Adherence with lipid-lowering, antihypertensive, and diabetes medications. Am J Pharm Benefits 2011; 3: 165-71.

[13]   Joki N, Hase H, Nakamura R, Yamaguchi T. Onset of coronary artery disease prior to initiation of haemodialysis in patients with end-stage renal disease. Nephrol Dial Transplant 1997; 12(4): 718-23.
[http://dx.doi.org/10.1093/ndt/12.4.718] [PMID: 9141000]

[14]   Schiffrin EL, Lipman ML, Mann JFE. Chronic kidney disease: effects on the cardiovascular system. Circulation 2007; 116(1): 85-97.
[http://dx.doi.org/10.1161/CIRCULATIONAHA.106.678342] [PMID: 17606856]

[15]   Rahman M, Xie D, Feldman HI, *et al.* Association between chronic kidney disease progression and cardiovascular disease: results from the CRIC Study. Am J Nephrol 2014; 40(5): 399-407.
[http://dx.doi.org/10.1159/000368915] [PMID: 25401485]

[16]   Elsayed EF, Tighiouart H, Griffith J, *et al.* Cardiovascular disease and subsequent kidney disease. Arch Intern Med 2007; 167(11): 1130-6.
[http://dx.doi.org/10.1001/archinte.167.11.1130] [PMID: 17563020]

[17]   Schillaci G, Reboldi G, Verdecchia P. High-normal serum creatinine concentration is a predictor of cardiovascular risk in essential hypertension. Arch Intern Med 2001; 161(6): 886-91.
[http://dx.doi.org/10.1001/archinte.161.6.886] [PMID: 11268234]

[18]   Sarnak MJ, Coronado BE, Greene T, *et al.* Cardiovascular disease risk factors in chronic renal insufficiency. Clin Nephrol 2002; 57(5): 327-35.
[http://dx.doi.org/10.5414/CNP57327] [PMID: 12036190]

[19]   Mann JF, Lonn EM, Yi Q, *et al.* Effects of vitamin E on cardiovascular outcomes in people with mild-to-moderate renal insufficiency: results of the HOPE study. Kidney Int 2004; 65(4): 1375-80.
[http://dx.doi.org/10.1111/j.1523-1755.2004.00513.x] [PMID: 15086477]

[20]   Pannier B, Guerin AP, Marchais SJ, Metivier F, Safar ME, London GM. Postischemic vasodilation, endothelial activation, and cardiovascular remodeling in end-stage renal disease. Kidney Int 2000; 57(3): 1091-9.
[http://dx.doi.org/10.1046/j.1523-1755.2000.00936.x] [PMID: 10720961]

[21]   Muntner P, Coresh J, Smith JC, Eckfeldt J, Klag MJ. Plasma lipids and risk of developing renal dysfunction: the atherosclerosis risk in communities study. Kidney Int 2000; 58(1): 293-301.
[http://dx.doi.org/10.1046/j.1523-1755.2000.00165.x] [PMID: 10886574]

[22]   Levey AS. Controlling the epidemic of cardiovascular disease in chronic renal disease: where do we start? Am J Kidney Dis 1998; 32(5) (Suppl. 3): S5-S13.
[http://dx.doi.org/10.1053/ajkd.1998.v32.pm9820463] [PMID: 9820463]

[23]   Anavekar NS, Pfeffer MA. Cardiovascular risk in chronic kidney disease. Kidney Int Suppl 2004; 66(92): S11-5.
[http://dx.doi.org/10.1111/j.1523-1755.2004.09203.x] [PMID: 15485401]

[24]   Keith DS, Nichols GA, Gullion CM, Brown JB, Smith DH. Longitudinal follow-up and outcomes among a population with chronic kidney disease in a large managed care organization. Arch Intern Med 2004; 164(6): 659-63.
[http://dx.doi.org/10.1001/archinte.164.6.659] [PMID: 15037495]

[25]   Astor BC, Coresh J, Heiss G, Pettitt D, Sarnak MJ. Kidney function and anemia as risk factors for coronary heart disease and mortality: the Atherosclerosis Risk in Communities (ARIC) Study. Am Heart J 2006; 151(2): 492-500.
[http://dx.doi.org/10.1016/j.ahj.2005.03.055] [PMID: 16442920]

CHAPTER 21

Newer Technologies in Cardiovascular Disease Detection and Management

Abstract: Cardiovascular diseases cause mortality and morbidity worldwide. The progression of cardiovascular disease is associated with several risk factors which include hypertension, diabetes mellitus, obesity, stress, kidney disease, smoking and alcohol increase the risk of developing cardiovascular complications. The newer health care technologies in the cardiovascular disease prevention include sensor devices, web-based strategies, smart phone applications, telemedicine; text message based mobile applications, stem cell therapy, robotic sleeve, artificial intelligence algorithms, big data technology, voice technologies, block chain technology, bioresorbable stents, leadless pacemaker, chatbots technology are used to prevent the progression of cardiovascular disease. The cardiovascular diseases are imposing huge health care expenditure burden on patients and their families. Health care innovations deal with the application of ideas, procedures, and novel concepts designed to promotes benefits to society. Advance health care information technologies are useful for the detection of cardiovascular disease risk at the earlier stages to provide better health care interventions to improve their quality of life. The innovative technologies are boosting the advances in cardiovascular health care. The novel health care technologies should focus on developing new innovations for improving the quality of patient care services in hospitals.

Keywords: Artificial Intelligence, Block Chain Technology, Diabetes Mellitus, Hypertension, Leadless Pacemaker, Sensor Devices.

INTRODUCTION

Cardiovascular disease is a major cause of death worldwide. Previous research studies stated that in 2001 16.6 million people died with the cardiovascular disease this count may rise to 25 million by 2025. The improper treatment leads to develop various complications such as coronary artery disease, hypertension, angina pectoris, and cerebrovascular disease. Cardiovascular disorders will be the largest cause of death and disability from developing countries. In developing countries, cardiovascular diseases are occurring from the age group of 30-64 years. The progression of cardiovascular disease is conjoined with various risk factors such as gender, diabetes mellitus, obesity, smoking, alcohol, and hypertension.

M.S. Umashankar & A. Bharath Kumar

The cardiovascular diseases are imposing huge health care expenditure burden on patients and their families. Health care innovations deal with the application of ideas, procedures, and novel concepts designed to promotes benefits to society. Innovative ideas are explored to confront serious health care issues in the community. Health care advancement technologies could significantly lower the progression of cardiovascular diseases in society.

TYPES OF CARDIOVASCULAR DISEASE [1, 2]

Coronary Artery Disease

Coronary artery disease is the circulatory disorder that consists of the supply of oxygen to the heart is narrowed. This condition is occurred due to the deposition of the fatty materials inside the coronary arteries that can raise the risk of coronary artery disease complications. The rupture of the plaques forms the clot in the blood vessels which leads to blockage in the coronary arteries. The clinical manifestations of coronary artery disease include chest pain, shortness of the breath, sweating, nausea, vomiting, dizziness, and irregular heartbeats. Angina pectoris is a disease in which the reduction in the blood supplies to the myocardium which creates a burning sensation at the sternum.

The coronary artery disease complications are diagnosed with electrocardiogram, chest x ray, echocardiogram, doppler studies, coronary angiogram is used to identify the progression of coronary artery disease risk complications. Previous research studies have been emphasized that several risk factors are associated with the origin of coronary artery disease risk which includes hypertension, abnormal cholesterol, smoking, alcohol, diabetes mellitus, and blood pressure. Regular prescribing pattern of statins, anti platelet drugs, beta blockers, calcium channel blockers, Angiotensin-converting enzyme (ACE) inhibitors, and angiotensin II receptor blockers (ARBs) can lower the acceleration of coronary artery disease risk complications.

Cerebrovascular Disease

It is a type of cardiovascular disease which is associated with the circulatory system, which supplies blood to the brain. The depleted level of blood supply to the brain causes the progression of the stroke. The major risk factors for stroke include physical inactivity, smoking, alcohol, obesity, blood pressure, diabetes mellitus, insomnia is greatly linked with the development of stroke. The uncontrolled levels of hypertension damages the artery lining in the cerebrum leads to block the oxygenated blood to the brain which causes thrombosis. The various types of cerebrovascular disease include subarachnoid hemorrhage, transient ischemic attack, and dementia.

Atrial fibrillation is a clinical condition where continuous atrial cell fibrillation without heart contraction of the atrial cells causes an irregular heartbeat that leads to the formation of blood clot in the arteries. The blood clot can restrict the blood supply to the heart results in increasing the risk of stroke. It is diagnosed with blood test, computerized tomography scan, cerebral angiogram; carotid ultra sound is used to detect the severity of stroke. Statins, anti platelets, thrombolytics, and ACE inhibitor is used to treat the progression of stroke complications.

Congenital Heart Disease

It is associated with the structural function of the heart. This condition is observed in newborn children. Congenital heart defects occur during the first eight weeks of fetus development that affects 8 out of 1,000 babies. It should be monitored with continuous treatment to prevent the risk of developing congenital heart defects. Congenital heart defects change the blood flow to the heart. The defect ranges from mild to severe clinical symptoms that can lead to develop life-threatening conditions. It is the most commonly occurring birth defect in newborns babies. The clinical manifestations of congenital heart disease are heart murmur, fatigue, and cyanosis, shortness of breath, and underdeveloped limbs. It is caused by several risk factors such as genetic predisposition, infections during pregnancy, alcohol, and tobacco, and poor nutrition. It is treated with Thrombolytic drugs, beta blockers, anti platelet drugs, ACE inhibitors, ARB's, calcium channel blockers, diuretics drugs *etc.* are used to reduce congenital heart disease burden among affected children.

Peripheral Arterial Disease

It is a widespread circulatory disorder in which narrowed arteries can condense blood flow to limbs. The accretion of fatty deposits in the arteries may lessen the blood flow to the heart, brain, legs which are called peripheral arterial disease. The progressive narrowing of the blood vessels may interfere with blood circulation to the various organs can lead to an increase in the risk of cardiovascular diseases.

The clinical manifestations of the peripheral arterial disease include cramps in hip and calf muscles, discoloration of legs, painful hips, leg weakness, numbness in the legs, and difficulty in finding a pulse in the leg or foot, coldness in lower leg or foot, change in the color of legs. The peripheral artery disease risk factors include smoking, diabetes, high blood pressure; high blood lipids increase the risk of peripheral artery disease. The management of peripheral artery disease includes the combined use of pharmacological treatment and lifestyle changes and revascularization procedures can lower the ischemic events among high risk profile patients.

NEWER TECHNOLOGIES FOR TREATING CARDIOVASCULAR DISEASES [3, 4]

Stem Cell Therapy

Stem cells are procured from various sources and that is used to treat degenerative disorders and neuromuscular disorders. The degenerative disorders are origin from the bone, cartilage, muscle, fat, muscle and damage the various essential organs in the body. The degenerative disorders are chronic renal failure, diabetes mellitus, osteoarthritis, chronic renal failure, stroke, myocardial infarction, parkinson's disease, and alzheimer's disease.

Skeletal Myoblasts

Skeletal myoblasts have effective plasticity to increases the conduction of cardiac muscles. The specimens collected from the cardiac muscle biopsies are used to regenerate the cardiac tissues.

Bone Marrow-derived Stem Cells

It consists of hematopoietic stem cells which are extensively used in tissue regeneration in clinical studies. Bone marrow cells are used to contribute to the regeneration of the cardiac cells. Mesenchymal stem cells: These cells are found in bone marrow, adipose tissue and umbilical cord blood and heart.

Hemopoietic Stem Cells and Erythropoietic Cells

Hemopoietic stem cells are present in the bone marrow which is likely to differentiate into myeloid and lymphoid cells. Erythropoietic cells are present in the peripheral blood they can separate into endothelial cells which increases the formation of neo vascularisation.

C-kit+ CSCs

It will produce a multi potent cell that is expressed in the kinase receptor c-kit and act as an initial source for new myocardial cells regeneration.

Robotic Sleeve

It was developed by Harvard University and Boston Children's Hospital, USA. This device can l hold the cardiac muscles and improves the heart beating during heart failure. It consists of a thin silicone sleeve with pneumatic actuators that can act on the cardiac muscle layers which can improve the heart rate. It is used to improve the weakened heart beats and to treat the risk of a heart attack. The robot syncs with heart through a thin silicone sleeve with soft pneumatic actuators that mimic the heart outer muscle layers.

Implantable Cardioverter Defibrillator

These devices are useful to treat continuous ventricular tachycardia or fibrillation. The new generation Implantable defibrillators may serve as a pacemaker, which can stimulate the heart beats when it is too slow. An implantable cardioverter defibrillator is a power device which is fixed under the skin for tracking the heart rate. It consists of thin wires which are attached to the implantable cardioverter defibrillator in the heart. During the abnormal heart rhythm the device will detect the abnormal heart rhythm and restore a normal heart beat.

3D Bioprinted Heart Tissue

It is a bioprint a human cardiac patch, which is placed on the heart muscles to improve the heart functions and faster the recovery from acute heart failure. It is used to reprogramme a patient's blood cells into stem cells to lower the progression of cardiovascular disease.

Artificial Intelligence Algorithms

This concept was designed by Google company. This method depends on the verily algorithm that is used to detect heart disease by observing the patients eye. The rear interior wall of the eye screens the network of blood vessels that reveals the future risk of developing cardiovascular disease.

TECHNOLOGICAL APPLICATIONS FOR PREDICTION OF CARDIOVASCULAR DISEASES

The application of technology in the health care field that enables the role of health care practitioner's to treat the various chronic diseases more efficiently. The recent advancement in health care technologies is data mining, and artificial intelligence is used to predict the future occurrence of disease severity.

Early prediction of the disease allows patients to receive more appropriate treatment for various cardiovascular diseases. Early stage of treatment can increase the life expectancy and also the quality of life of the affected population.

Data Mining

Data mining is a computational process which analyzes the large data and helps for designing new treatment pattern. It consists of descriptive and predictive tasks. The predictive task is used to assess the future risk of developing various diseases in the community.

Mobile Health Advances in Physical Activity, Fitness and Atrial Fibrillation

Cardiovascular disease prevention consist of regular physical activity, medication adherence, consumption of healthy diet, and stress management and maintaining controlled levels of blood sugar, lipid levels, hypertension could lower the progression of the disease complications. This can performed with mobile devices such as wearable devices [5 - 9].

CARDIOVASCULAR HEALTH TECHNOLOGIES IN 2019

Big Data Technology

It used to analyze and predict the future risk of cardiovascular diseases. The data technology is used to solve the specific problems associated with various medical conditions. The data models are used to deign disease risk assessment tools which include clinical investigations and lifestyle and disease, drug safety to predict the risk of various diseases.

Artificial Intelligence Technology

Artificial intelligence is a health care technology that allows the more clinical data fed into the algorithms can help physician's ineffective clinical decision making about the health status of the disease patients.

The artificial intelligence is known as Ultronics. The AI represents the artificial intelligence in the cardiology field. This system uses topological analysis to evaluate the huge patients clinical data obtained from an echocardiogram to identify coronary artery disease at an early stage. The ultronics is associated with cardiovascular research. AI can interpret the more patient's data and helps for prompt detection and prevention of cardiovascular diseases to provide continuous health care to disease patients. The reinforcement of algorithms in hospitals and enables the risk categorization of the patients and finally improves the clinical services in health care areas.

Voice Technologies

It is used to improve the health outcomes of cardiac disease patients. The detection of patient's health status is based on the voice commands to identify the systemic changes in the body which helps for measuring cardiac disease risk.

Block Chain Technology

The block chain technology is slowly developing technology in the health care world. The computer generated protocol is used to store the patient's clinical data in a digital ledger. Block chain technology is a reliable and timely collection is used to improve the patient diagnostic and treatment care service to affected patients. The electronic health care record system is used to record the patient's clinical data.

Chatbots Technology

Chatbots are artificial intelligence messaging technologies which is designed to collect the information from users to give answers based on consumer input. These are automated channels are used to collect the information from doctors who can check the health status of the disease patients. A chatbot can collect routine information from a patient and then pass that information directly to the primary physician. A chatbot technique is used to collect the patient's routine clinical information and the physician can verify the patient's health status. This technology can easily connect with other software systems to improve the standards in current health care practices. Mobile health care applications are used to track of health status of the patent, collecting patient's feedback, encouraging the disease patient's regular adherence to physical activity, and life style change for better health care.

Telemedicine Apps Technology

Telehealth technology contains a smart phone application and online video conference software. The telehealth devices are incorporated in the sophisticated devices which can measure the patient's clinical manifestations without the need of medical professional. This includes a remote or video based interaction with the patient and collecting patient health information from medical records with other health care provider for a medical opinion on the patient from another locality.

Tele medicine involves a health care professional who can use tele communication technology to deliver health care treatment to the patient. Remote monitoring of the patients with cardiac devices results in timely diagnosis and management of cardiovascular disease clinical symptoms leads to achieving better clinical outcomes [10 - 19].

Automated Texts Technology

Text messages technology is one of the simple techniques for health care practitioners to improve patient care. The prevention of cardiac diseases based on the text message interventions which includes diet based counseling, disease counseling, alcohol and smoking cessation counseling, weight management, medication adherence, physical activities, risk factors control and drug based information can improve the patients health related outcomes.

Sensor Technology

The sensor technology is based on the Bluetooth scales with an interactive voice response system to connect with cardiac disease patients and to assess the health sickness of the patients. The interactive voice response system consists of a list of questions which is more specific to the cardiac disease.

The interactive voice response system questions deal with patient's clinical manifestations like swelling, appetite, shortness of breath, and prescription drug details used to sense the patients cardiovascular risk status. To initiate this technology it needs proper mobile phone service to transmit the signals *via* the Bluetooth enabled scales and to receive the interactive voice response system calls. Patients who are affected with cardiovascular diseases are likely to improve their health condition from digitally-connected health care technologies that help to manage their health condition [20 - 23].

Google Glass

It is a wearable computing technology which consists of a head set located on a face like a pair of eye glass. Google glass is used to observe the blockages of the coronary arteries during the coronary angiographic examination.

Bioresorbable Stents

During the artery open heart surgery the clinicians usually place the tiny mesh tube in the heart which is called stent. The prevention of clot formation in the coronary arteries may need long term drug treatment. A new type of stent which is dissolves within a year to solve the problem which is known as bio resorbable stents. Currently, available bioresorbable stents are less flexible and harder to place inside the coronary arteries.

Leadless Pacemaker

Pacemaker having a small battery with sufficient power supply which is placed on the skin. It consists of leads which supply electrical impulses to the cardiac muscles to establish normal heart beats. Pacemakers are reliable; few people had anatomical difference that causes difficult to implant the leads in the heart walls. The leadless is a pacemaker is a unit which is placed on the heart walls to generate the heart beats [24, 25].

Valve-in-valve Procedure

Heart valves are made from the animal tissues which is called a bioprosthetic valve that is used to replace the damaged aortic valves. The bioprosthetic valve is fixed into the heart with the help of catheter. Bioprosthetic valves have a lower risk of clot formation as compared with mechanical valves. Currently, valve-i--valve procedure is more preferred which is used to avoid the high risk of surgery.

Protein Patch for Heart Muscle Growth

The low level of oxygen and blood supply to the heart muscles and damage of the heart muscles leads to develop heart failure. A patch based proteins were placed on the damaged heart muscles results in regrow of damaged cardiac muscles which makes the heart function normally.

ADVANCES IN CARDIOVASCULAR DIAGNOSTIC DEVICES

The recent trends in cardiovascular diagnostics consist of portable monitors, wearables, telemetry, and remote patient monitoring. Cardiac innovations are used to increase the accuracy of the diagnosis speed and to improve patient compliance.

ECG Devices

It is used to record and detect the electrical activity and abnormal rhythms of the heart. A new ECG diagnostic device provides high display, and novel softwares data management for effective detection of cardiovascular abnormalities.

Example: Cardiolyse is a newer device which is developed by UK based health care company. It is used to detect the cardiovascular investigation parameters and abnormalities of the heart.

Heart Check Pen

It is developed by cardio comm solutions, canda. It is a hand held ECG device which is used to record the heart rhythm during the attack of cardiovascular diseases. It has been approved by U.S. food and drug administration for patient care. The data acquired by using bluetooth connectivity to link with android mobile phones.

Holter Monitors

It is a battery-operated continuous heart rate monitoring device that can record the abnormal cardiac abnormalities. Body Guardian Holter: It is developed by Preventice Solutions, Texas. It consists of rechargeable device, adhesive patches attached to skin and to record the cardiac abnormalities.

Implantable Cardiac Monitors

It is an implantable loop recorder that is placed subcutaneous region and ECG device is implanted in the left para sternal region to record cardiovascular abnormalities like arrhythmias, atrial fibrillation, and myocardial infarction *etc.* The implants are placed in the left upper chest area and left breast area to improve the device working performance.

Endotronix

It is developed by the endotronix company, Lisle, United States. It consists of a battery-less sensor device that can analyze the pulmonary artery pressure and to detect the future risk of developing cardiovascular disease.

CONCLUSION

Cardiovascular diseases are causing more health care burden to the affected population. The development of cardiovascular disease is associated with various risk factors and ineffective control of these factors may increase the risk of cardiovascular complications. The cardiovascular diseases are imposing huge health care burden on patients and their families. The advance health care technologies in cardiovascular disease include sensor device, mobile application with specific lifestyle modifications includes diet, lipid control, risk detection, blood pressure control and cessation of alcohol and smoking can improve the health condition of the patients.

Health care innovations deal with the application of ideas, procedures, and novel concepts designed to promotes benefits to society. Health care technology tools such as internet sources, mobile applications; sensor equipment's can identify the risk of cardiovascular disease and to improve the health condition of the patient. Digital health care technologies are used to better understanding the risk factors and control of risk status to lower the occurrence of cardiovascular disease severity in health care. Mobile health care technologies are used to send the message based interventions for risk factors control and to prevent the progression of cardiovascular disease burden. Effective implementation of health care technologies in the cardiology patient care areas could reduce the health care cost and also improve the health related outcomes among cardiac disease patients. The application of technology in the health care field that enables the role of health care practitioner's to treat the various chronic diseases more efficiently. The recent advancement in health care technologies is data mining, and artificial intelligence is used to predict the future occurrence of cardiovascular disease severity in the disease patients.

REFERENCES

[1]   Groves PH, Pomfrett C, Marlow M. Review of the role of NICE in promoting the adoption of innovative cardiac technologies. Heart 2018; 104(22): 1817-22.
       [http://dx.doi.org/10.1136/heartjnl-2018-313256] [PMID: 29773657]

[2]   Campbell B. The NICE Medical Technologies Advisory Committee and medical technologies guidance. Heart 2011; 97(8): 674-5.
       [http://dx.doi.org/10.1136/hrt.2010.219741] [PMID: 21335447]

[3]   Campbell B, Dobson L, Higgins J, Dillon B, Marlow M, Pomfrett C. A new health technology assessment system for devices: the first five years. Int J Technol Assess Health Care 2017; 33(1): 19-24.
       [http://dx.doi.org/10.1017/S0266462317000253] [PMID: 28502278]

[4]   Campbell B, Knox P. promise and plausibility: health technology adoption decisions with limited evidence. Int J Technol Assess Health Care 2016; 32(3): 122-5.
       [http://dx.doi.org/10.1017/S0266462316000234] [PMID: 27530151]

[5]   Golzar M, Fotouhi-Ghazvini F, Rabbani H, Zakeri FS. Mobile cardiac health-care monitoring and notification with real time tachycardia and bradycardia arrhythmia detection. J Med Signals Sens 2017; 7(4): 193-202.
       [http://dx.doi.org/10.4103/jmss.JMSS_17_17] [PMID: 29204376]

[6]   Haberman ZC, Jahn RT, Bose R, *et al.* Wireless smartphone ECG enables large-scale screening in diverse populations. J Cardiovasc Electrophysiol 2015; 26(5): 520-6.
       [http://dx.doi.org/10.1111/jce.12634] [PMID: 25651872]

[7]   Chung HU, Kim BH, Lee JY, *et al.* Binodal, wireless epidermal electronic systems with in-sensor analytics for neonatal intensive care. Science 2019; 363(6430): 1-12.
       [http://dx.doi.org/10.1126/science.aau0780] [PMID: 30819934]

[8]   Kim J, Campbell AS, de Ávila BE-F, Wang J. Wearable biosensors for healthcare monitoring. Nat Biotechnol 2019; 37(4): 389-406.
       [http://dx.doi.org/10.1038/s41587-019-0045-y] [PMID: 30804534]

[9]   Blaya JA, Fraser HSF, Holt B. E-health technologies show promise in developing countries. Health Aff (Millwood) 2010; 29(2): 244-51.
       [http://dx.doi.org/10.1377/hlthaff.2009.0894] [PMID: 20348068]

[10]   Green BB, Cook AJ, Ralston JD, *et al.* Effectiveness of home blood pressure monitoring, Web communication, and pharmacist care on hypertension control: a randomized controlled trial. JAMA 2008; 299(24): 2857-67.
       [http://dx.doi.org/10.1001/jama.299.24.2857] [PMID: 18577730]

[11]   McDermott MM, Spring B, Berger JS, *et al.* Effect of a home-based exercise intervention of wearable technology and telephone coaching on walking performance in peripheral artery disease. JAMA 2018; 319(16): 1665-76.
       [http://dx.doi.org/10.1001/jama.2018.3275] [PMID: 29710165]

[12]   Bumgarner JM, Lambert CT, Hussein AA, *et al.* Smartwatch algorithm for automated detection of atrial fibrillation. J Am Coll Cardiol 2018; 71(21): 2381-8.
       [http://dx.doi.org/10.1016/j.jacc.2018.03.003] [PMID: 29535065]

[13]   Li X, Dunn J, Salins D, Zhou G, *et al.* Digital health: tracking physiomes and activity using wearable biosensors reveals useful health-related information. PLoS Biol 2017; 15(1): e2001402.
       [http://dx.doi.org/10.1371/journal.pbio.2001402]

[14]   Scheuner MT. Genetic predisposition to coronary artery disease. Curr Opin Cardiol 2001; 16(4): 251-60.
       [http://dx.doi.org/10.1097/00001573-200107000-00006] [PMID: 11574787]

[15]   DeFilippis AP, Young R, Carrubba CJ, *et al.* An analysis of calibration and discrimination among multiple cardiovascular risk scores in a modern multiethnic cohort. Ann Intern Med 2015; 162(4): 266-75.
       [http://dx.doi.org/10.7326/M14-1281] [PMID: 25686167]

[16]   Senecal C, Widmer RJ, Johnson MP, Lerman LO, Lerman A. Digital health intervention as an adjunct to a workplace health program in hypertension. J Am Soc Hypertens 2018; 12(10): 695-702.
       [http://dx.doi.org/10.1016/j.jash.2018.05.006] [PMID: 29908726]

[17]   Lakshminarayan K, Westberg S, Northuis C, *et al.* A mHealth-based care model for improving hypertension control in stroke survivors: Pilot RCT. Contemp Clin Trials 2018; 70: 24-34.
       [http://dx.doi.org/10.1016/j.cct.2018.05.005] [PMID: 29763657]

[18]   Terry M. Medical apps for smartphones. Telemed J E Health 2010; 16(1): 17-22.
       [http://dx.doi.org/10.1089/tmj.2010.9999] [PMID: 20070172]

[19]   Bosworth HB, Powers BJ, Olsen MK, *et al.* Home blood pressure management and improved blood pressure control: results from a randomized controlled trial. Arch Intern Med 2011; 171(13): 1173-80.
       [http://dx.doi.org/10.1001/archinternmed.2011.276] [PMID: 21747013]

[20]   Honeyman E, Ding H, Varnfield M, Karunanithi M. Mobile health applications in cardiac care. Interv Cardiol (Lond) 2014; 6(2): 227-40.
       [http://dx.doi.org/10.2217/ica.14.4]

[21]   Wu O, Briggs A, Kemp T, *et al.* Mobile phone use for contacting emergency services in life threatening circumstances. J Emerg Med 2017; 42(3): 291-8.
       [http://dx.doi.org/10.1371/journal.pbio.2001402]

[22]   Alnosayan N, Chatterjee S, Alluhaidan A, Lee E, Houston Feenstra L. Design and usability of a heart failure mHealth system: a pilot study. JMIR Human Factors 2017; 4(1): e9.
       [http://dx.doi.org/10.2196/humanfactors.6481] [PMID: 28341615]

[23]   McConnell MV, Turakhia MP, Harrington RA, King AC, Ashley EA. Mobile health advances in physical activity, fitness, and atrial fibrillation: moving hearts. J Am Coll Cardiol 2018; 71(23): 2691-701.
       [http://dx.doi.org/10.1016/j.jacc.2018.04.030] [PMID: 29880130]

[24]   Walsh JA III, Topol EJ, Steinhubl SR. Novel wireless devices for cardiac monitoring. Circulation 2014; 130(7): 573-81.
       [http://dx.doi.org/10.1161/CIRCULATIONAHA.114.009024] [PMID: 25114186]

[25]   Dang W, Manjakkal L, Navaraj WT, Lorenzelli L, Vinciguerra V, Dahiya R. Stretchable wireless system for sweat pH monitoring. Biosens Bioelectron 2018; 107: 192-202.
       [http://dx.doi.org/10.1016/j.bios.2018.02.025] [PMID: 29471280]

CHAPTER 22

Clinical Pharmacist Intervention in Management of Cardiovascular Diseases

Abstract: Cardiovascular diseases are the disorders of the cardiovascular system which include coronary heart disease, hypertension, myocardial infarction, angina pectoris, rheumatic heart disease, cerebrovascular disease. The development of cardiovascular diseases is associated with complex risk factors such as smoking, alcohol, obesity, unhealthy diet, physical inactivity, stress, family history of cardiovascular disease; hypertension and diabetes mellitus can increase the risk of cardiovascular disease complications. Recent health care statistics revealed that cardiovascular diseases are causing 17.3 million deaths every year and this count will extends 23.6 million by the end of 2030. Clinical pharmacy practice is one of the greatest professions among other health care disciplines in the hospital practice. The clinical pharmacist has a vital role in enhancing the care of patients through providing primary care services such as diet counseling, disease counseling, lifestyle modification counseling, medication counseling which includes uses, indications, warnings, precautions, side effects, dose, time of intake of medications, risk factors identification, risk screening, drug related problems reporting, awareness on pharmacovigilance, conducting awareness programmes on cardiovascular disease prevention, control of lipid, glycemic levels, blood pressure, stress management, weight control, physical exercise, low salt intake, cessation of smoking, alcohol and early implementation of clinical pharmacist services in the hospitals could lower the progression of cardiovascular disease risk incidences.

Keywords: Clinical Pharmacist, Clinical Pharmacy Practice, Coronary Heart Disease, Diabetes Mellitus, Hypertension.

INTRODUCTION

Pharmacy is a life-saving health care discipline that deals with compounding and dispensing of medications, and offering clinical services to the community. It connected with health sciences with pharmaceutical sciences to promote the safe and effective use of the medications. Recently, the pharmacy profession has been shifted from compounding and dispensing of medications to enhance the patient care services in the community. Pharmaceutical care is defined as the need for providing pharmacotherapy to improve the individual patient's quality of life and helps in reaching defined outcomes.

M.S. Umashankar & A. Bharath Kumar

Clinical pharmacists coordinate with health care professionals to design, and implementing the therapeutic plan will increase the health related outcomes of diseased patients [1 - 4]. Pharmacy practice has a vital role in building the trust of disease patients on health care services to reduce the health related cost, treatment associated problems, medication side effects and effective practice of drug regimen could improve the health outcomes among disease patients. The clinical pharmacy field not only targets on medications but also relies on patient oriented care services. Clinical pharmacists will be positioned in this practice to interact with patients and to solve the various health care issues and finally to achieve the better health status of the patients. Currently, clinical pharmacy practice is one of the greatest professions among other health care disciplines in the hospital practice. The clinical pharmacist has an essential role in health care that includes assessing patient medication records, detection of medication errors, dispensing of medications, solving of drug related problems and encouraging the individualized drug regimen and delivering evidence based information to the health care professionals could reduce the health care associated problems among disease patients. The classification of the pharmacist according to the various working departments includes academic pharmacist, hospital pharmacist compounding pharmacist, clinical pharmacist, retail pharmacist, industrial pharmacist, community pharmacist and oncology pharmacist to improve the quality of health care services in society. The creativity of clinical pharmacists may improve through accepting the challenges, developing proper therapeutic plans, new methods to improve communication skills to get knowledge on health care. Clinical pharmacists should have good personnel skills, intellectual skill, creative thinking, handling the risk situations, good honesty and have good clinical problems solving capability.

Clinical pharmacist must have excellent research knowledge and strong medical background to reach the advanced technologies in health care to increase the patient oriented quality care services. The clinical pharmacist must have a subject background in anatomy, physiology, pharmacology, pathology, biochemistry, medicinal chemistry, biopharmaceutics, biostatistics, and clinical pharmacy to create innovative ideas that helps for enhancing the standards in health care research.

A clinical pharmacist is a liaison between doctor and patient and effectively communicates with various health care professionals about treatment plan, counseling, diet, drug shift, health care policy, and to promote patient safety in health care. The regular advance clinical training programmes to clinical pharmacists on communication skills, disease screening, risk factors prevention and management could lower the disease burden. Clinical pharmacist should be competent person and acquire leadership qualities. He has to take accurate decisions and create a solution for serious health care issues that can help for reducing health care related problems in the hospitals. The clinical pharmacist has a strong therapeutic knowledge of assessing patient medication history and minimizing drug related problems, medication errors, dose adjustment, lowering health care cost to affected patients that can help for reaching desired patient health related outcomes.

Clinical pharmacy is an integral part of the health care system. Clinical pharmacists in the ward rounds helping to doctors in the recommendation of treatment regiment to the patients. Clinical pharmacists positioned in the hospitals to address several health care issues to improve the safe prescribing pattern of the drugs to the disease patients.

Clinical pharmacy practice guides the health care team to prescribe the best quality of medications to the public. The clinical pharmacist has an effective role in the management of coronary artery disease includes identification and solving of drug problems, risk factors identification, and control to improve the adherence in medications. Coronary artery disease is a leading cause of death worldwide as per the statement from world health organization in 2011. World health organization estimated that 17 million people died from coronary artery diseases annually. About 80% of the cardiovascular deaths are occurring from the low and middle income countries. Clinical pharmacist should educate the patients about their medications to use in an effective schedule to improve the health status and reduce the need of readmission in the hospitals. Clinical pharmacist have a vital role in enhancing the care of patients through providing primary care services such as medication counseling which includes uses, indications, warnings, precautions, side effects, dose, time of intake of medications to promote the better quality of life and medication adherence among high cardiovascular risk profile patients. The clinical pharmacist services were shown in Fig. (1). Health care providers have complex challenges in the patient care areas includes patients with complex disease condition, shifting drug regimens, drug problems management, disease management, improving medication adherence can promote the effective health status to the cardiovascular disease patients [5 - 11]. Advanced disease prevention and management training to the clinical pharmacist on advanced patient counseling for various diseases, medication problems management, drug information services and effective implementation of the clinical pharmacist care services in the patient care areas could lower the progression of cardiovascular diseases in health care.

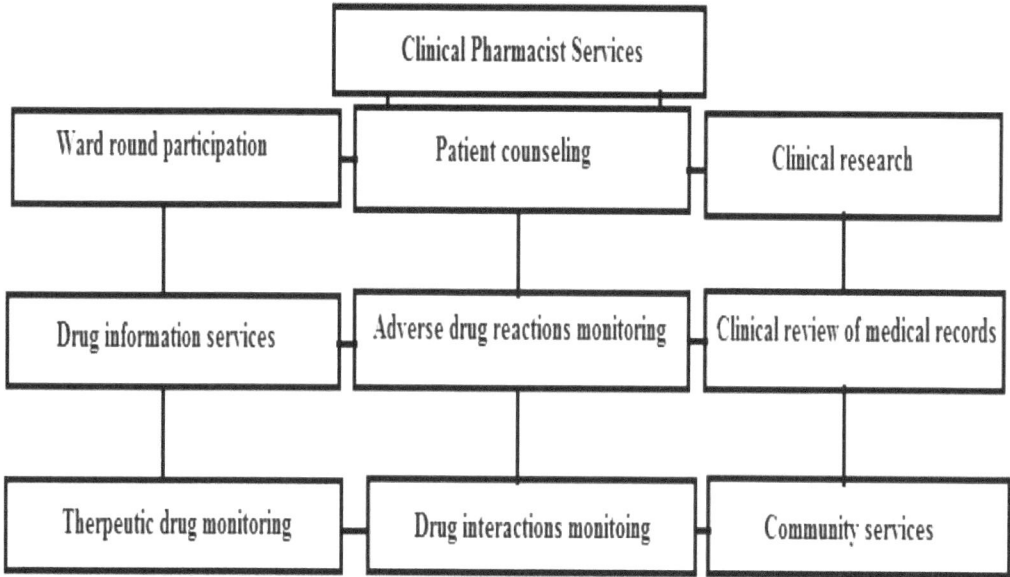

Fig. (1). Clinical Pharmacist services.

KNOWLEDGE, SKILLS, AND ABILITIES

• Ability to read, write and communicate in English to other health care professionals

• Knowledge of ethical issues and regulatory laws

• Exhibit honesty and professionalism

• Excellent customer service, good relation with patients, and co-workers

• Ability to maintain confidentiality of patient details

• Research skills to initiate the research porgrammes in health care

• Knowledge of disease state management

• Ability to interpret laboratory values

• Ability to suggest changes in medication therapy

BASIC KNOWLEDGE OF HOSPITAL PHARMACY PRACTICE AREAS

• Ability to demonstrate competence in the following areas

• Compounding of sterile products as per official pharmacopoeia standards

• Ability to do the pharmacokinetic dosing

• Knowledge on medical record review

• Preparation of total parenteral nutrition

• Ability to initiate the clinical interventions in the patient care areas

• Determination of appropriate selection of antibiotics

• Anticoagulation management and medication reconciliation

• Adverse drug reaction reporting in health care

CLINICAL PHARMACIST REQUIREMENTS

It is shown in Fig. (2).

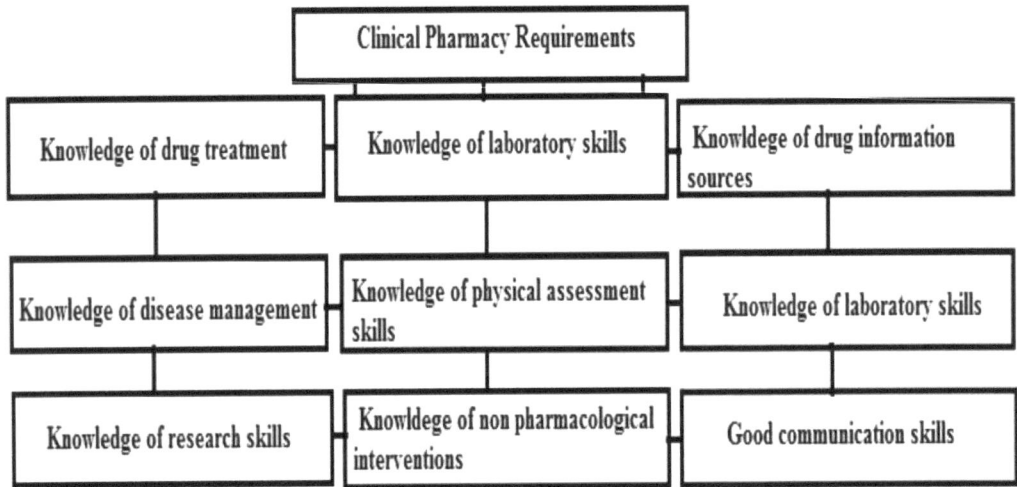

Fig. (2). Clinical pharmacy requirements.

• Hands-on training on patient care services

• Residency training in clinical pharmacy

• Previous working experience as clinical pharmacist

• Outstanding communication skills

• Experience in drug administration and safety procedures of medications

• Knowledge of computers applications

• Excellent interpersonal skills

• Good subject knowledge in Pharmacy, Pharmacology

• Knowledge of medications software

• Problem-solving capability

CLINICAL PHARMACIST DUTIES

• Development of clinical pharmacy programs

• Design of health care policies and regulations

• Analysis of patients medication records

• Evaluation of appropriateness of medication therapy

• Assessment of patients laboratory investigations

• Solving patients health care issues

• Identification of health care problems

• Development of effective treatment medication plans

• Minimizing the risk of adverse side-effects

• Medication dosage adjustment

• Prevention of drug interactions

• Patient counseling services

• Participates in quality assurance initiatives

• Reduction of health care cost

• Designing new medication problems assessment software's

• Advise on effective administration of drugs

• Patient follow-up care services

• Maintaining the patients medication records

CARDIOVASCULAR DISEASE PREVENTION IN THE CLINICAL SETTINGS: A ROLE OF PHARMACIST

Introduction

Cardiovascular diseases include coronary heart disease, hypertension, myocardial infarction, angina pectoris, rheumatic heart disease, cerebrovascular disease, and other conditions. The lack of risk factors screening and treatment patterns raise the incidences of cardiovascular disease events in the practice. Regular medication adherence, healthier life style practices and newer diagnostic tests could lower the cardiovascular disease occurrences in the community. The American Heart Association guideline strongly recommends that newer therapeutic approaches and individualized treatment practices prevent the progression of coronary artery disease complications [12 - 14]. The hypertension is controlled by adhering to the regular treatment, less salt intake, smoking and alcohol cessation, and lifestyle modifications can prevent the development of hypertensive complications in the community [15 - 18].

Risk Factors for Cardiovascular Disease [19, 20]

• Hypertension
• Alcohol
• Smoking
• Diabetes mellitus
• Obesity
• Family history of cardiovascular disease
• Age
• Gender

Clinical Symptoms of Various Cardiovascular Diseases

• Chest pain
• Chest tightness
• Chest discomfort
• Shortness of breath
• Swelling of the legs, ankles and feet
• Fatigue
• Irregular heartbeats
• Fever

Detection Test for Cardiovascular Diseases

• Chest X-rays
• Echocardiogram

- Doppler studies
- Electrocardiogram
- Coronary Angiography

Lifestyle Modifications for Prevention of Cardiovascular Diseases [21-24]

- Stress management
- Smoking and alcohol cessation
- Regular medication adherence
- Regular meditation practice
- Intake of healthy diet
- Regular physical exercise for about 30 minutes every day

Cardiovascular Disease Management Drugs [25]

Angiotensin II Receptor Blockers

- Candesartan
- Telmisartan
- Valsartan
- Losartan

Angiotensin Converting Enzyme Inhibitors

It includes:

- Captopril
- Lisinopril
- Fosinopril
- Ramipril
- Enalapril

Calcium Channel Blockers

These drugs include:

- Diltiazem
- Verapamil
- Nifedipine
- Nimopidine
- Amlodipine

Beta Blockers

- Atenolol
- Bisoprolol
- Propranolol
- Metoprolol

Cholesterol Lowering Medications Include

<u>*Statins*</u>

- Atorvastatin
- Rosuvastatin
- Simvastatin

<u>*Diuretics*</u>

- Furosemide
- Chlorothiazide
- Hydrochlorothiazide
- Acetazolamide
- Amiloride
- spironolactone

<u>*Anti-platelet Drugs*</u>

- Aspirin
- Dipyridamole
- Clopidogrel
- Ticagrelor

<u>*Thrombolytic Drugs*</u>

It includes:

- Streptokinase
- Alteplase
- Urokinase

CLINICAL PHARMACIST CARE SERVICES IN THE PREVENTION AND MANAGEMENT OF CARDIOVASCULAR DISEASE

- Execution of Patient counseling and disease education services in the community.

• Identification, documentation and management of drug related problems (adverse drug reactions, drug interactions, over dose, improper indications).

• Monitoring and promoting medication adherence to prescribed drugs in practice.

• Conducting awareness programmes in the community to prevent chronic diseases.

• Conducting medical camps and participate in health screening programmes to vanish disease burden to society.

• Educate the health care professionals involved in improving patient care services in the practice.

• Interacting with health care team to evaluate and develop guidelines for the prevention and management of cardiovascular diseases.

• Develop; evaluate patient risk tools for prevention and management of cardiovascular diseases

• Participate in the development of research protocol, antibiotic and hospital policy regulations.

• Collaboration with community pharmacist to detect cardiovascular disease risk factors prevention and control, conduct research and to improve the quality of patient care services at community level.

• Providing updated drug information services to the health care team.

• Monitoring the cardiovascular diseases patient follow care services at regular intervals.

• Participate in the formulation of hospital formulary.

• Monitoring the therapeutic drug monitoring practices.

• Conducting Research in the field of Pharmacy practice, pharmacoepidemiology and Health economics related to cardiovascular diseases

• Participate in professional services and audits in hospital settings.

CONCLUSION

Cardiovascular disease incidence is spontaneously rising in each part of the world and significantly impacts the high health care cost and poor health care outcomes to the individuals. The clinical pharmacy field not only targets on medications but also relies on patient oriented care services. Clinical pharmacists will be positioned in this practice to interact with patients and to solve the various health care issues and finally to achieve the better health status of the patients. A clinical pharmacist must have excellent research knowledge and a strong medical background to reach the advanced technologies in health care to increase patient oriented quality care services. The reduction of cardiovascular disease incidences can be lowered by adhering to the medications, approaching healthier life style practices and novel diagnostic approaches can helpful for the reduction of cardiovascular incidences in health care. The strategic therapeutic management of cardiovascular diseases causative factors and early need for amalgamation of clinical pharmacist care services such as diet counseling, disease counseling, lifestyle modification counseling, medication usage counseling, risk screening, physical exercise, stress management, weight reduction, termination of smoking, alcohol, control of lipid, glycemic, blood pressure, stress management, patient referral services, drug policy and guidelines designing; drug problems identification and management could ultimately improve the patient health status and also lowers progression of cardiovascular disease burden in cardiology practice.

REFERENCES

[1]   Hepler CD, Strand LM. Opportunities and responsibilities in pharmaceutical care. Am J Hosp Pharm 1990; 47(3): 533-43.
        [PMID: 2316538]

[2]   Morgado MP, Morgado SR, Mendes LC, Pereira LJ, Castelo-Branco M. Pharmacist interventions to enhance blood pressure control and adherence to antihypertensive therapy: Review and meta-analysis. Am J Health Syst Pharm 2011; 68(3): 241-53.
        [http://dx.doi.org/10.2146/ajhp090656] [PMID: 21258029]

[3]   Cai H, Dai H, Hu Y, Yan X, Xu H. Pharmacist care and the management of coronary heart disease: a systematic review of randomized controlled trials. BMC Health Serv Res 2013; 13: 461.
        [http://dx.doi.org/10.1186/1472-6963-13-461] [PMID: 24188540]

[4]   Swieczkowski D, Merks P, Gruchala M, Jaguszewski MJ. The role of the pharmacist in the care of patients with cardiovascular diseases. Kardiol Pol 2016; 74(11): 1319-26.
        [http://dx.doi.org/10.5603/KP.a2016.0136] [PMID: 27714709]

[5]   McDonough RP, Doucette WR. Drug therapy management: an empirical report of drug therapy problems, pharmacists' interventions, and results of pharmacists' actions. J Amer Pharm Assn 2003; 43: pp. (4)511-8.

[6]   Santschi V, Chiolero A, Burnand B, Colosimo AL, Paradis G. Impact of pharmacist care in the management of cardiovascular disease risk factors: a systematic review and meta-analysis of randomized trials. Arch Intern Med 2011; 171(16): 1441-53.
        [http://dx.doi.org/10.1001/archinternmed.2011.399] [PMID: 21911628]

[7]   Koshman SL, Charrois TL, Simpson SH, McAlister FA, Tsuyuki RT. Pharmacist care of patients with heart failure: a systematic review of randomized trials. Arch Intern Med 2008; 168(7): 687-94.
        [http://dx.doi.org/10.1001/archinte.168.7.687] [PMID: 18413550]

[8]   Mosca L, Barrett-Connor E, Wenger NK. Sex/gender differences in cardiovascular disease prevention:

what a difference a decade makes. Circulation 2011; 124(19): 2145-54.
[http://dx.doi.org/10.1161/CIRCULATIONAHA.110.968792] [PMID: 22064958]

[9]   Al Hamarneh YN, Rosenthal M, Tsuyuki RT. Glycemic control in community-dwelling patients with type 2 diabetes. Can Pharm J 2012; 145(2): 68-69.e1.
[http://dx.doi.org/10.3821/145.2.cpj68] [PMID: 23509504]

[10]   Ritchey MD, Wall HK, Gillespie C, George MG, Jamal A. Million hearts: prevalence of leading cardiovascular disease risk factors--United States, 2005-2012. MMWR Morb Mortal Wkly Rep 2014; 63(21): 462-7.
[PMID: 24871251]

[11]   Vivian EM. Improving blood pressure control in a pharmacist-managed hypertension clinic. Pharmacotherapy 2001; 2: 1337-44.
[PMID: 12495164]

[12]   Santschi V, Chiolero A, Burnand B, Colosimo AL, Paradis G. Impact of pharmacist care in the management of cardiovascular disease risk factors: a systematic review and meta-analysis of randomized trials. Arch Intern Med 2011; 171(16): 1441-53.
[http://dx.doi.org/10.1001/archinternmed.2011.399] [PMID: 21911628]

[13]   Hackam DG, Quinn RR, Ravani P, et al. The 2013 Canadian Hypertension Education Program recommendations for blood pressure measurement, diagnosis, assessment of risk, prevention, and treatment of hypertension. Can J Cardiol 2013; 29(5): 528-42.
[http://dx.doi.org/10.1016/j.cjca.2013.01.005] [PMID: 23541660]

[14]   Genest J, McPherson R, Frohlich J, et al. 2009 Canadian guidelines for the diagnosis and treatment of dyslipidemia and prevention of cardiovascular disease in the adult–2009 recommendations. Can J Cardiol 2009; 25: 567-79.
[http://dx.doi.org/10.1016/S0828-282X(09)70715-9] [PMID: 19812802]

[15]   Mc Namara KP, George J, O'Reilly SL, et al. Engaging community pharmacists in the primary prevention of cardiovascular disease: protocol for the Pharmacist Assessment of Adherence, Risk and Treatment in Cardiovascular Disease (PAART CVD) pilot study. BMC Health Serv Res 2010; 10: 264-71.
[http://dx.doi.org/10.1186/1472-6963-10-264] [PMID: 20819236]

[16]   Babb J, Downs K. Fighting back: pharmacists' roles in the federal response to the September 11 attacks. J Am Pharm Assoc (Wash) 2001; 41(6): 834-7.
[http://dx.doi.org/10.1016/S1086-5802(16)31331-6] [PMID: 11765108]

[17]   Bouvy ML, Heerdink ER, Urquhart J, Grobbee DE, Hoes AW, Leufkens HG. Effect of a pharmacist-led intervention on diuretic compliance in heart failure patients: a randomized controlled study. J Card Fail 2003; 9(5): 404-11.
[http://dx.doi.org/10.1054/S1071-9164(03)00130-1] [PMID: 14583903]

[18]   Singh PS, Singh G, Singh SK. Clinical profile and risk factors in acute coronary syndrome. J Indian Acad Clin Med 2013; 14: 130-2.

[19]   Rainville EC. Impact of pharmacist interventions on hospital readmissions for heart failure. Am J Health Syst Pharm 1999; 56(13): 1339-42.
[http://dx.doi.org/10.1093/ajhp/56.13.1339] [PMID: 10683133]

[20]   Reta A, Dashtaei A, Lim S, Nguyen T, Bholat MA. Opportunities to improve clinical outcomes and challenges to implementing clinical pharmacists into health care teams. Prim Care 2012; 39(4): 615-26.
[http://dx.doi.org/10.1016/j.pop.2012.08.005] [PMID: 23148954]

[21]   Taveira TH, Wu WC, Martin OJ, Schleinitz MD, Friedmann P, Sharma SC. Pharmacist-led cardiac risk reduction model. Prev Cardiol 2006; 9(4): 202-8.
[http://dx.doi.org/10.1111/j.1520-037X.2006.05339.x] [PMID: 17085982]

[22]   McConnell KJ, Denham AM, Olson KL. Pharmacist-led interventions for the management of cardiovascular disease opportunities and obstacles. Dis Manag Health Outcomes 2008; 16(3): 131-44.
[http://dx.doi.org/10.2165/00115677-200816030-00001]

[23]   Mehos BM, Saseen JJ, MacLaughlin EJ. Effect of pharmacist intervention and initiation of home blood pressure monitoring in patients with uncontrolled hypertension. Pharmacotherapy 2000; 20(11): 1384-9.
[http://dx.doi.org/10.1592/phco.20.17.1384.34891] [PMID: 11079287]

[24]   Vivian EM. Improving blood pressure control in a pharmacist-managed hypertension clinic. Pharmacotherapy 2002; 22(12): 1533-40.
[http://dx.doi.org/10.1592/phco.22.17.1533.34127] [PMID: 12495164]

[25]   Omboni S, Sala E. The pharmacist and the management of arterial hypertension: the role of blood pressure monitoring and telemonitoring. Expert Rev Cardiovasc Ther 2015; 13(2): 209-21.
[http://dx.doi.org/10.1586/14779072.2015.1001368] [PMID: 25578090]

ABBREVIATIONS

AV valve	Atrioventricularvalve
AV node	Atrioventricular node
ACTA2	Actin alpha 2
ARNIs	Angiotensin receptor-neprilysin inhibitors
ARB	Angiotensin II receptor blockers
ACEI	Angiotensin converting enzyme inhibitors
ACAT	Acyl-CoA cholesterol acyl transferase inhibitors
AI	Artificial intelligence
cTnI	Cardiac troponin I
cTnT	Cardiac troponin T
CAD	Coronary artery disease
CyPA	Cyclophilin A
CT scan	Computerized tomography
CCTA	Coronary computed tomography angiography
CETP	Cholesteryl ester transfer protein
cGMP	Cyclic guanosine-3′,5′-monophosphate
CABG	Coronary artery bypass graft
COX	Cycloxygenase
CRRT	Continuous renal replacement therapy
DHA	Docosahexaenoic acid
DCM	Dilated cardiomyopathy
DMARDs	Disease modifying anti-rheumatic drugs
DM	Diabetes mellitus
DPP	Dipeptidyl peptidase 4
DGAT	Diacyl glycerol acyl transferase
DVT	Deep vein thrombosis
ECG	Electrocardiogram
ET-1	Endothelin-1
EP	Electrophysiology
EF	Ejection fraction
EPA	Eicosapentaenoic acid
FBN1	Fibrillin-1

GDF-15 Growth differentiation factor-15

GLP1 Glucagon-like peptide-1

hs-cTn High-sensitivity cardiac troponin

H-FABP Heart-type fatty acid binding protein

Hs-CRP High-sensitivity C-reactive protein

H-FABP Heart-type fatty acid binding protein

HDL High-density lipoprotein

HMG CoA β-hydroxy β-methylbutyryl-CoA

H2O2 Hydrogen peroxide

HIV Human immune deficiency virus

IVC Inferior Vena Cava

JNC Joint National Committee

LDL Low-density lipoprotein

LSS-inhibitors Lanosterol synthase inhibitors

LV Left ventricular

Lp-PLA2 Lipoprotein-associated phospholipase A2

miRNAs MicroRNAs

MPO Myeloperoxidase MPO

MTP Microsomal triglyceride transfer protein

MRI Magnetic resonance imaging

NAD Nicotinamide adenine dinucleotide

NADH Nicotinamide adenine dinucleotide hydrogen

NIACR-receptors Niacin receptors

NO Nitric oxide

NPC1L1 Niemann-Pick C1-Like 1

NSAIDs Nonsteroidal anti-inflammatory drugs

PAI-1 Plasminogen activator inhibitor 1

PPARγ Peroxisome proliferator-activated receptor-γ

PAPP-A Pregnancy-associated plasma protein-A

PCI Percutaneous Coronary Intervention

PDE5 Phosphodiesterase type 5

PE Pulmonary embolism

PCSK9 Proproteinconvertasesubtilisin/kexin type 9

sPLA2 Secretory phospholipase A2

sCD40L Soluble CD40 ligand

TAVR Transcatheter aortic valve replacement

tPA Tissue plasminogen activator

TNF-alpha Tumor necrosis factor alpha

SGLT2 Sodium-glucose co-transporter-2

UDP Uridinediphosphate

VLDL Very-low-density lipoprotein

SUBJECT INDEX

I

J

K

L

intake of 268, 284
loss of 81, 118, 137, 204, 217, 238, 286
Sodium reabsorption 65, 81, 118, 138, 204, 217, 238, 286
  aldosterone-sensitive 81, 118, 138, 204, 217, 238, 286, 324
Spiral computed tomography 88
Stenosis 37, 38, 42, 151, 197, 243, 245
  moderate 42
  valvular 37
Stenosis of artery 74
Steroids 47, 49, 233
  anabolic 233
Steroids narcotic analgesics 249
Sterol biosynthesis 54
streptococcus pyogenes 243
Streptokinase 79, 92, 116, 136, 168, 199, 236, 267
Stress management 28, 32, 63, 66, 69, 75, 102, 105, 143, 157, 249, 253, 268, 269
  practices 143
  programmes 157
Stretching 128, 247
  intense valvular tissue 247
  of muscle fiber 128
Stroke 17, 50, 69, 108, 109, 110, 111, 157
  developing 157
  incidence of 110, 111
  ischemic 17, 50, 69, 108, 109
Stroke risk 121
  factors 121
Stromelysins 18
Surgery 39, 41, 42, 84, 86, 92, 222, 304, 305
  cardiac 42, 222
  open heart 304
  traditional heart valve 39
Surgical risk 42
Syndrome 19, 89, 130, 195
  acute coronary artery 19
  adult respiratory 130
  post phlebitic 89
Syphilis 37, 74
System 1, 10, 20, 40, 129, 232, 242, 243, 251, 278, 303
  adrenergic 232
  cardiac 1, 20
  chronic sympathetic 10
  electronic health care record 303
  immune 242, 251
  musculoskeletal 243

renin-angiotensin 40, 278
renin angiotensin aldosterone 129
renin angiotensionogen aldosterone 62
Systole 1, 8, 9, 10, 38, 193, 197, 198
  atrial 8
  ventricular 8, 9, 10
Systolic function 129, 229

T

Tachycardia 65, 128, 141, 148, 149, 152, 169, 205, 239, 261, 280
  paroxysmal 149
  supraventricular 141, 149, 152, 205, 239
Technology 297, 301, 303, 304, 306
  block chain 297, 303
  sensor 304
Telehealth technology 303
Telemedicine apps technology 303
Test 17, 29, 30, 31, 32, 74, 75, 84, 88, 101, 114, 121, 154, 256, 283
  blood sugar 29, 256
  blood urea 283
  blood urea nitrogen 283
  creatinine clearance 283
  hemoglobin 283
  invasive 88
  magnetic resonance imaging 84
  noninvasive 31
  proteomics 121
  regular hypertension screening 114
Therapy 41, 86, 91, 92, 110, 115, 257, 292, 297, 300, 312, 314
  anticoagulation 91, 92
  antiplatelet 115
  diabetic 115
  gene 240
  hormonal 110
  medication 86, 257, 312, 314
  stem cell 297, 300
  thrombolytic 92
Thromboembolism 157, 197
Thrombogenesis 259
Thrombolytic agents 92
Thrombosis 69, 71, 84, 91, 260, 298
Thyroid 60, 232
  disease 232
  problems 60
Thyrotoxicosis 125, 131
Tissue 89, 92

www.ingramcontent.com/pod-product-compliance
Lightning Source LLC
Chambersburg PA
CBHW080019240326
41598CB00075B/117